FUNDAMENTALS *for* PUBLIC HEALTH PRACTICE

SAGE was founded in 1965 by Sara Miller McCune to support the dissemination of usable knowledge by publishing innovative and high-quality research and teaching content. Today, we publish over 900 journals, including those of more than 400 learned societies, more than 800 new books per year, and a growing range of library products including archives, data, case studies, reports, and video. SAGE remains majority-owned by our founder, and after Sara's lifetime will become owned by a charitable trust that secures our continued independence.

Los Angeles | London | New Delhi | Singapore | Washington DC | Melbourne

FUNDAMENTALS *for* PUBLIC HEALTH PRACTICE

AMANDA HOLLAND
KATE PHILLIPS
MICHELLE MOSELEY
LORRAINE JOOMUN

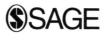

Los Angeles | London | New Delhi
Singapore | Washington DC | Melbourne

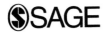

Los Angeles | London | New Delhi
Singapore | Washington DC | Melbourne

SAGE Publications Ltd
1 Oliver's Yard
55 City Road
London EC1Y 1SP

SAGE Publications Inc.
2455 Teller Road
Thousand Oaks, California 91320

SAGE Publications India Pvt Ltd
B 1/I 1 Mohan Cooperative Industrial Area
Mathura Road
New Delhi 110 044

SAGE Publications Asia-Pacific Pte Ltd
3 Church Street
#10-04 Samsung Hub
Singapore 049483

Editor: Alex Clabburn
Assistant Editor: Ruth Lilly
Production Editor: Zoheb Khan
Copyeditor: Solveig Gardner Servian
Indexer: Cathryn Pritchard
Marketing Manager: Ruslana Khatagova
Cover Design: Sheila Tong
Typeset by KnowledgeWorks Global Ltd.
Printed in the UK

Library of Congress Control Number: 2022935614

British Library Cataloguing in Publication data

A catalogue record for this book is available from the British Library

ISBN 978-1-5264-9626-3
ISBN 978-1-5264-9625-6 (pbk)

At SAGE we take sustainability seriously. Most of our products are printed in the UK using FSC papers and boards. When we print overseas we ensure sustainable papers are used as measured by the PREPS grading system. We undertake an annual audit to monitor our sustainability.

CONTENTS

ABOUT THE EDITORS

Amanda Holland is a senior lecturer at the School of Healthcare Sciences, Cardiff University, and joined the University in 2015. Amanda is a registered health visitor, adult nurse and nurse educator. She teaches undergraduate nurses and midwives and postgraduate healthcare students. Her specialist area is in Specialist Community Public Health Nursing, Health Visiting. Amanda is programme manager of the Specialist Community Public Health Nursing (SCPHN) Programme for Health Visiting, a role she has held since 2018. In 2019, the SCPHN team were awarded the SNTA Post-Registration Educators of the Year. Amanda was awarded Senior Fellowship of the Higher Education Academy in 2021 and was jointly awarded the RCN Wales Nurse Educator of the Year 2021 runner up. Amanda leads SCPHN programme modules and has taught international students, leading a health promotion module in Oman. She is the Community Practitioner and Health Visitor Association Executive Chair for Wales, and previous Vice Chair, roles she has held since 2016. Amanda co-developed the all-Wales Health Visitor Observation and Assessment of the Infant (HOAI) and is currently undertaking a PhD exploring this aspect of health visitor practice. Amanda is a published author, and she has spoken at national and international conferences.

Kate Phillips is an NMC-registered Adult & Child Nurse, as well as a professionally NMC-registered Specialist Community Public Health Nurse (Health Visitor). Her clinical experience includes practising as a Flying Start Health Visitor in Wales for eight years where she promoted the health and wellbeing of families and communities. Her career moved into higher education at Cardiff University in 2015 due to her passion for teaching and supporting the development of the future nursing workforce. She currently works as a Child Nursing lecturer at the University of Leeds. Her subjects of interest are public health, health promotion and the importance of fathers and their engagement in health services. She is also a member of the Community Practitioner and Health Visitor Association Executive Committee.

Michelle Moseley is the Education and Lifelong Learning Adviser at RCN Wales. Michelle is a registered general nurse, sick children's nurse, health visitor, and nurse educator. Her specialist area of teaching and learning is associated with public health nursing where she managed the Specialist Community Public Health Nursing (SCPHN) programme (health visiting) within the School of Healthcare Sciences (HCARE) at Cardiff University, as well as undertaking other roles including undergraduate education lead and director of learning in practice. Michelle is passionate about safeguarding and was awarded the RCN Wales Nurse of the year Award for Safeguarding in 2018. Also in 2019, the SCPHN team at HCARE were awarded the SNTA Post-registration educators of the year. In 2020 Michelle was awarded Senior Lecturer and Senior Fellow of the Higher Education Academy. Michelle continues to write and teach, delivering public health and safeguarding sessions at Cardiff University as well as within her role within the RCN. Michelle commenced a PhD in 2018 on a part-time basis and is exploring how supportive safeguarding supervision is for health visitors. Michelle is currently seconded into Welsh Government as Professional Lead for clinical supervision working within the Chief Nursing Officer team.

Lorraine Joomun is a qualified nurse and health visitor and has been working in healthcare education at Cardiff University for 24 years. During this time Lorraine managed and led the Specialist Community Public Health Nurse (Health Visitor) Programme, while also undertaking an additional role as Professional Head of Primary Care and Public Health Nursing. Lorraine currently leads the health promotion module within the SCPHN programme; she has previously led the global public health modules within the school and health promotion modules in Oman. Lorraine has a special interest in homelessness, which developed while undertaking her PhD.

ABOUT THE CONTRIBUTORS

Alex Nute is a lecturer and programme manager for undergraduate mental health nursing in Cardiff University School of Healthcare Sciences. He spent his clinical career in South Wales working in acute admissions, psychiatric intensive care services and the regional neuropsychiatry service where he led the in-patient and day services before moving into quality improvement and clinical education, joining the University full time in 2013.

Caroline Bradbury-Jones is a registered nurse, midwife and health visitor and has extensive experience of working directly with families, particularly those with high levels of need. Her research work has focused broadly within the scope of addressing inequalities and more specifically on issues of family violence.

Cathryn Smith is a lecturer in primary care and public health with 11 years of clinical experience in community nursing and primary care. Cathryn has an MSc in Community Health Studies and is currently undertaking a PhD in healthcare professionals decision making in end of life for patients with dementia.

Dana Summut is a registered nurse and part-time research associate at the University of Birmingham. Her research interests include gender-based violence and healthcare education. Since her undergraduate degree she has worked closely with Professor Caroline

Bradbury-Jones on a number of projects including research papers and the development of an e-learning resource.

Dave Clarke currently works at the University of the West of England as Associate Dean for Partnerships and Head of the School of Health and Social Wellbeing. As well as being a senior academic Dave has an interest in LGBT+ activism and health, which developed while undertaking his PhD. Dave has led a number of LGBT+ projects with a focus on developing student and staff awareness of LGBT+ health inequalities and enhancing allyship.

David Evans OBE is a National Teaching Fellow and Professor in Sexualities and Genders: Health and Well-being at the University of Greenwich. A registered nurse, former Catholic priest, he has a professional doctorate (EdD) researching sexual health education for nurses across England. David has been a sexual health and HIV educator since 1990. He has published widely and presented at conferences across the UK and abroad. His various websites can be accessed via https://en.gravatar.com/davidtevans @ David_T_Evans

Deb McNee is a Child Nursing Lecturer at Swansea University. Her background is in child health with over 30 years, experience as both a Children's nurse and Health Visitor. She holds an MSc in Specialist Community Public Health Nursing and was previously a Specialist Health Visitor for Gypsies and Travellers.

Dianne Watkins OBE is a registered nurse, midwife, health visitor (SCPHN) and educator. She is currently the Director of International and Civic Mission, School of Healthcare Sciences, Cardiff University having held numerous strategic international positions. Dianne has worked with Welsh Government on the introduction of degree nurse education, non-medical prescribing and advanced practice. Her international education and research include development and delivery of nurse degree education for the Sultanate of Oman and advising their Ministry of Health on community nursing services. She has worked with the University of Namibia on development of a BSc in Public Health and nurse leadership programmes. Dianne has established a 'practice development unit' in a Malawian hospital to deliver evidence-based care and was awarded an OBE in June 2020 for her services to nurse education and research.

Emma Senior is a programme and module lead in the Department of Nursing, Midwifery and Health at Northumbria University. Emma holds NMC registration in adult nursing and is a Specialist Community Public Health Nurse in Health Visiting and Sexual Health Advisor. Emma's academic and research interests are wide ranging, but focus broadly on Military families, Public Health and Technology Enhanced Learning.

Fatima Husain is an applied policy researcher with over 23 years' experience of conducting research to better understand disadvantage and discrimination, in particular, at the interface of service provision. Her research has focused on child poverty, parenting and minority ethnic families, the welfare system, health and social care, and education.

Iain McPhee began his addiction career working in treatment and rehabilitation services in the 1990s, delivering psychological interventions to problem users of alcohol and controlled drugs. Iain is a senior interdisciplinary Researcher and Lecturer based at University of the West of Scotland. He is a consultant drug expert witness, and contributes to local, national and international drug policy.

Ian Bond was born into a smoking family and a smoking world and not surprisingly was diagnosed with COPD at the age of 60, almost 20 years ago. It was a time when 'Big Tobacco' was recognised for what it was and that the addiction to smoking was manipulated and monetised for profit at the expense of health services and individuals across the world. Since then Ian has become a contributor and speaker for ASH (Action on Smoking and Health), a committee member with the British Lung Foundation and has built a successful business using the latest technology to support COPD patients.

Jane Hanley is the CEO of Perinatal MH Training CIC. For almost 40 years Jane has been interested in the perinatal mental health of parents. She has written articles, papers and four books, been involved in research projects, and is a former President of the International Marcé Society for Perinatal Mental Health. Jane is an Honorary Senior Lecturer in PMH and Public Health, Swansea University.

Joanne McEwan works for Health Education England as a Public Health Development Manager. Previous roles include breast cancer service development in Egypt, research nurse at the Oxford Vaccine Group and health visitor. She has an MA in Geography on water and health, and is a Mary Seacole Scholar and creator of the *Let's talk FGM* app.

John Watkins is a Consultant Epidemiologist with Public Health Wales and Cardiff University. His research and teaching include epidemiology and infectious diseases, particularly influenza and the COVID-19 pandemic. He is an adviser to UK and Welsh governments on pandemic planning and the challenges of SARS-CoV-2. He has also chaired the Welsh Government's Influenza Advisory Group. Working with the WHO and others, he helped develop the WHO Global Research Agenda for Influenza in 2009 and in 2013 participated in updating the UK's Influenza Pandemic Plan. John presents internationally and publishes extensively in the field of infectious respiratory disease, the effectiveness of vaccines in prevention and the historical impact of influenza pandemic disease and more recently on SARS-CoV-2 and COVID-19.

Linda Mages is recently retired. Prior to retirement Dr Mages worked as a health visitor/team leader/practice educator for nearly 15 years before accepting a senior lecturer post. As a health visitor she worked with colleagues and other health and social care professionals towards reducing the impact of health inequalities on diverse families, including the early prevention of poor nutrition and obesity. In the role of senior lecturer Dr Mages led SCPHN programmes at the Universities of West of England, South Wales and Northumbria. With the outbreak of COVID-19, Dr Mages returned to practice at the Cumberland Infirmary Carlisle where she continues to work as a 'bank' and dermatology nurse.

Lucy Holland is a Higher Scientific Officer at the Department for Environment, Food and Rural Affairs, currently working within science-policy interface on ecosystem assessment. Lucy holds a BSc in Anthropology and an MRes in Conservation Research. Lucy is a Trustee and Ambassador for Gwent Wildlife Trust.

Lynette Harland Shotton is Head of Subject in the Department of Social Work, Education and Community Wellbeing at Northumbria University. Lynette is a registered adult nurse and Specialist Community Public Health Nurse in the health visiting field. Lynette's academic and research interests are varied, but focus broadly on understanding and addressing health and educational inequality.

Nadine Littler has a special interest in obesity and Public Health, following her role working as a SCPHN (School Nurse) which highlighted the major implications this disease can have on an individual's life course. Currently she is working as a National Clinical Practice Facilitator and is completing a PhD in Public Health.

Philip Tremewan is a Registered Nurse, BSc (Hons). He qualified as a Registered Nurse in 1994 and has worked in the older people's environment of long-term conditions, intermediate care and end-of-life care. Philip has worked within the area of Safeguarding since 2009 for both NHS provider and commissioning organisations; he is currently employed as Nurse Consultant for Safeguarding at South East Coast Ambulance Service NHS Foundation Trust.

Shirley Willis is a Queen's Nurse and lecturer in Primary Care and Public Health and Programme Manager for the PgDip Community Health Studies Specialist Practice District Nursing/Practice Nursing Programme with Nurse Prescribing at the School of Healthcare Sciences at Cardiff University. Shirley holds an External Examiner role for Specialist Practice programmes at the University of Suffolk and Swansea University.

Susan Greening is a Registered Nurse, specialising in Learning Disabilities and Mental Health, who qualified in 1996. Susan has an MSc in Advanced Professional Practice majoring in Dementia and End-of-life Care. She retired from her role of Deprivation of Liberty Safeguards and Mental Capacity Act Co-ordinator in August 2020 but returned as a Best Interests Assessor and has also been involved in the COVID-19 vaccine rollout as Clinical Supervisor in a Community Vaccination Team.

FOREWORD

As a public health professional for 30 years, academic, and Vice President of the Community Practitioners and Health Visitors Association (CPHVA) in the United Kingdom (UK) and Co-Director of the International Collaboration on Community Health Care and Research (ICCHNR), it is my very great privilege to craft the foreword for this impressive and vital text. My public health knowledge and practice arises both in the UK and North American context where I served as a Canada Research Chair in Ethnicity and Health. My connection to the editors of this textbook is via our professional practice as health visitors in the UK and members of the CPHVA.

As we move further in to the 21st Century in the post-pandemic world, public health practice has risen to increasing global prominence and significance. Although the Fundamentals of Public Health Practice focuses on the United Kingdom professional audience our country-specific public health experience in the era of international travel is inextricably linked to other nation states. It is no longer possible to secure national and state boundaries as a means to the protection and promotion of public health. Coupled with the phenomena of international migration and population diversity in all high income nation states, alongside our globally connected economies and dependency that confirm our public health, promotion and practice is locally and globally connected. In this sense the text creates transferrable knowledge and learning beyond the four nation states of the United Kingdom establishing international reach and pedagogical relevance.

A strength of the text is the ability to appeal to and have relevance for a wide range of professional groups including interdisciplinary students in health and social care, nursing, midwifery, allied health professionals, social work, alongside qualified health professionals. I regard the text as seminal and fundamental reading for all those involved in promoting and protecting public health globally. The chapters within the book create comprehensive and wide-ranging coverage of the topics intrinsically linked to public health practice.

The credentials of all the contributors are impressive. The editors have convened a superlative cadre of inter-disciplinary public health specialists. As public health experts with international lenses, their knowledge and perspectives are contemporary and address significant public health topics which combined, constitute a critical public health 'crisis' requiring imperative governmental action, policy and practice responses in almost all low income, middle income and high income countries. Regardless of the country context, the human health experience is often shared globally and manifests great commonality. Indeed our recent experience of the pandemic has demonstrated that no nation state holds the ability to be a 'public health island' devoid of external global influences and globalisation.

The topics addressed in the text such as health literacy, obesity, child development, mental health, substance misuse, gender-based violence, inequalities in health, sexual health, gender identity issues and ethno-cultural diversity constitute a critical lexicon of public health issues that are globally relevant and pertinent for all practitioners, facilitators of learning and students.

This influential textbook is critical and significant as we continue to face major public health challenges globally. Never has the field of public health practice been more valued by international, national and local decision makers than now in the post-pandemic era.

Professor Gina Awoko Higginbottom MBE
5th May 2022

1

INTRODUCTION: OVERVIEW OF GLOBAL HEALTH POLICY AND HEALTH POLICY ACROSS THE FOUR UK NATIONS

AMANDA HOLLAND

Public health

Public health is not easy to define and comprehend. There is no single definition of public health and leaders in the field have themselves struggled to agree on what public health is, why it is important and what it should do (Fleming and Parker 2015, Schneider 2017). Definitions have varied over time and from country to country. The World Health Organization (WHO 2012) accept Sir Donald Acheson's definition as, 'the art and science of preventing disease, prolonging life and promoting health through the organized efforts of society' (Public Health England 1988, p.1). Prior to this definition the term 'public health' was associated with a rather narrow view of sanitary health and epidemic disease prevention; however, this definition allows for a focus on the wider determinants of health associated with lifestyle, the environment, societal and behavioural influences, and health system delivery. We live in an ever-changing society where social structures and health priorities continually shift, highlighting the need for knowledge and evidence to support an understanding of current challenges to public health and the impact it has on individual health and society as a whole.

At the time of writing this textbook the world was in the grips of a global pandemic as a novel coronavirus, causing the disease COVID-19, spread across the world resulting in widespread illness and death (WHO 2020). National governments and public health policy responded by limiting civil liberties of citizens and shutting down borders and economies to counter the impact of COVID-19, with the most urgently shared public health agenda focusing on globally accessible vaccination. Evidence has emerged indicating how populations have been and continue to be subjected to unprecedented hardships as a result of the pandemic, impacting on all aspects of public health, the likes of which have never been seen in peace times (United Nations 2020). The long-term impact of COVID-19 is yet to be understood as people face continuous threats to their health and wellbeing, with the most vulnerable in society disproportionately affected by ever persistent health inequalities impacting on mental health, physical health, and the social determinants of health.

Before COVID-19 the world was making good progress towards achieving objectives set out in the health-related Sustainable Development Goals (SDGs) and WHO's Triple Billion Targets, which by 2023 aims to achieve:

- one billion more people enjoying better health and wellbeing,
- one billion more people benefiting from universal health coverage (covered by health services without experiencing financial hardship),
- one billion more people better protected from health emergencies.

(WHO 2021a)

Data from The World Health Statistics 2021 report (WHO 2021b) identified health trends from 2000–2019 across countries, regions and income groups for more than 50 health-related indicators for the SDGs and WHO's Triple Billion Targets. Data showed that life expectancy at birth increased from 66.8 years in 2000 to 73.3 years in 2019, and healthy life expectancy increased from 58.3 years to 63.7 years. Reduction in the numbers of deaths caused by communicable disease have significantly declined in comparison to non-communicable disease. For example, the number of deaths from malaria fell from 736,000 in 2000 to 409,000 in 2019, HIV infection rates reduced by 40% since its peak in 1998; however, deaths from non-communicable diseases such as cancer, cardiovascular diseases, diabetes and chronic respiratory diseases have increased from 60.8% in 2000 to 73.6% in 2019 (WHO 2021b). While global tobacco use has decreased by 33% since 2000, the prevalence of adult obesity is increasing, with nearly one-quarter of the population in high-income countries reported to be obese. In upper-middle income countries people are more susceptible to being overweight; however, in low- to lower-middle-income countries the risk of children and women experiencing malnutrition, stunting, wasting and anaemia in pregnancy remains high (WHO 2021a).

Before the pandemic, countries in all income groups and across different healthcare services were reported to be making good progress towards universal health coverage; however, the WHO (2021a) reports financial protection to support services has deteriorated particularly in the poorest countries, countries affected by conflict, and as a result of focus shifting to respond to the COVID-19 pandemic. Despite an increased focus on global health security, the WHO (2021a) identified a critical need for well-coordinated, multisectoral health emergency capacity and preparedness at all levels within all countries to mitigate, maintain, manage and improve public health risks within a national context and worldwide pandemic context.

Since the pandemic global activity focuses on 'Building Back Better' with the United Nations (UN 2020) leading the way with recommendations on how governments can seize opportunities to build back better. In a policy brief by the High-Level Committee on Programmes Inequalities Task Team, *COVID-19 Inequalities and Build Back Better* (UN 2020), the unequal impact of the pandemic and underinvestment in public health is discussed with evidence indicating worsened health inequalities within and between countries and a fully-fledged economic and social crisis. Key messages include recognition of how the impact of the pandemic is threatening to derail progress towards the SDGs. Key messages and recommendations include:

- Avoid a downward spiral that intensifies economic damage and catalyzes a broader humanitarian crisis, addressing inequalities should be a core part of implementing the UN system's framework for the immediate socioeconomic response to COVID-19.
- Governments and the global community have a once-in-a-generation opportunity to 'build back better', to transform economies and create more equitable societies that allow everyone to enjoy the full range of their human rights, without discrimination.
- To achieve this, bold action is needed to build stronger, equity-focused health systems; to strengthen social protection and public services; to forge a job-intensive

recovery for people-centred and environmentally sustainable economies; to implement gender responsive economic policies, based on international solidarity and multilateral collaboration; and to ensure social cohesion and community resilience.

(United Nations 2020, p. 1).

In the UK the Government's Build Back Better Plan pledges significant investment in health and social care to benefit all four nations: Wales, England, Scotland and Northern Ireland. The plan aims to level out health outcomes across the UK, with prevention being the central principle in delivering sustainable services. Addressing and fixing the underlying causes of ill health that contribute to worsening health outcomes and increased financial burden on the NHS is vital to improving public health and resilience against future health threats (HM Government 2021). Across the UK national governments have set out strategic plans to improve public health and address the increasing demands and challenges on the health and wellbeing of individuals and communities. In Wales, the long-term future vision is for a whole-system approach. The policy document *A Healthier Wales: Our Plan for Health and Social Care* (Welsh Government 2021) details aspirations for Welsh Government, NHS Wales and local government to work in partnership to design and deliver health and social care service together, meeting individual needs and preferences with an emphasis on keeping people healthy and well.

In Scotland, *Public Health Scotland's (PHS) Strategic Plan 2020–2023* also pledges a new approach to public health with an ambitious vision where everybody thrives (PHS 2020). The plan discusses the need for people, organisations and groups to join forces to promote and support individuals and communities to flourish.

In Northern Ireland a whole systems approach for public health was proposed in 2013 with a 10-year strategic framework set out in the *Making Life Better* charter (Department of Health, Social Services and Public Safety 2013). Good progress was reported in 2015 on a number of strategic actions such as work towards strengthening universal and targeted provision to promote and support parenting, early years education and learning, and empowering healthy living and healthy communities; however, no further reports on progress have been published since (Department of Health, Social Services and Public Safety 2015).

In November 2021 the UK hosted the 26th United Nations Climate Change Conference, (Conference of the Parties (COP) 26) (UN 2021). For nearly 30 years countries have come together for global climate summits, and during this time climate change has gone from a fringe issue to a global priority. Climate change can negatively impact physical health, biological and ecological systems. For example, air pollution, pollen concentrations, diseases borne by vectors such as mosquitos, food and waterborne diseases, flooding, droughts, increased temperatures, and food security are all examples of threats to public health that have intensified as a result of climate change (Center for Disease Control and Prevention 2021). The goals of COP 26 seek to reduce and secure global carbon emissions to net zero and keep within 1.5 degrees' reach, to adapt communities, protect and restore ecosystems, mobilise finances and work together through collaboration between governments, businesses and civil society to accelerate action and tackle the climate crisis (UN 2021). The COP 26 health programme includes initiatives to build climate resilient and low carbon sustainable health systems and raise the voice of health professionals as advocates on climate change (WHO 2021c).

Table 1.1 is a useful summary of key UK and national policy and legislation relevant to public health. This will be discussed further throughout the chapters of this textbook as it provides an overview of the most contemporary key public health priorities.

Table 1.1   Table of key national strategies, policy and legislation relevant to public health

UK.
- Working Together to Safeguard Children. A guide to inter-agency working to safeguard and promote the welfare of children (HM Government, 2018)
- Modern Slavery Act 2015 (Legislation.gov.uk, 2015)
- Coronavirus Act 2020 (Legislation.gov.uk, 2020)

Wales
- Social Services and Well-being (Wales) Act 2014 (Legislation.go.uk, 2014)
- Wellbeing of Future Generations (Wales) Act 2015 (Welsh Government, 2015)
- Violence against Women, Domestic Abuse and Sexual Violence (Wales) Act 2015 (Legislation. gov.uk, 2015)
- Nurse Staffing Levels (Wales) Act 2016 (Legislation.gov.uk, 2016)
- Working to achieve a healthier future for Wales. Public Health Wales Long Term Strategy 2018-30 (Public Health Wales 2018)
- A Healthier Wales – Our plan for Health and Social Care (Welsh Government, 2021)
- The Health and Social Care (Quality and Engagement) (Wales) Act (Legislation.gov.uk, 2021)

England
- Global Health Strategy 2014 – 2019 (Public Health England, 2014)
- Safeguarding Policy (NHS England and NHS Improvement, 2015)
- LGBT Action Plan: Improving the Lives of Lesbian, gay, bisexual and transgender people (Government Equalities Office, 2018)
- Healthy Children: Transforming child health information (NHS England, 2016)
- Wellbeing and Mental Health: Applying All Our Health (Office for Health Improvement and Disparities 2022)
- Public Health England Strategy 2020-2025 (Public Health England, 2020)

Scotland
- Mental Health Scotland Act 2015 (Scottish Government, 2015)
- Human Trafficking and Exploitation (Scotland) Act (Scottish Government, 2015)
- Health and Social Care Delivery Plan (Scottish Government, 2016)
- Child Poverty Scotland Act (Legislation.gov.uk, 2017)
- A Fairer Healthier Scotland. A Strategic Framework for Action 2017-2022 (NHS Scotland, 2017)
- Public Health Scotland's Strategic Plan 2020-2023 (Public Health Scotland, 2020)

Northern Ireland
- Making Life Better (Department of Health, Social Services and Public Safety, 2013)
- The Mental Capacity Act (Northern Ireland) 2016 (Legislation.gov.uk, 2016)
- Health and Wellbeing 2026 – Delivering Together (Department of Health, 2017)

How this book is organised

This textbook is tailored to all health and social care students such as nurses and midwives, allied health care professionals, social care workers, qualified health and social care practitioners and anyone who plays a role in understanding, promoting and protecting public health. Taking a life-span approach, it discusses cultural and societal change, and directly links to health and social care contextualised to all four nations in the UK, whilst also considering global health debates. Each chapter begins with a list of learning outcomes to inform the reader about knowledge that can be gained from reading the chapters, why the chapter is relevant and how it can influence future practice. At the end of each chapter questions are posed to encourage and support reflection on learning. Further reading is recommended to explore topic areas and each chapter provides a list of recommendations.

The textbook begins with a chapter discussing the most relevant topic of COVID-19. It considers lessons learnt and makes recommendations for future practice. The impact of COVID-19 is also considered throughout the book in relation to specific aspects of public health. The textbook is then presented in five sections.

Section one focuses on identifying and addressing the health needs of communities and wider society, targeting health promotion and prevention strategies to promote health and reduce health inequalities. It provides the reader with a theoretical understanding of health promotion theories, models and approaches that enable practitioners to recognise the challenges of promoting health, directing resources and developing appropriate health promotion strategies to meet the ever changing health needs of society. Then, a discussion of health literacy enables practitioners to understand the importance of identifying individuals' capacity, knowledge and understanding of healthcare messages and services as active partners in their care so that they can make appropriate health decisions. This knowledge base will underpin discussions in the chapters that follow as contemporary public health priorities are discussed.

Section two explores child development and the influence of early relationships from conception, it considers how this lays the foundations for human development and long-term health and wellbeing, for better or for worse. Perinatal mental health is explored from the perspective of both mothers and fathers. Critical discussions within this section stimulates an understanding of how early relationships and childhood experiences influence health outcomes.

Section three focuses on inequalities in health. The key topics of obesity, health of the older person, substance misuse, mental health, oral health and sexual health are considered, supported by discussions of evidence, policy guidelines and early intervention and prevention strategies to promote health and reduce inequalities. Discussions will enable practitioners to critically consider the appropriateness and effectiveness of public health care approaches and to tailor individualised care.

Section four explores aspect of safeguarding children and adults. Safeguarding individuals from risk of harm is a key public health priority and is everyone's business. This section discusses safeguarding issues, and presents key legislation and policy aimed at protecting individuals from harm. It also addresses the multifaceted issues of domestic abuse and honour-based violence. This will enable practitioners to gain a clear understanding of their roles and responsibilities to safeguard individuals.

Section five discusses how, in an every changing society contemporary public health must always consider the influence of culture, equality and diversity on health. This is examined with a focus on the health and social inequalities of homelessness, travellers and LGBTQ+ community. The importance of cultural awareness and sensitivity is explored.

A variety of authors from across the UK have contributed to this book sharing their experiences and expertise within their fields of practice. The editors wish to thank everyone for their incredible contributions, making this valuable textbook possible. The royalties of this book will be donated to Noah's Ark Children's Hospital charity fund, Cardiff, Wales.

References

Center for Disease Control and Prevention. 2021. *Climate and Health.* Available at: www.cdc.gov/climateandhealth/effects/default.htm [Accessed 05.10.2021].

Department of Health, Social Services and Public Safety. 2013. *Making Life Better. A Whole System Strategic Framework for Public Health.* Available at: www.health-ni.gov.uk/publications/making-life-better-strategy-and-reports [Accessed 10.10.2021].

Department of Health, Social Services and Public Safety. 2015. *Making Life Better. 1st Progress Report 2014/15.* Available at: www.health-ni.gov.uk/publications/making-life-better-strategy-and-reports [Accessed 10.10.2021].

Department of Health. 2017. *Health and Wellbeing 2026 – Delivering Together.* Available at: https://www.health-ni.gov.uk/publications/health-and-wellbeing-2026-delivering-together [Accessed 10.10.2021].

Fleming, M. L., Parker, E. 2015. *Introduction to Public Health.* (5th edn.) Elsevier: Australia.

Government Equalities Office. 2018. *LGBT Action Plan: Lives of Lesbian, Gay, Bisexual and Transgender People.* Available at: https://www.gov.uk/government/publications/lgbt-action-plan-2018-improving-the-lives-of-lesbian-gay-bisexual-and-transgender-people [Accessed 10.10.2021].

HM Government. 2018. *Working Together to Safeguard Children. A Guide to Inter-professional Working to Safeguard and Promote the Welfare of Children.* Available at: https://www.gov.uk/government/publications/working-together-to-safeguard-children–2 [Accessed 10.10.2021].

HM Government. 2021. *Build Back Better: Our Plan for Health and Social Care.* Presented to Parliament by the Prime Minister by Command of Her Majesty. Available at www.gov.uk/government/publications/build-back-better-our-plan-for-health-and-social-care [Accessed 07.10.2021].

Legislation.gov.uk. 2014. *Social Services and Well-being (Wales) Act 2014.* Available at: https://www.legislation.gov.uk/anaw/2014/4/contents [Accessed 10.10.2021].

Legislation.gov.uk. 2015. *Modern Slavery Act 2015.* Available at: https://www.legislation.gov.uk/ukpga/2015/30/contents/enacted [Accessed 10.10.2021].

Legislation.gov.uk. 2015. *Violence against Women, Domestic Abuse and Sexual Violence (Wales) Act 2015*. Available at: https://www.legislation.gov.uk/anaw/2015/3/contents/enacted [Accessed 10.10.2021].

Legislation.gov.uk. 2015. *Human Trafficking and Exploitation (Scotland) Act (Scottish Government, 2015)*. Available at: https://www.legislation.gov.uk/asp/2015/12/contents/enacted [Accessed 10.10.2021].

Legislation.gov.uk. 2016. *Nurse Staffing Levels (Wales) Act 2016*. Available at: https://www.legislation.gov.uk/anaw/2016/5/contents/enacted [Accessed 10.10.2021].

Legislation.gov.uk. 2016. *The Mental Capacity Act (Northern Ireland) 2016*. Available at: https://www.legislation.gov.uk/nia/2016/18/contents/enacted [Accessed 10.10.2021].

Legislation.gov.uk. 2017. *Child Poverty (Scotland) Act 2017*. Available at: https://www.legislation.gov.uk/asp/2017/6/contents/enacted [Accessed 10.10.2021].

Legislation.gov.uk. 2020. *Coronavirus Act 2020*. Available at: https://www.legislation.gov.uk/ukpga/2020/7/contents/enacted [Accessed 10.10.2021].

Legislation.gov.uk. 2021. *The Health and Social Care (Quality and Engagement) (Wales) Act 2021*. Available at: https://www.legislation.gov.uk/anaw/2014/4/contents [Accessed 10.10.2021].

NHS England and NHS Improvement. 2015. *Safguarding Policy*. Available at: https://www.england.nhs.uk/publication/safeguarding-policy/ [Accessed 10.10.2021].

NHS England. 2016. *Healthy Children: Transforming Child Health Information*. Available at: https://www.england.nhs.uk/wp-content/uploads/2016/11/healthy-children-transforming-child-health-info.pdf [Accessed 10.10.2021].

NHS Scotland. 2017. *A Fairer Healthier Scotland: A Strategic Framework for Action 2017–2022*. Available at: http://www.healthscotland.scot/publications/a-fairer-healthier-scotland [Accessed 21.04.2021].

Office for Health Improvement and Disparities. 2022. *Wellbeing and Mental Health: Applying All Our Health*. Available at: https://www.gov.uk/government/publications/wellbeing-in-mental-health-applying-all-our-health/wellbeing-in-mental-health-applying-all-our-health [Accessed 21.04.2022].

Public Health England. 1988. *The Report of the Committee of Inquiry into the Future Development of the Public Health Function*. HMSO: London.

Public Health England. 2014. *Global Health Strategy 2014–2019*. Available at: https://assets.publishing.service.gov.uk/government/uploads/system/uploads/attachment_data/file/354156/Global_Health_Strategy_final_version_for_publication_12_09_14.pdf [Accessed 10.10.2021].

Public Health England. 2020. *Public Health England Strategy 2020–2025*. Available at: https://www.gov.uk/government/publications/phe-strategy-2020-to-2025 [Accessed 10.10.2021].

Public Health Scotland. 2020. *Public Health Scotland's (PHS) Strategic Plan 2020–2023*. Available at: https://publichealthscotland.scot/our-organisation/a-scotland-where-everybody-thrives-public-health-scotland-s-strategic-plan-2020-to-2023/ [Accessed 10.10.2021].

Public Health Wales. 2018. *Working to Achieve a Healthier Future for Wales. Public Health Wales Long Term Strategy 2018–30*. Available at: https://business.senedd.wales/documents/s77112/Paper%202%20-%20Public%20Health%20Wales%20-%20Long%20Term%20Strategy.pdf [Accessed 10.10.2021].

Schneider, M. J. 2017. *Introduction to Public Health*. (5th edn). Jones and Bartlett Learning: Burlington, MA.

Scottish Government. 2015. *Mental Health Scotland Act 2015*. Available at: https://www.gov.scot/publications/mental-health-scotland-act-2015-key-provisions/ [Accessed 10.10.2021].

Scottish Government. 2016. *Health and Social Care Delivery Plan*. Available at: https://www.gov.scot/publications/health-social-care-delivery-plan/ [Accessed 10.10.2021].

United Nations. 2020. *COVID-19 Inequalities and Building Back Better. Policy Brief by HLCP Inequalities Task Team*. Available at: HLCP-policy-brief-on-COVID-19-inequalities-and-building-back-better-1.pdf (un.org) [Accessed 09.09.2021].

United Nations Climate Change Conference. 2021. *COP26 Goals*. Available at: https://ukcop26.org/cop26-goals/ [Accessed 10.10.2021].

Welsh Government. 2015. *Well-being of Future Generations (Wales) Act 2015*. Available at: https://gov.wales/well-being-of-future-generations-wales [Accessed 10.09.2021].

Welsh Government. 2021. *A Healthier Wales: Our Plan for Health and Social Care*. Available at: https://gov.wales/healthier-wales-long-term-plan-health-and-social-care [Accessed 10.10.2021].

World Health Organization. 2020. *WHO Director-General's remarks at the media briefing on 2019-nCoV on 11 February*. Available at: www.who.int/dg/speeches/detail/who-director-general-s-remarks-at-the-media-briefing-on-2019-ncov-on-11-february-2020 [Accessed 09.09.2021].

World Health Organization. 2021a. *The Impact of COVID-19 on Global Health Goals*. Available at: The impact of COVID-19 on global health goals (who.int) [Accessed 09.09.2021].

World Health Organization. 2021b. *World Health Statistics 2021*. Available at: World Health Statistics 2021: A visual summary (who.int) [Accessed 09.09.2021].

World Health Organization. 2021c. *COP26 Health Programme*. Available at: www.who.int/initiatives/cop26-health-programme [Accessed 05.12.2021].

2

THE COVID-19 PANDEMIC – LESSONS LEARNT AND FUTURE PRACTICE

JOHN WATKINS AND DIANNE WATKINS

LEARNING OUTCOMES

By the end of this chapter you will be able to:

- Provide a historical overview of COVID-19 and its clinical features.
- Discuss the public health response and vaccination programmes.
- Discuss the wider implications of COVID-19 on health and wellbeing.
- Outline opportunities for health and social care practice in a pandemic.

Introduction

In December 2019 news emerged from the city of Wuhan, in the Chinese province of Hubei, of a novel respiratory virus causing widespread illness and deaths (Phelan et al. 2020). By early January 2020 it became clear this new and yet unnamed virus was a 'coronavirus', a group of viruses that cause common cold symptoms known to spread from person to person (Li et al. 2020). SARS-CoV-2 was identified as the coronavirus that causes the disease known as 'COVID-19'. Within weeks of identification it was demonstrated that the virus was transmitted person to person and by mid-January cases were starting to appear outside mainland China (Li et al. 2020). Seven attendees at an international conference in Singapore held on 20th–22nd January, also attended by a resident of Wuhan, were later seen to be possible sources for outbreaks in Singapore, Malaysia, South Korea and the UK (Hodcroft 2020). The UK conference attendee went on to infect 13 other people linked to a chalet in a French ski resort. An outbreak on the *Diamond Princess* cruise liner, subsequently quarantined in Yokohama for a month, is thought to be linked to an 80-year-old passenger who embarked the ship in Yokohama on 20th January and was later admitted to hospital with COVID-19 symptoms in Hong Kong in early February (Mizumoto et al. 2020). In total over 700 out of 3,711 passengers/crew tested positive for the virus and 14 died.

By late January, the World Health Organization (WHO) heightened its alert level (WHO 2020a) and the USA's Centers for Disease Control and Prevention (CDC) expressed the view that the current global circumstances suggested this new virus was likely to cause a pandemic (US CDC 2020). On the 11th February WHO formally named the new virus 'SARS-CoV-2' and the disease it caused 'COVID-19' and declared a worldwide pandemic on the 11th March 2020 (WHO 2020b).

In August 2020 there were 24 million cases worldwide and 900,000 deaths linked to COVID-19 (Johns Hopkins Coronavirus Resource Center 2020). By January 2022 this figure rose to 307 million cases and 5.49 million deaths worldwide (Worldometer Coronavirus 2022), with UK deaths reaching a total of 150,000 (BBC 2022). By comparison in 1918, with a world population much smaller than today, there were 50 to 100 million estimated deaths from so-called 'Spanish flu' (2% of the population at the time), and approximately 29,000 people lost their lives to seasonal influenza in the UK in 1989 (Ashley et al. 1991).

Vaccines were developed in the autumn of 2020, offering high levels of immunity to the disease, although infection rates remained high worldwide, death and hospitalisation from serious COVID-19 were greatly reduced following the introduction of vaccines (Christie 2021).

This chapter will provide a historical overview of the virus SARS-CoV-2 responsible for causing COVID-19 and explore public health policy and national governments' decision making in limiting civil liberties of citizens and shutting down vibrant economies to counter the impact of COVID-19. It will discuss the emergence of a vaccine, and the effects of government restrictions and COVID-19 on health. Mitigation measures put in place by national governments have affected the physical and mental health of populations, with future generations left to pick up the impact on the UK economy (Brien and Keep 2021).

Pandemics and the emergence of SARS-CoV-2

Pandemics have historically been defined as worldwide epidemics caused by a novel emergent pathogen that spreads readily from person to person and affects every country and every continent within a single year. The 21st century has witnessed emergent global threats caused by other coronaviruses such as SARS-CoV (Droston et al. 2003), and MERS-CoV (Zaki et al. 2012), and now SARS-CoV-2. SARS-CoV caused Severe Acute Respiratory Syndrome (Drosten et al. 2003), a disease linked to Asian Palm Civets sold in live animal markets in Guangdong China. The civets were probably intermediary hosts that carried the virus from cave dwelling bats in the wild. In 2012 a second coronavirus emerged in the Middle East, MERS-CoV (Zaki et al. 2012), that resulted in approximately 2,500 cases with a case fatality rate of 30%. Unlike SARS-CoV-2 this virus does not transmit readily from person to person and again probably arose from bats, with camels as an intermediate host. While speculation remains as to the exact mechanism by which the SARS-CoV-2 virus jumped the species barrier, the evidence points to human interaction: either directly from bats, or again via intermediate hosts in fish markets, or research laboratories (Cyranoski 2020). The likely common source for all coronavirus infections in humans seem to be linked to bats, and as a species they harbour many more strains of coronavirus than the three that have caused Severe Acute Respiratory Syndrome (SARS) symptoms to date.

Clinical features of COVID-19

Zhou et al. (2020) published a complete review of 191 cases admitted to hospitals in Wuhan up to the 31st January 2020, drawn from the first cohort of 813 hospitalised patients (see Table 2.1). This early study highlighted many of the features that are seen with COVID-19.

The majority of individuals who contract SARS-CoV-2 have very mild symptoms, or none at all, accounting for around 80% of all cases (Tenforde et al. 2020). Approximately 5% of cases need hospitalisation, 1% assisted ventilation and mortality is about 0.15%. Age, underlying chronic conditions, obesity, being male and of Black and Asian origin are also related to poor prognosis (Michaud et al. 2020).

SARS-CoV-2 enters the body via the respiratory tract, the eye and the oropharynx (Weiss and Leibowitz 2011). On entry to the body the virus attaches itself to cell walls via a spike protein to Angiotensin Converting Enzyme 2, ACE-2, binding sites (Michaud et al. 2020), which are found in many organs of the body, principally the lungs and gastrointestinal tracts. The age-specific distribution of ACE-2 binding sites in the body drives the age-based

Table 2.1 Clinical picture (Zhou et al. 2020)

Clinical feature	Days from illness onset and symptoms
Fever	1
Cough	1 (range 1 to 4)
Shortness of breath	4 to 10
Sepsis	7 to 14
Acute Respiratory Distress Syndrome	8 to 15
ICU admission	8 to 15
Death or discharge	15 to 25
Duration of viral shedding	15 to 24 (longest duration 37 days in survivors, or to death)

difference in the attack rates seen with clinical disease. Children have relatively fewer ACE-2 receptors compared to adults, resulting in generally fewer symptoms, of much lower severity and lower transmission rates (Tenforde et al. 2020). This is in stark contrast to influenza where children have a key role in driving epidemic spread (Reichert et al. 2001).

The other key feature of COVID-19 seems to be that there is very little difference in the initial levels of viral excretion between those who remain asymptomatic, or with mild disease and those who have more severe outcomes (Zhou et al. 2020). Maximum viral shedding occurs in the 24 to 48 hours before and after symptoms appear, some 4 to 5 days after contracting the virus (He et al. 2020). Viral antigen is detectable 4 to 5 weeks after symptom onset but the epidemiological importance of this is unclear. Those who go on to develop more life threatening and debilitating disease generally start to deteriorate 7 days after symptom onset (Zhou et al. 2020). 80% of infected individuals have little, or no symptoms of disease. This poses a particular challenge for public health containment measures, such as 'Tracking and Tracing' cases and contacts.

In terms of treatment of COVID-19, drugs such as Dexamethasone (RECOVERY Collaborative Group 2021a), Fluvoxamine (Reis et al. 2021) and ACE inhibitors (Safizadeh et al. 2022) have been shown to reduce the impact of SARS-CoV-2 infection in terms of hospitalisation and deaths. In addition, new therapies such as the monoclonal antibodies, Casirivimab, Imdevimab (RECOVERY Collaborative Group 2021b), Tocilizumab (Salama et al. 2021) and Sotrovimab (Mahase 2021) are proving effective. The first of these new antiviral agents to gain approval in the UK was Molnupiravir, a drug that increases the number of mutations in the SARS-CoV-2 virus RNA, hence disrupting its ability to replicate, but serious safety concerns about its long-term side effects and teratogenicity remain, which will no doubt limit its use (Bernal et al. 2021).

Public health pandemic response

Based on the experiences of the 2009 H1N1pv Influenza pandemic, the UK produced an Influenza Pandemic Preparedness Plan (Department of Health 2011). It set out a phased response to any future pandemic by Influenza: the initial phase covered Detection and Assessment; followed by a Treatment and Escalation phase; and a Recovery phase. This plan was modified to address the threat posed by COVID-19, which, at its onset, had no treatment or vaccine and an unpredictable clinical course. Active interventions in the COVID-19 plan related to non-pharmaceutical interventions such as closing schools, universities, places of social gathering and so on, and self-isolation of suspected cases and contacts.

During the early stages of the pandemic, depicted on UK news bulletins, were images of critical care facilities in Italy and Spain unable to cope with demand and normally stoical doctors and nurses brought to tears by fatigue and feelings of hopelessness in trying to deal with COVID-19 cases. This led British politicians to develop strategies to protect the NHS and frontline services. Against this backdrop of foreboding, the flames of fear that were ripping through the corridors of power were fuelled by mathematical models, produced by Imperial College London. These models predicted that unless draconian lockdown measures were imposed in the UK the national death toll could exceed 500,000 (Flaxman et al. 2020).

On the 23rd March 2020, faced with this unpalatable prospect the Prime Minister activated primary, emergency legislation (DoH 2020) and plunged the UK into total lockdown limiting civil liberties, free movement of people, the closure of all non-essential businesses, hospitality and entertainment, with only essential services being allowed to continue. Total lockdown was imposed for several months and started to ease in late summer 2020, with regional partial lockdowns re-introduced in the autumn to try to curtail increasing cases. Alongside these draconian measures the UK imposed a total travel ban for all non-essential travel to and from the UK and severe limitations in movement away from home except for essential workers. Many Western countries, driven by the same mathematical models, followed suit plunging the global economy into a recession not seen since the 1920s (Centre for Economics and Business Research 2020).

To define social distancing measures the UK government introduced designated Alert levels ranging from Alert Level 5 to Alert Level Zero. Level 5 is full population lockdown whilst Level 0 is where life returns to near normal. In the UK alert levels were raised and lowered on several occasions in line with infection rates. In December 2021, as Omicron variant (see below) infections rose, social distancing measures were reintroduced and mask wearing again became mandatory in some settings, such as retail, theatres, transport and schools.

Face masks and social distancing

Prior to vaccination the main public health intervention with COVID-19 was non-pharmaceutical interventions such as social distancing and the wearing of face coverings. In trying to reopen economies and make educational, retail, entertainment and hospitality venues viable, one of the major impediments to this was an arbitrary 2-metre social distancing rule, which was out of step with that imposed in other countries. To address this problem, the Department of Health in England introduced what they described as a 1-metre plus rule (BBC 2020). This stated that it was desirable to maintain a 2-metre separation between people at all times (other than household contacts); however, in those situations where this rule could not be easily adhered to (e.g. school corridors, public transport etc.) face coverings should be worn. While having wide public support, the evidence base underpinning this decision was solely lacking. Chu et al. (2020) have addressed the benefits of wearing face masks and social distancing in risk reduction. This study found that in periods of low population prevalence of the virus and hence low risk of transmission, the added benefit of a 2-metre social distancing rule, as opposed to 1-metre, while reducing the risk of transmission by 50%, the absolute risk reduction was of the order of 0.25% (1 extra case in 400 contacts). With population carriage of approximately one per hundred individuals being infected, this translates to one extra case per 4,000 contacts.

Vaccines

By the summer of 2020 cases in the UK had fallen, but effective vaccines were still in clinical trials. In autumn 2020 two novel vaccines, first from the Oxford/AstraZeneca group (Voysey et al. 2021) and then Pfizer/BioNTech (Amit et al. 2021) showed remarkable results, with trials demonstrating an efficacy of over 90% in preventing serious disease and deaths after two doses. In December 2020 mass vaccination programmes started in most Western Nations with uptake rates of up to 90% in the elderly and vulnerable in the UK. As time went on further strains of SARS-CoV-2 emerged, in turn, each replacing earlier variants, the most significant being the Alpha and Delta strains followed by the Omicron strain first identified in South Africa in November 2021, the latter being highly infectious but causing much milder symptoms (BBC 2021). The vaccines gave protection against all the strains identified and reduced the threat of death, serious disease and hospitalisations in those who had received two vaccines. As a precaution, third booster doses were administered in many countries, and this proved to be an effective means of maintaining low population mortality rates.

It is beyond the scope of this chapter to cover the rollout and subsequent impact of vaccination on the course of the pandemic, but it is important to note that most developed nations had, by late 2020, embarked on the most ambitious vaccine rollout in history. For example, by the autumn of 2021 the UK had offered all adults over the age of 18 years two doses of vaccine and over 80% had taken up this offer. With the emergence of the Omicron variant in November 2021 a third dose of vaccine was offered to this group and again over 80% of all those over 70 years had taken up this offer by January 2022.

Vaccines had broken the link between cases and deaths and had proven, with booster doses, they could reduce the chances of symptomatic illness by 70% and hospitalisations and deaths by over 90% (UK Health Security Agency 2022).

While throughout 2021 vaccine coverage rates increased, anti-vaccine groups emerged, opposed to receiving the vaccine; the consequence of this was that by the third wave of the pandemic the vast majority of those suffering serious disease and hospitalisation were unvaccinated. For this reason, the major focus for national governments, not just in the UK, was a drive for all adults to receive a third booster of one of the mRNA vaccines (UK Health Security Agency 2022).

Immunity

Prior to the SARS-CoV-2 pandemic, despite the ubiquitous nature of coronaviruses in the human population, known for decades, there remained a considerable number of unanswered questions relevant to public health. It was unclear whether immunity gained against a specific strain of coronavirus offers any protection against different strains, and there was little evidence to support this. In addition, it was not known how long strain specific immunity may last, or whether it reduced over the longer term. It was also unclear as to whether individuals could become re-infected with the same virus, although early in the pandemic there were a few anecdotal reports of individuals contracting SARS-CoV-2 a second time.

As the pandemic progressed evidence started to emerge that reinfection with SARS-CoV-2, even after vaccination, was indeed taking place. Longitudinal studies showed that over time protective antibody levels declined especially over a period of up to 12 months (Xiang et al. 2021), this level of decline resulting in susceptibility to new infection with the original, or mutated virus. However, these reinfections carried with them the risk of much milder disease and it emerged that the more serious complications, hospitalisations and deaths were averted by either vaccine or infection and generated specific B and T-cell immune responses (Dan et al. 2021).

In the early phase of the pandemic most tests of immunity were based on the search for SARS-CoV-2 specific antibodies, which generally are short lived and may not answer the question as to whether exposure to SARS-CoV-2 confers long-term protection, a significant public health question. Immunity to viruses, for example influenza, generates not only antibody but also T-cell mediated immunity which has been shown to be long lived, probably life-long, and have a much broader spectrum of action against viruses than antibodies. As the pandemic progressed and more people were either infected, or vaccinated, against SARS-CoV-2, it became apparent that vaccines and natural infection generated long-lasting protection against the many variants of the virus. In addition, prior exposure to other common cold causing coronaviruses generated protective T-cell responses, giving a glimmer of hope that vaccines and treatments could be developed that would protect mankind against all known and emerging variants in the future (Grifoni et al. 2020, Mateus et al. 2020).

Impact on health and wellbeing

The implementation of societal lockdown to reduce the transmission of infection came at great cost economically and in relation to its effects on individual health and wellbeing. The Office of Budget Responsibility estimated the economic impact of lockdown to the UK economy would be £260 billion, some 10% of GDP (Office of Budget Responsibility 2020, Watkins 2020), a figure revised upwards to within the range of £315 to 410 billion in 2021 (Brien and Keep 2021).

In the first 9 months of the new emergent pandemic it was becoming clear that 80% of cases were either mild or asymptomatic, and most deaths occurred in vulnerable groups (the elderly, those with chronic disease and those of ethnic origin of colour) with an overall mortality rate approaching that of seasonal influenza, at or below 0.1%. A blanket ban on the civil liberties of the population, many of whom will never suffer the ill effects of this virus, are profound and long-lasting, much of this burden being carried by the young and those in deprived communities with insecure employment. Douglas et al. (2020) explored the broader impact that the SARS-CoV-2 pandemic has had on various sectors of the population. While Chin et al. (2020) questioned the robustness of the models used to influence lockdowns and other restrictive social interventions.

Underpinning the findings of Douglas et al. (2020), Leigh-Hunt et al. (2017) published evidence on the association between social isolation, loneliness and increased all-cause mortality with an odds ratio of 1.29 (95% CI; 1.06, 1.56), conversely good social networks were protective odds ratio 0.87 (95% CI; 0.82, 0.91). Findings supported by Rico-Uribe et al. (2018) identified loneliness as a risk factor for all-cause mortality. Leigh-Hunt et al. (2017) also identified associations between loneliness and poorer mental health outcomes. While loneliness, social isolation and depression are long-term problems in many Western societies, where the extended family support network is fragmented, the COVID-19 pandemic, the imposed rules on social distancing and the limitation/outright ban on visiting to health and social care settings exacerbated this problem (National Health Library & Knowledge Service, 2020).

The opportunities for health and social care practice in the aftermath of a pandemic

The effects of a pandemic such as COVID-19 on society are far reaching and could not have been predicted. Nations across the globe were forced to make decisions to control spread of the pandemic from a limited evidence base and health and social care practitioners were thrown into unknown territory. Whilst this dealt with the immediate physical health issues, the long-terms effects are yet to be fully experienced. As outlined in Table 2.2, various groups in society are more at risk and practitioners have needed to predict how practice may change, based on the emerging evidence and effects on society. COVID-19 has had an adverse effect on the way societies, families and individuals

Table 2.2 Groups at risk of COVID-19 (Douglas et al. 2020)

- Older people—highest direct risk of severe COVID-19, more likely to live alone, less likely to use online communications, at risk of social isolation
- Young people—affected by disrupted education at critical time; in longer term most at risk of poor employment and associated health outcomes in economic downturn
- Women—more likely to be carers, likely to lose income if need to provide childcare during school closures, potential for increase in family violence for some
- People of East Asian ethnicity—may be at increased risk of discrimination and harassment because the pandemic is associated with China
- People with mental health problems—may be at greater risk from social isolation
- People who use substances or in recovery—risk of relapse or withdrawal
- People with a disability—affected by disrupted support services
- People with reduced communication abilities (eg. learning disabilities, limited literacy or English language ability)—may not receive key governmental communications
- Homeless people—may be unable to self-isolate or affected by disrupted support services
- People in criminal justice system—difficulty of isolation in prison setting, loss of contact with family
- Undocumented migrants—may have no access to or be reluctant to engage with health services
- Workers on precarious contracts or self-employed—high risk of adverse effects from loss of work and no income
- People on low income—effects will be particularly severe as they already have poorer health and are more likely to be in insecure work without financial reserves
- People in institutions (care homes, special needs facilities, prisons, migrant detention centres, cruise liners)—as these institutions may act as amplifiers

function, affecting the most vulnerable such as the elderly, those with underlying physical or mental health problems, and families living in abusive households. Increased numbers of domestic violence cases are evidenced through a 25% rise in calls to the UK Domestic Violence Hotline and 150% increase in visits to refuges (Bradbury-Jones 2020). Home is not always a safe place for adults or children, and crisis support is essential where families are living with an abuser in a locked-down, socially isolated situation as part of government rules and regulations to control the spread of this virus. Whilst the focus was on dealing with the acute nature of the disease, the wider implications of social control measures has had a devasting effect on other groups in society. Calls to child help lines increased and UNICEF (2020) warned of the risk to children, stating that

> Evidence from previous infectious disease outbreaks indicate that existing child protection risks are exacerbated, and new ones emerge as a result of the epidemic as well as of the socioeconomic impacts of prevention and control measures. (UNICEF 220, p.1)

Health visitors, school nurses and social workers need to be particularly vigilant during a pandemic, recognising the adverse effects on vulnerable children. Although remote support can be offered it does not replace one-to-one support for individuals and families. Health and social care practitioners should search for health needs, stimulate an awareness of health needs at all levels, and facilitate health enhancing activities during and after any future pandemic the world may face. Children form the future generation and their health and wellbeing is of paramount importance. In the face of adversity, families living in poverty will be subjected to greater situational stress, worsened by a pandemic. Community practitioners are well placed to offer help, support and advice, ensuring the most vulnerable are protected.

The psychological impact of the COVID-19 pandemic and the resultant social isolation is adversely affecting the general population and will particularly influence those with pre-existing mental health issues or substance abuse concerns. These problems coupled with fear of the unknown, of contracting the disease, anxiety and distress can lead to suicidal behaviour and COVID-19 survivors may be at increased risk (Sher 2020). They may peak following a pandemic, as well as during, and therefore it is imperative for practitioners to be alert to such issues, offering extra help and support to survivors and to those with a known mental health problem or addiction.

The numbers of deaths from COVID-19 alluded to earlier in this chapter leave an unmet need in terms of bereavement support required. Huge segments of the 'at risk' population (elderly and Black and minority groups) and practitioners involved in the acute care and death of COVID-19 patients face psychological trauma. Health and social care workers must care for their peers, recognise the effects of a pandemic upon them and offer counselling, when appropriately skilled to do so. Efforts to address post-traumatic stress and promote coping mechanisms should form part of their work.

Professional practice during and post pandemic should include working at meso through to micro levels. Practitioners can engage with policy makers to ensure needs of the most vulnerable are considered and assist in protocol development that ensures required workplace infection control measures are implemented. Involvement in population-based initiatives such as mass-vaccination programmes and track and trace may also form part of their role, as would media campaigns to ensure that messages to the population are accurate and understandable, with attention given to those individuals with communication difficulties.

The practice surrounding a pandemic presents endless opportunities for those working in a community setting, as well as practitioners offering front-line care in acute environments. The focus of working through and in the aftermath of a pandemic must include meeting the needs of society as a whole, realising that new health issues will surface and practitioners must be ready and willing to adopt practice to meet such needs. They should work with populations to empower them to look after their own health and play a part in reducing spread. Practitioners should act as advocates, ensuring that those most at need receive appropriate health and social care during a pandemic.

Conclusion

At the time of writing, the COVID-19 pandemic is far from over, particularly in the developing world and emerging economies where vaccine availability and distribution is limited. It has often been said that 'no one is safe until we are all safe', and hence a united global response is necessary. Although COVID-19 has helped develop a template for dealing with a pandemic, not all lessons learnt are positive. This is understandable when the blueprint for practice is being developed on a day-by-day basis as problems arise. What we have learnt is that the needs of society are far reaching and extend beyond the physical presence of the disease. Longer-term problems are yet to materialise, and only then will we have learnt what has worked well and how future generations can be helped to survive.

It will be essential for future successful management of pandemics that the following is considered:

- A robust process by which threats posed by human encroachment on nature are recognised, quantified and evaluated globally, and international legally binding agreements developed to reduce pandemic zoonotic infections occurring.
- The upscaling of vaccine production, vaccine programmes and treatments made available to all nations, regardless of where they are developed or ability to pay.
- An evaluation of national and international responses to the COVID-19 pandemic, particularly the effectiveness of face masks, social distancing, locking-down of society and border control, to assess the benefits and adverse effects on health and wellbeing.
- A review of mathematical modelling and epidemiological data used to drive national public health responses to a pandemic, using lessons learnt from COVID-19.
- An evaluation of UK health and social care systems and their ability to upscale to meet the challenges of a pandemic.

Future research into the effects of a pandemic on health to inform the evidence base for practice. Consider the following questions

1. Thinking globally, what actions are needed going forward, to reduce the chances of a future pandemic occurring and those measures that need to be put in place to mitigate its impact if one occurs?
2. What do you see as the priorities for nation states, in the early phases, post pandemic, to ensure the worst impacts on the health of its citizens can be reduced?
3. What do you see as the key indirect harms of the SARS-CoV-2 pandemic, in the UK, that were a consequence of public policy and how have these impacted on society as a whole and individuals in particular?

Key terms

COVID-19: The disease caused by the coronavirus SARS-CoV-2.

Immunity: The condition of being able to resist a particular disease, especially through preventing development of a pathogenic microorganism or by counteracting the effects of its products.

Lockdown: A restriction policy for people or community to stay where they are, usually due to specific risks to themselves or to others if they were to move and interact freely. During the COVID-19 pandemic, the term 'lockdown' was used for actions related to mass quarantines or stay-at-home orders.

Monoclonal antibodies: Laboratory-made proteins that mimic the immune system's ability to fight off harmful pathogens such as viruses. Casirivimab and imdevimab are monoclonal antibodies that are specifically directed against the spike protein of SARS-CoV-2, designed to block the virus' attachment and entry into human cells.

Pandemic: An epidemic of a disease that has affected large numbers of people in every country and continent throughout the world over a 12-month period.

SARS-CoV-2: The coronavirus that can cause the disease called COVID-19.

Social distancing: In public health, social distancing, also called physical distancing, is a set of non-pharmaceutical interventions or measures intended to prevent the spread of a contagious disease by maintaining a physical distance between people and reducing the number of times people come into close contact with each other.

Vaccine: A biological preparation that provides active acquired immunity to a particular infectious disease. A vaccine typically contains an agent that resembles a disease-causing microorganism and is often made from weakened or killed forms of the microbe, its toxins or one of its surface proteins.

Further reading

Ashton, J. 2021. *Blinded by Corona*. Gibson Square Books: London.

Krakauer, D., West, G. (Eds). 2021. *The Complex Alternative – Complexity Scientists on the COVID-19 Pandemic*. The SFE Press: Santa Fe, NM.

Miller, J., Sahin, U., Tureci, O. 2022. *The Vaccine: Inside the Race to Conquer the COVID-19 Pandemic*. Macmillan: New York.

References

Amit, S., Regev-Yochay, G., Afek, A., Kreiss, Y., Leshem, E. 2021. Early rate reductions of SARS-CoV-2 infection and COVID-19 in BNT162b2 vaccine recipients. *Lancet.* doi: 10.1016/S0140-6736(21)00448-7

Ashley, J., Smith, T., Dunnell K. 1991. Deaths in Great Britain associated with the influenza epidemic of 1989/90. *Pop Trends*; 65: 16–20.

BBC. 2020. Coronavirus: could social distancing of less than two metres work? *BBC News*; 23 June. Available at: www.bbc.co.uk/news/science-environment-52522460 [Accessed 09.03.2022].

BBC. 2021. Omicron wave appears milder, but concern remains. *BBC News*; 22 December. Available at: www.bbc.co.uk/news/health-59758784 [Accessed 09.03.2022].

BBC. 2022. COVID-19: UK surpasses 150,000 deaths, and how rapid tests changed the pandemic. *BBC News*; 10 January. Available at: www.bbc.co.uk/news/uk-59925446 [Accessed 09.03.2022].

Bernal, A. J., Gomes da Silva, M. M., Musungaie, D. B., Kovalchuk, E., et al. 2021. Molnupiravir for oral treatment of COVID-19 in non-hospitalized patients. *NEJM*. Available at: doi: 10.1056/NEJMoa2116044 [Accessed 09.03.2022].

Bradbury-Jones, C. 2020. The pandemic paradox: the consequences of COVID-19 on domestic violence. *Journal of Clinical Nursing*. Available at: doi: 10.1111 JOCN 15296 [Accessed 09.03.2022].

Brien, P., Keep, M. 2021. *Public Spending during the COVID-19 Pandemic*. House of Commons Library: No. 09309. Available at: https://researchbriefings.files.parliament.uk/documents/CBP-9309/CBP-9309.pdf [Accessed 09.03.2022].

Centre for Economics and Business Research. 2020. Estimates of daily economic impact of the UK's lockdown by sector. *Cebr*; 6 April. Available at: https://cebr.com/reports/as-the-uk-remains-in-lockdown-government-may-need-to-target-more-support-at-manufacturing-sector/ [Accessed 09.03.2022].

Chin, V., Ioannidis, J. P. A., Tanner, M. A. & Cripps, S. 2020. Effects of non-pharmaceutical interventions on COVID-19: a tale of three models. *medRxiv* 2020.07.22.20160341.

Christie, B. 2021. COVID-19: vaccines are highly effective in preventing deaths from delta variant, study indicates. *BMJ*; 375: n2582. Available at: http://dx.doi.org/10.1136/bmj.n2582 [Accessed 09.03.2022].

Chu, D. K., Akl, E. A., Duda, S., Solo, K., Yaacoub, S., et al. 2020. *Physical distancing, face masks, and eye protection to prevent person-to-person transmission of SARS-CoV-2 and COVID-19: a systematic review and meta-analysis*. Available at: https://doi.org/10.1016/S0140-6736(20)31142-9 [Accessed 09.03.2022].

Cyranoski, D. 2020. Mystery deepens over animal source of Coronavirus. *Nature*; 579 (7797), 18–19.

Dan, J. M., Mateus, J., Kato, Y., Hastie, K. M., et al. 2021. Immunological memory to SARS-CoV-2 assessed for up to 8 months after infection. *Science*. doi: 10.1126/science.abf4063

Department of Health. 2011. *Pandemic Influenza Preparedness Team. UK Influenza Pandemic Preparedness Strategy 2011*. Department of Health: London.

Department of Health. 2020. *What the Coronavirus Bill will do?* Available at: www.gov.uk/government/publications/coronavirus-bill-what-it-will-do/what-the-coronavirus-bill-will-do [Accessed 09.03.2022].

Douglas M., Katikireddi S. V., Taulbut M., McKee M., McCartney G. 2020. Mitigating the wider health effects of COVID-19 pandemic response. *BMJ*; 369:m1557. doi: 10.1136/bmj.m1557

Drosten, C., Gunther, S., Preiser, W., et al. 2003. Identification of a novel coronavirus in patients with severe acute respiratory syndrome. *New England Journal of Medicine*; 348: 1967–76. doi: 10.1056/NEJMoa030747

Flaxman, S., Mishra, S., Gandy, A., Unwin, H. J. T., et al. 2020. Estimating the effects of non-pharmaceutical interventions on COVID-19 in Europe. *Nature*. doi: 10.1038/s41586-020-2405-7

Grifoni, A., Weiskopf, D., Ramirez, S. I., Mateus, J., et al. 2020. Targets of T-cell responses to SARS-CoV-2 coronavirus in humans with COVID-19 disease and unexposed individuals. *Cell*; 181, 1489–1501. doi: 10.1016/j.cell.2020.05.015

He, X., Lau, E. H. Y., Wu, P., Deng, X., Wang, J., et al. 2020. Temporal dynamics in viral shedding and transmissibility of COVID-19. *Nature Medicine*. doi: 10.1038/s41591-020-0869-5

Hodcroft, E. 2020. Preliminary case report on the SARS-CoV-2 cluster in the UK, France, and Spain. *Swiss Med. Wkly*; 150,w20212

Johns Hopkins Coronavirus Resource Center. 2020. *COVID-19 Data*. Available at: https://coronavirus.jhu.edu/ [Accessed 17.09.2020].

Leigh-Hunt, N., Bagguley, D., Bash, K., et al. 2017. An overview of systematic reviews on the public health consequences of social isolation and loneliness. *Public Health*; 2017;152:157–171. doi: 10.1016/j.puhe.2017.07.035

Li, Q., Guan, X., Wu, P., et al. 2020. Early transmission dynamics in Wuhan, China of novel coronavirus-infected pneumonia. *N. Engl. J. Med*. published online 29th January. doi: 10.1056/NEJMoa2001316

Mahase, E. 2021. COVID-19: UK approves monoclonal antibody sotrovimab for over 12s at high risk. *BMJ*; 375, n2990. http://dx.doi.org/10.1136/bmj.n2990

Mateus, J., Grifoni, A., Tarke, A., Sidney, J., et al. 2020. Selective and cross-reactive SARS-CoV-2 T cell epitopes in unexposed humans. *Science*; 370: 89–9.

Michaud, V., Deodhar, M., Arwood, M., Al Rihani, S. B., et al. 2020. ACE2 as a therapeutic target for COVID-19; its role in infectious processes and regulation by modulators of the RAAS system. *J. Clin. Med*.; 9, 2096. doi: 10.3390/jcm9072096

Mizumoto, K., Kagaya, K., Zarebski, A., Chowell, G. 2020. Estimating the asymptomatic proportion of coronavirus disease 2019 (COVID-19) cases on board the Diamond Princess cruise ship, Yokohama Japan 2020. *Eurosurveillance*; 25(10):pii=2000180. https://doi.org/10.2807/1560-7917

National Health Library & Knowledge Service, Madden, A., Leen, B. 2020. Evidence summary: what is the impact of the coronavirus pandemic on the mental health of elderly nursing home residents? [V1.0]. *Health Service Executive*. Available at: www.lenus.ie/handle/10147/627785 [Accessed 24.06.2020].

Office of Budget Responsibility. 2020. *The OBR's Coronavirus Analysis*; April 14. Available at: https://cdn.obr.uk/The_OBRs_coronavirus_analysis.pdf [Accessed 16.06.2022].

Phelan, A. L., Katz, R., Gostin, L. O. 2020. The novel coronavirus originating in Wuhan, China: challenges for global health governance. *JAMA*. doi: 10.1001/jama.2020.1097

RECOVERY Collaborative Group. 2021a. Dexamethasone in hospitalized patients with COVID-19. *N. Engl. J. Med*. 2021; 384:693–704. doi: 10.1056/NEJMoa2021436

RECOVERY Collaborative Group. 2021b. Casirivimab and imdevimab in patients admitted to hospital with COVID-19 (RECOVERY): a randomised, controlled, open-label, platform trial. *medRxiv preprint*. doi: 10.1101/2021.06.15.21258542

Reichert, T. A., Sugaya, N., Fedson, D. S., Glezen, W. P., et al. 2001. The Japanese experience with vaccinating school children against influenza. *New England Journal*; 344, 889–896.

Reis, G., Moreira-Silva, E., Silva, D., Thabane, L., et al. 2021. Effect of early treatment with fluvoxamine on risk of emergency care and hospitalisation among patients with COVID-19: the TOGETHER randomised, platform clinical trial. *Lancet Glob. Health*. doi: 10.1016/S2214-109X(21)00448-4

Rico-Uribe, L. A., Caballero, F. F, Martín-María, N., Cabello, M., Ayuso-Mateos, J. L., Miret, M. 2018. Association of loneliness with all-cause mortality: a meta-analysis. *PloS One*.13(1):e0190033. doi:10.1371/journal.pone.0190033

Safizadeh, F., Nguyen, T. N. M., Brenner, H., Schöttker, B. 2022. Association of Renin–Angiotensin–Aldosterone System inhibition with COVID-19 hospitalization and all-cause mortality in the UK Biobank. *Brit. J. Clinical Pharma* (in press). doi: 10.1002/BCP.15192

Salama, C., Han, J., Yau, L., Reiss, W. G., et al. 2021. Tocilizumab in patients hospitalized with COVID-19 pneumonia. *NEJM*; 384, 20–30. doi: 10.1056/NEJMoa2030340

Sher, L. 2020. The impact of the COVID-19 pandemic on suicide rates. *QJM An International Journal of Medicine*; hcaa202, https://doi.org/10.1093/qjmed/hcaa20

Tenforde, M., Kim, S., Lindsell, C. J., Rose, E. B., et al. 2020. Symptom duration and risk factors for delayed return to usual health among outpatients with COVID-19 in a Multistate Health Care Systems Network — United States, March–June 2020. *MMWR Morb. Mortal Wkly. Rep.*; 69, 993–998.

UK Health Security Agency. 2022. Boosters continue to provide high levels of protection against severe disease from Omicron in older adults. *GOV.UK Press Release*; 7th January. Available at: www.gov.uk/government/news/boosters-continue-to-provide-high-levels-of-protection-against-severe-disease-from-omicron-in-older-adults [Accessed 09.03.2022].

UNICEF. 2020. *Protection of children during the COVID-19 pandemic: children and alternative care immediate response measure*. Available at: www.unicef.org/media/68506/file/COVID-19-Alternative-Care-Technical-Note.pdf [Accessed 14.09.2020].

US CDC 2020. US Centers for Disease Control and Prevention. *Coronavirus disease 2019 (Covid-19): situation summary*. https://doi.org/10.1016/S0140-6736(20)31142-9

Voysey, M., Clement, S., Madhi, S., Weckx, L., et al. 2021. Single dose administration, and the influence of the timing of the booster dose on immunogenicity and efficacy of ChAdOx1 nCoV-19 (AZD1222) vaccine. *Lancet Preprints*. Available at: https://papers.ssrn.com/sol3/papers.cfm?abstract_id=3777268 [Accessed 09.03.2022].

Watkins, J. 2020. COVID-19 Lockdown – Time to find an exit strategy and reflect on the costs and benefits! *Gen. Int. Med. Clin. Innov.* doi: 10.15761/GIMCI.1000194

Weiss, S. R., Leibowitz J. L. 2011. Coronavirus pathogenesis. *Adv. Virus Res.*; 81: 85–164.

World Health Organization. 2020a. *Statement on the first meeting of the International Health Regulations Emergency Committee regarding the outbreak of novel coronavirus (2019-nCoV)*. 23 January 2020 Statement Geneva, Switzerland. Available at: www.who.int/news-room/detail/23-01-2020-statement-on-the-meeting-of-the-international-health-regulations-(2005)-emergency-committee-regarding-the-outbreak-of-novel-cor-onavirus-(2019-ncov) [Accessed 09.03.2022].

World Health Organization. 2020b. *WHO Director-General's remarks at the media briefing on 2019-nCoV on 11 February*. Available at: www.who.int/dg/speeches/detail/who-director-general-s-remarks-at-the-media-briefing-on-2019-ncov-on-11-february-2020 [Accessed 09.03.2022].

Worldometer Coronavirus. 2022. Available at: www.worldometers.info/coronavirus/ [Accessed 09.03.2022].

Xiang, T., Liang, B., Fang, Y., Lu, S., et al. 2021. Declining levels of neutralizing antibodies against SARS-CoV-2 in convalescent COVID-19 patients one year post symptom onset. *Front. Immunology*. Available at: https://doi.org/10.3389/fimmu.2021.708523 [Accessed 09.03.2022].

Zaki, A. M., van Boheemen, S., Bestebroer, T. M., Osterhaus, A. D., Fouchier, R. A. 2012. Isolation of a novel coronavirus from a man with pneumonia in Saudi Arabia. *N. Engl. J. Med.*; 367, 1814–1820. doi: 10.1056/ NEJMoa1211721

Zhou, F., Yu, T., Du, R., Fan, G., et al. 2020. Clinical course and risk factors for mortality of adult inpatients with COVID-19 in Wuhan, China: a retrospective cohort study. *Lancet*; 28;395(10229), 1054–1062. doi: 10.1016/S0140-6736(20)30566

Section 1:

HEALTH PROMOTION AND PREVENTION

3

HEALTH PROMOTION

LORRAINE JOOMUN

═══════════ LEARNING OUTCOMES ═══════════

By the end of this chapter you will be able to:

- Have an understanding of health promotion approaches and models.
- Recognise the complexities of delivering health promotion when considering people's beliefs and values, and how salutogenesis supports health and wellbeing.
- Discuss the barriers to health promotion, how these affect behaviour change and how to overcome these barriers.
- Have an awareness of cultural competency and how this is essential when working in multicultural communities.

Introduction

'Health promotion' theory draws on the knowledge base from sociology, psychology, community development and the political sciences (Laverack 2014). 'Health promotion' is an umbrella term for a broad collection of strategies to tackle the wider determinants of health. It is the process of enabling people to increase control over and to improve their health. It moves beyond a focus on individual behaviour towards a wide range of social and environmental interventions.

The focus of this chapter will raise awareness of the building blocks of health promotion first by giving an overview of what is health promotion and where health promotion sits within public health. The main aspect of the chapter will discuss models and approaches to health promotion. Included in this discussion is the concept of 'making every contact count' (MECC), salutogenesis, marginalisation and barriers to health promotion. The social, psychological and cultural awareness of health promotion including values and beliefs in underpinning behaviour change have been discussed and links made to COVID-19.

Health promotion

Health promotion has been scrutinised and debated since the early 1970s; the Lalonde Report in 1974 focused on the health of Canada's population, raised concerns about health education and individual's responsibility on health behaviour. The emergence of what is known as 'The New Public Health' was adopted alongside the introduction of global public health conferences that raised the profile of health promotion. The first of these conferences saw the declaration of Alma Ata in 1978, the need for urgent action globally by all governments to protect and promote the health of all people. It was acknowledged that inequalities in health are unacceptable, and that people should be involved in the planning of their own health care. Health services should be redefined to include: agriculture, animal husbandry, food, industry, education, housing, public works and communications. Another milestone in health promotion was the Ottawa Charter in 1986 (WHO 1986). Five criteria were set out, building health public policy, strengthening community action, creating supporting environments, developing personal skills and reorienting health services. The charter advocates 'a socio-ecological approach to improve health in which people and their environments are considered to be inextricably linked' (WHO 1986, p. 3). Following on from the Ottawa Charter, the Jakarta Declaration went a step further in recognising the importance of taking health promotion into the 21st century:

> Health promotion, through investment and action, has a marked impact on the determinants of health and can be used to create the greatest gain for people, to contribute significantly to the reduction of inequalities in health, to further human rights, and to build social capital. (WHO 1997)

There were other global public health conferences that followed, and each added to the list of changes that should be brought about to improve the Nation's health. Health promotion covers a range of strategies to tackle health determinants of the wider population. There are a variety of definitions that have been proposed, such as

> raising the health status of individuals and communities. Promotion in the health context means improving, advancing, supporting, encouraging and placing health higher on personal and public agendas. (Scriven 2010)

Some definitions focus on activities and others on values and principles like the definition above. These definitions are forever changing and developing to encompass health and wellbeing in the 21st century.

Health promotion approaches

There are five approaches to health promotion (Ewles and Simnett 2003), these approaches offer different kinds of activities, and more than one approach is advocated.

There is no consensus on what the right approach is or set of activities for health promotion and public health practice. Health promoters need to work out for themselves which approach and which activities they use, in accordance with professional codes of conduct, professional values and an assessment of client's needs. Different approaches to promoting health are useful tools of analysis, which can help to clarify aims and values. A framework of five approaches is suggested in Table 3.1 with the values implicit in any approach identified.

Of the five approaches, behavioural change was one of the first approaches to be used and is still used within health campaigns. Behavioural change focuses on lifestyle activities that impact on health. Its purpose is to use persuasive messages to promote healthy lifestyle behaviours and for individuals to take responsibility for their own wellbeing. Disadvantages of using this approach are that it does not consider the social factors that affect health, including cultural, political, economic and social influences. A further aspect is victim blaming; this approach is centred on the fact that if individuals are provided with information they will act on this information and change their behaviour (Ewles and Simnett 2003).

The self-empowerment or self-actualisation approach enables the individual to make choices and have control over their own health where possible. This approach focuses on raising confidence and self-esteem and promoting self-efficacy. The client-centredness of this approach is conducive to working in partnership with clients, to enable decision making and problem solving in facilitation of the individual taking control of their own life. This approach is based on the individual and not targeted at groups or populations.

An educational approach is where information is provided to update knowledge and understanding of health issues. However, this approach assumes that information attainment will lead to a change in behaviour, although using this approach alone is not always effective. The inclusion of three learning styles – affective, cognitive and

Table 3.1 The five approaches to health promotion

Medical/Preventative	Behaviour change
• This approach is concerned with compliance, to ensure that patients take up and comply with procedures, such as screening and immunisation. • Methods are encouraged, and professionals are paternalistic in using this approach. • Includes three levels of prevention: primary, secondary and tertiary.	• Change individual attitudes or behaviour adapt a healthy lifestyle. • Makes use of persuasion as a technique. • Assumes that people are able to make changes. • Ignores complexity associated with behaviour change. • Views health as a property of individuals. • Victim blaming.
Educational	**Client centred/Empowerment**
• Inform knowledge and understanding of health issues, help people to explore values and attitudes. • Respect individual's choice to choose. • To include learning styles: affective, cognitive and behavioural • Provides unbiased information. • Assumes that knowledge will lead to change in behaviour.	• Working in partnership with clients, make their own decisions and choices according to their own interests and values. • Clients valued as equals, raising self-esteem and confidence and promoting self-efficacy. • Leads to own ability to control and make choices. • Health promoter becomes a facilitator whose role is to act as a catalyst whilst promoting a public health intervention.
Social change	
• Focus on changing society not behaviour of individuals, targeted towards groups and populations. • Known as a radical approach to health promotion. • Focus on legislation and the environment.	

behavioural – within this approach aids the health promoter in identifying attitudes, skills and reasoning to inform health promotion interventions.

Where compliance in relation to treatments is required for the health and wellbeing of individuals, the medical/preventative approach is recommended. This approach incorporates three levels of prevention: primary, secondary and tertiary. Professionals usually take a paternalistic attitude to this approach, which is often persuading parents to uptake immunisation for their children or women to uptake cervical cytology screening (Scriven 2017).

The final approach is social change, which focuses on how changes to society can support health by tackling social and environmental situations. From a political perspective, professionals can influence policy decisions and focus on resource distribution. This approach is directed at groups and populations rather than an individual approach such as behavioural. Empowerment plays a part in this approach as this is about giving people a voice regarding their health and care needs (Edelman et al. 2010).

Health promotion models

There are a variety of health promotion models and theories that offer frameworks to aid understanding of the complexities of health promotion. These models provide a theoretical base and guidance when delivering health promotion messages. Some examples of these models are the Health Belief model, Transtheoretical model, Social Cognitive theory, Theory of Reasoned Action, Tannahill's and Beattie's, that are often used within healthcare. No one model fits all individuals and communities, so practitioners will need to develop a programme that is specific to the requirements of each individual or group. In early childhood, habits are formed that are often lifelong unless these habits are broken. Habits are often embedded in domestic practices and need changing as early as possible before they become well established. It is important to remember that in the case of children and adolescents, managing emotional fallout and stress for behaviour change needs to be prioritised as education on health alone will not give them the skills and self-efficacy to change habits.

Professionals working with families and communities when initiating these health promotion programmes will likely be more successful. Each individual will need a different programme according to their internal or external locus of control. Having an internal locus of control is the belief that your actions determine success or failure, that is an individual has control of what choices they make in relation to lifestyle choices. Whereas an external locus of control is believed to be related to fate or luck, here individuals believe they have no control over the outcome. For this reason, individuals with an external locus of control do better connecting to group programmes rather than an individualised programme. One such model where internal and external locus of control has some influence is the Health Belief model. This model consists of four areas of beliefs: perceived susceptibility, perceived severity, perceived benefits and perceived barriers. There are also constructs such as self-efficacy and cues to action. These cues are particularly relevant in determining whether action takes place or not. Influencing factors may be environmental, the media or internal. Cues to action for people with internal locus of control may be breathlessness on exertion for lifestyle factors such as smoking or obesity. These indicators will not be a determining factor for people with external locus of control, however appointment reminders via messaging or email may be helpful.

From a cognitive perspective, perceptions of health alongside self-efficacy and the benefits of health are significant factors to health promoting behaviours. These factors along with personal and environmental all function synergistically as determinants of each other as suggested by Social Learning Theory (Bandura 1977). The basis of this theory focuses on how people understand their environments and themselves and how they behave in such circumstances. Therefore, if health is not an important or valued concept for them or their family, then it is unlikely that health promotion messages will be acted upon. Lifestyle change is one of the more common health promotion messages that practitioners may plan and deliver. A model often used for behaviour change (e.g. smoking, obesity, alcohol or drug misuse) is the Transtheoretical model by Prochaska and DiClemente (1983). The client's current stage of change must be ascertained before interventions can be considered. There are five stages within this model, precontemplation, contemplation, preparation, action, and maintenance, not forgetting that relapse can occur during action or maintenance. Individuals can present at any stage and progress forward or even stay at a particular stage for a long period of time. Each stage has concepts and interventions to aid the individual in making a life-style change. These concepts are: considering whether to make a change; identifying the pros and cons of changing behaviour; the impact of the change; and support while actioning the change.

It is pertinent that first, health promoters need to understand the supportive struc-tures that are available in the community, namely policy, behaviours and norms for a particular lifestyle factor. For example, obesity, access to low-cost healthy food or exercise options if unavailable in a particular community may compromise individuals' attempts to take on a healthier lifestyle. However, the health promoter can reasonably offer interventions to try to overcome these barriers. When individuals commit to a life-style change, in so doing their self-efficacy improves and gives them the motivation and power to continue. What is also apparent is that as self-efficacy strengthens, the barriers to lifestyle changes reduce. Nevertheless, if individuals do not maintain motivation to succeed, they will relapse. It is not as simple as just concentrating on lifestyle factors, although these are a major player in health. Social determinants of health must be con-sidered as these equally influence health across the life course. It is well documented that one of the wider determinants, namely poverty, is a much stronger predictor of health status than behavioural factors.

Making every contact count

Improving and promoting healthy lifestyles by advocating and supporting behaviour change with the aim of lowering the risk of chronic disease is the focus of making every contact count (MECC). This method of health promotion is targeted at all health service staff to empower them to take responsibility in supporting behaviour change. Discus-sion of health and wellbeing should be integral to everyday practice as a health care practitioner and not seen as a separate public health role. The purpose is to maximise each contact with a patient, client or any individual, whether family or friends, to offer appropriate intervention to support behaviour change (Nelson et al. 2013).

Interventions can occur at different levels of intensity, these are brief advice, brief intervention and motivational interviewing (Public Health Wales 2020, Public Health England 2020). Some staff may be competent and confident to deliver all three levels. It depends on the role and competence at what level you feel comfortable at deliver-ing. MECC is an approach to behaviour change that uses day-to-day interactions which organisations and people have with other people to support them in making positive changes to their physical and mental health and wellbeing.

Salutogenesis

The term **salutogenesis** is an approach that focuses on factors that support health and wellbeing, rather than disease. The term was developed by Antonovsky (1979), who rejected the dichotomy separating health and illness, suggesting that health and ill health was part of a continuum with one at either end. To differentiate between the salutogenic approach and a pathogenic approach to health promotion, the latter is a reactive approach where the response is to illness or disease, whereas salutogenic is where the professional is more proactive and moves the individual towards optimum health (Becker et al. 2010). Antonovsky's studies were focused on stress and how people managed stress and stayed healthy. He concluded that not all people who are stressed have negative health outcomes, some maintained their wellbeing. Antonovsky's theory is that generalised resistance resources (GRR) are a coping mechanism that is effective in combating stressors. These GRR allow individuals to manage and make sense of events in their lives. This led to the emergence of the sense of coherence (SOC) construct and is associated with how individuals make sense of the world. SOC incorporates three elements: comprehensibility (understanding the challenge, that you understand the events in your life), manageability (that you have the skills and ability and available resources, your health decisions are within your control) and meaningfulness (motivation and coping, that your health is worth making changes for and there is purpose in doing this). The strength of one's SOC determines the drive towards health (Antonovsky 1996). If a person believes there is no point in changing and is not motivated to change, they are unlikely to change their behaviour. Therefore, salutogenesis is influenced by experiencing a robust SOC (Janssen et al. 2014).

Barriers

Health promotion messages delivered by health professionals are not always taken up by individuals who may choose to maintain their unhealthy behaviours. Professionals often label these individuals as 'non-compliant'; this is seen as individuals not following advice. Although the professionals want people to choose health promotion recommendations, they sometimes fail to understand that individuals have the right to choose their course of action (Edelman et al. 2010). Changing behaviour through education alone is not always successful, and using persuasive messages in informing their health choices is sometimes futile as the individual's beliefs and values, stressors within their lives and low self-esteem can prevent changes in lifestyle being made. So, an understanding of the individual situation in respect of these factors and the health promotion messages conveyed may inform behaviour change. Financial constraints could be another important barrier to changing behaviour. People may not have the resources to fund travel to clinics or other venues, or indeed gym membership and so on. Therefore, realistic interventions should be considered, and in accordance with the 'convenience factor' as often these are not considered.

Professionals often voice that individuals are making excuses as to why they cannot change behaviour, but must respect the choice that the individual has made. Often these are not excuses but real-life factors that make it difficult for people to see beyond their current situation. Working through some of these issues can be helpful and give the individual options which may then progress to changes in lifestyle.

Marginalisation

Marginalisation is a process and a condition that prevents individuals or groups from full participation in social, economic and political life, and can prevent individuals from actively participating (Marshall 1998). Marginalisation can contribute to low self-esteem and exclusion from health promotion programmes; these are usually groups that are often vulnerable such as the homeless, travellers, ethnic minorities and so on. Individuals will feel powerless and find difficulty accessing resources and/or health care services (Laverack 2014). It is imperative that marginalised populations have opportunities to identify their own health needs and health promotion activities either individually or as a group. Especially those groups or individuals that have no voice due to being socially excluded, disempowered or ostracised by society (Roguski and McBride-Henry 2020). Society often marginalises individuals according to their status and social structure (Chaturvedi 2014). The dignity of marginalised groups is often violated through being unfairly treated, or in receipt of a poor service (Parker 2012).

Social, psychological and cultural factors

Social and psychological factors influence health behaviours, which can be reactive such as eating more when stressed or proactive, deciding to eat more healthily. Often behaviour is based on lay health beliefs and conceptions of health. How much choice do individuals have when dealing with stressful living or working conditions and unemployment? Lifestyle issues such as smoking and unhealthy eating are often used as a coping mechanism in these circumstances. It is so easy to blame individuals for their unhealthy habits and lifestyle when they may be victims of socioeconomic circumstances (Scriven 2017).

Culture may impact people's health and is centred on beliefs, values and perceived causes of illness and disease. All cultures have their own models of illness and belief systems regarding health, including treatments. In promoting health, interventions will need to be adapted to be more compatible with the cultural beliefs and values. The synergy between spirituality and culture could potentially be powerful. Spirituality, including values, beliefs and practices can be based on a connection to a higher or sacred power. This is often witnessed when individuals have the belief that their health is out of their control, such as in external locus of control when they see their health as down to fate or in 'the lap of the gods'.

Language and communication can affect access to health information and services if these are not available in the person's primary language, which is essential for quality accessible health care. It is important to offer participants interventions in their preferred language, occasionally available as information leaflets, to allow the participants choice. Interpreters and translators are often used to overcome the language barrier between health care professionals and the client. However, the interpretation of what the professional indicates and the translator's version is sometimes incorrect. Therefore, miscommunication can relate to a lack of shared understanding around basic health concepts (Jongen et al. 2017).

COVID-19 and health promotion

At the time of writing, with the COVID-19 pandemic being a major public health issue since the beginning of 2020, it is fundamentally important to consider the role of health promotion. The need to increase people's control over their health is a necessity to protect themselves and others. Health messages that have been formulated on sound scientific evidence, not only in protecting against the virus but also in encouraging exercise and fresh air to improve social resilience. Health promotion activities of healthy eating and exercise, mental health promotion and other aspects of behaviour change all lead to improved wellbeing and resilience for individuals and populations (Saboga-Nunes et al. 2020). The salutogenic approach to wellbeing by maintaining equilibrium is very much in tune with the public health response. Being cognisant of marginalised groups or individuals that are socially isolated should be inclusive of health promotion interventions.

Conclusion

'Health promotion' is an umbrella term for a wide range of strategies to tackle wider health determinants in improving populations' health. Frameworks for practice have been developed for professionals to deliver health promotion messages; these are numerous and varied and are classified as models of health promotion and approaches to health promotion. Health promotion is complex and needs to be individually tailored to the person. Awareness of social, psychological and cultural factors that impact on people's lifestyle must be taken into consideration, alongside barriers. Without recognition of these factors it is unlikely individuals will change behaviour. Other aspects of health promotion include strategies such as MECC to empower health professionals in promoting health and wellbeing. Antonovsky's theory of salutogensis offers a different perspective on people's values and beliefs and why health promotion is not always successful. Since 2020 all Nations have been living through the COVID-19 global pandemic and health promotion has been a driving force to try to improve the population's health and wellbeing.

Consider the following questions

1. There are many different models and theories of health promotion. How would you choose between them and tailor them to each individual?
2. People have complex lives. How would you ensure that you are not victim blaming when individuals make a choice to not change their lifestyle?

3. Assessment of the person's needs is essential before delivery of health promotion intervention. When and how would you undertake this?
4. Influencing policy is a key aspect of health promotion. Identify how you could be more effective in planning, networking and negotiating your skills.
5. Communication is an important aspect of the delivery of health promotion messages. What are the key elements of being culturally competent, and how would you ensure that these are addressed when working within a multi-diverse population?

Key terms

Behavioural change: The focus is on lifestyle behaviours that impact health. It seeks to persuade individuals to adopt healthy lifestyle behaviours, to use preventative health services and to take responsibility for their own health.

Empowerment: The process of becoming stronger and more confident, especially in controlling one's life and claiming one's rights.

Generalised Resistance Resources (GRR): relates to the characteristics of a person, a group, or a community that facilitate the individual's abilities to cope effectively with stressors and contribute to the development of the individual's level of sense of coherence (SOC).

Health promotion approaches: There are five approaches, each necessitating the use of different kinds of activities. These are medical/preventative, behavioural, educational, empowerment/client-centred and societal change.

Health promotion models: The aim is to explain the factors underlying motivation to engage in health promoting behaviours and focuses on people's interactions with their physical and interpersonal environments during attempts to improve health.

Health promotion: The process of enabling people to increase control over and to improve their health. It moves beyond a focus on individual behaviour towards a wide range of social and environmental interventions.

Making every contact count (MECC): An approach to behaviour change that uses day-to-day interactions that organisations and people have with other people to support them in making positive changes to their physical and mental health and wellbeing.

Marginalisation: Persons are socially excluded, in which individuals or groups are relegated to the fringes of a society, being denied economic, political and or symbolic power. They can be denied access to health care services.

Persuasive messages: Used to convince or persuade the individual that they need to change their lifestyle behaviour to improve their health and wellbeing.

Salutogenesis: An approach focusing on factors that support health and well being rather than on factors that cause disease. More specifically concerned with the relationship between health, stress and coping.

Sense of Coherence (SOC): reflects a coping capacity of people to deal with everyday life stressors and consists of three elements: comprehensibility, manageability and meaningfulness.

Further reading

Naidoo, J., Wills, J. 2016. *Foundations for Health Promotion.* (4th edn). Elsevier: Edinburgh.
Scriven, A. 2017. *Promoting Health: A Practical Guide.* (7th edn). Elsevier: Edinburgh.
South, J., White, J., Gamsu, M. 2013. *People-centred Public Health.* Policy Press: Bristol.
Tones, A., Green, J., Cross, R., Woodall, J. 2015. *Health Promotion: Planning & Strategies.* Sage: London.

References

Antonovsky, A. 1979. *Health, Stress and Coping.* Jossey-Bass Publishers: San Francisco, CA.
Antonovsky, A. 1996. The salutogenic model as a theory to guide health promotion. *Health Promotion International*; 11(1), 11–18.
Bandura, A. 1977. *Social Learning Theory.* Prentice Hall: Englewood Cliffs, NJ.
Becker, C., Glascoff, M., Felts, W. 2010. Salutogenesis 30 years later: where do we go from here. *International Electronic Journal of Health Education*; 13, 25–32.
Chaturvedi, S. 2014. Homelessness, identity and the therapeutic space. *BACP Children and Young People and Families Journal*; Sept., 26–29.
Declaration of Alma Ata. 1978. *American Journal of Public Health*; 105(6), June 2015. pp. 1094–1095.
Edelman C., Kudzma E., Mandle C. 2010. *Health Promotion Throughout the Life Span.* (8th Edn). Elsevier: Maryland Heights, MO.
Ewles, L., Simnett, I. 2003. *Promoting Health: A Practical Guide.* Bailliere Tindall: Edinburgh.
Janssen, B., Regenmortel, T., Abma, T. 2014. Balancing risk prevention and health promotion: towards a harmonizing approach in care for older people in the community. *Health Care Analysis*; 22, 82–102.
Jongen, C., McCalman, J., Bainbridge, R. 2017. The implementation and evaluation of health promotion services and programmes to improve cultural competency: a systematic scoping review. *Frontiers in Public Health*; 5, 1–14.
Lalonde, M. 1974. *A New Perspective on the Health of Canadians.* Ottawa. Available at: http://www.phac-aspc.gc.ca/ph-sp/pdf/perspect-eng.pdf [Accessed 06.04.2022].
Laverack, G. 2014. *The Pocket Guide to Health Promotion.* Open University Press: Maidenhead.
Marshall, G. 1998. *A Dictionary of Sociology.* Oxford University Press: Oxford.
Nelson, A. 2013. Making every contact count: an evaluation. *Public Health*. Available at: www.makingeverycontactcount.co.uk/media/1063/article-on-mecc-evaluation-2013.pdf [Accessed 03.01.2022].
Parker, J. 2012. Self-concepts of homeless people in an urban setting: processes and consequences of the stigmatised identity. *ScholarWorks @ Georgia State University*. Available at: https://scholarworks.gsu.edu/cgi/viewcontent.cgi?article=1064&context=sociology_diss [Accessed 20.09.2021].

Prochaska, J., DiClemente, C. 1983. Stages and processes of self-change of smoking: toward an integrative model of change. *Journal of Consulting and Clinical Psychology*; 51(3), 390–395.

Public Health England. 2020. *Making Every Contact Count*. PHE: London.

Public Health Wales. 2020. *Making Every Contact Count Wales*. PHW. Available at: www.mecc.publichealthnetwork.cymru/en/ [Accessed 14.12.2021].

Roguski, M., McBride-Henry, K. 2020. The failure of health promotion for marginalised populations. *Australian and New Zealand Journal of Public Health*; 44(6), 446–448.

Saboga-Nunes, L., Levin-Zamir, D., Bittlingmayer, U., et al. 2020. *A health promotion focus on COVID-19; keep the Trojan horse out of our health systems: promote health for ALL in times of crisis and beyond!* EUPHA-HP, IUHPE, UNESCO Chair Global Health & Education. Available at: https://eupha.org/repository/sections/hp/A_Health_Promotion_Focus_on_COVID-19_with_S.pdf [Accessed 02.02.2022].

Scriven, A. 2010. *Promoting Health: A Practical Guide*. Bailliere Tindall: London.

Scriven, A. 2017. *Ewles & Simnett's Promoting Health; A Practical Guide*. (7th edn). Elsevier: Edinburgh.

World Health Organization. 1986. *Ottawa Charter for Health Promotion: First International Conference on Health Promotion*. Ottawa. Available at: www.healthpromotion.org.au/images/ottawa_charter_hp.pdf [Accessed 06.02.2021].

World Health Organization. 1997. *Jakarta declaration on leading health promotion into the 21st century*. Available at: https://www.who.int/teams/health-promotion/enhanced-wellbeing/fourth-conference/jakarta-declaration#:~:text=Health%20promotion%2C%20through%20investment%20and,and%20to%20build%20social%20capital [Accessed 06.04.2022].

4

HEALTH LITERACY

LYNETTE HARLAND SHOTTON AND EMMA SENIOR

━━━━━━━━━━ LEARNING OUTCOMES ━━━━━━━━━━

By the end of this chapter you will be able to:

- Understand the key concepts and features of health literacy.
- Provide a brief overview of the UK policy response.
- Consider and introduce some of the strategies to measure and address health literacy.

Introduction

The purpose of this chapter is to provide an overview of health literacy and insight into some of the key concepts and features of health literacy. These include an overview of literacy and numeracy, as well as consideration of the scope of health literacy. The chapter refers to some of the approaches to understand, measure and address health literacy, taking into account both the policy and practical response across the four nations of the UK.

Health literacy

Health and social care professionals may generally assume that information and advice given to service users is understood, however, in reality this is not the case and very often it is misunderstood, in some cases resulting in harm (Cornett 2018). When service users do not comply with instructions or information given to them, it is often associated with low levels of health literacy rather than non-compliance (Cornett 2018). Health literacy is not a new concept and has featured in health and health promotion literature since the second half of the 20th century (Nutbeam 2000). Nutbeam (2008) refers to it as an evolving concept in that it is increasingly recognised and understood. The term builds on the notion that both health and literacy are critical resources for everyday living, and as such it is not surprising that efforts to improve health literacy feature highly in the national and international policy landscape (Rowlands et al. 2020). Although there are a number of definitions, the key focus of improving health literacy is to ensure that individuals have the right knowledge, skills, understanding and confidence to be able to access, understand, use, evaluate and navigate the increasingly complex health and social care arena (Public Health England 2015).

Literacy

Literacy is key in the development of health literacy and is the end result of the process of learning to read and write, to communicate effectively and make sense of our social context (Literacy Trust 2020). Across the UK all four nations report significant numbers of the adult population with poor literacy levels. It is estimated that in England 16.4% or 1 in 6 adults can be described as having poor literacy skills (Literacy Trust 2020). In Scotland, whilst a recent survey indicates that 73.3% of the working population have a level of literacy on a par with other developed countries, it also found that about a quarter or 1 in 4 (26.7%) had literacy difficulties, which occasionally presented challenges for them and of these 3.6.% experienced serious challenges because of low levels of literacy (Scottish Government 2020). In Northern Ireland around 17.9% or 1 in 5 adults have very poor literacy skills and in Wales the rates are 1 in 8 adults or 12% of the population (Literacy Trust 2020). Literacy is often referred to in terms of levels, and whilst there are variations in how these are defined, in England a Skills for Life Survey (Department for Business, Innovation and Skills (DBIS) 2012) commissioned by the UK Government identified the following five. Entry level 1 is the equivalent to literacy levels at age 5–7; at this level adults may struggle to read a road sign or to write short messages. Entry level 2 is equal to levels at age 7–9; at this level an adult may struggle to read a label. Entry level 3 is comparable to literacy levels at age 9–11; at this level individuals may struggle to read food labelling or utility bills.

Level 1 is equivalent to GCSE grades D–G/new GCSE 3–1 and adults at this level may struggle to understand a payslip. Level 2 is equivalent to GCSE grades A*–C/new GCSE 9–4. According to DBIS (2012) those with skills below Level 2 may struggle to critically evaluate information, for example, being able to identify bias in written materials or to spot fake news. For those individuals across the UK identified as having poor literacy skills, this would equate to being at Level 1 or below and are likely to face struggles in many aspects of their daily lives (Literacy Trust 2020). Despite this we must concede that even basic literacy skills provide a platform for individuals to further develop and improve, and as such literacy is a gateway to enabling individuals to participate more fully in society and the economy (Nutbeam 2015).

Numeracy

Numeracy is also an important feature of health literacy. This relates to the ability and confidence to be able to use numbers and mathematical techniques and is often considered to be as important a life skill as literacy (National Numeracy Organisation, (NNO) 2020). In real-world situations numeracy is required not only for doing sums but also to help individuals to interpret data, solve problems, process information, critically evaluate and make decisions (NNO 2020). This is particularly true for health data, where information often requires the ability to read qualitative text with numerical data embedded in it (Smith et al. 2015). On this basis poor numeracy is life-limiting, and those with poor numeracy are more likely to be unemployed or face difficulties with career progression (NNO 2019). As with literacy, across the UK levels of numeracy skill have been identified. Entry level 1 equates to the skill expected at age 5–7 and refers to the ability to recognise and select coins, order numbers up to 10. Entry level 2 equates to the skill expected aged 7–9; examples of skills at this level include being able to calculate basic costs and change required in cash transactions and the ability to add and subtract 2-digit numbers. At entry level 3 the individual would be able to divide two digits by one digit and compare weights using standard units. This would be expected at the age of between 9 and 11 years. Those at level 1 would be at the same stage as new GCSE 3–1/old GCSE D–G and would be able to do simple percentages and convert units of measure. At level 2 individuals would be at new GCSE 9–4/old GCSE A*–C and would be able to understand mathematical information for a range of purposes and show the ability to select and compare information in different formats, including graphic, numerical and written forms (NNO 2020). Across the UK it is accepted that numeracy levels have deteriorated, with the proportion of working age adults with numeracy skills equivalent to old GCSE grade C or above dropping from 26% in 2003 to 22% in 2011 (NNO 2020). 2019 figures estimate that over 49% of adults in the UK have the numeracy level expected of a primary school child (NNO 2019). More concerning is that a recent survey by Ipsos Mori in preparation for National Numeracy Day found that many adults in the UK (25%) do not wish to improve their numeracy skills and 30% felt they did not need to use numbers within the context of their working lives (Ipsos Mori 2019). In relation to health, those with lower numeracy skills are less likely to trust health data and their understanding of data means they often minimise risk in relation to health (Smith et al. 2015).

The impact of poor literacy and numeracy extends beyond the realm of employment and is of particular concern in the health and social care context. Education is a key social determinant of health and those with lower levels of literacy, numeracy and language skills are much more likely to experience the worst health outcomes (Crossley 2015), but also show higher rates of use of health care services (Heijmans et al. 2015). Whilst this is partially attributed to these individuals being more likely to be living in disadvantaged socio-economic circumstances, some of the adverse effects on health are also related to being less able to manage long-term health conditions and also being less receptive to and responsive to health education and intervention (Rowlands and Nutbeam 2013). Health literacy impacts on the ability of individuals to interact with providers of health services, their ability to take care of their own health and that of others and, importantly, their ability to participate in discussions and decisions about their health and the health of those they care for (NHS Scotland 2017). Health literacy also governs individuals' ability to use health information to make judgements and decisions in every-day life concerning health care, disease prevention, management and health improvement throughout the life course (Rowlands et al. 2020). Limited health literacy is also linked to unhealthy behaviours, which increase the risk of morbidity and mortality, such as smoking and alcohol misuse (Roberts 2015), as well as increased use of health services, emergency care and hospitalisation connected to reduced ability to self-care as outlined above (Protheroe et al. 2015). Berry (2016) suggests that the financial cost of low levels of health literacy are between 3–5% of the annual UK health budget, therefore it is not surprising that improving health literacy is a global concern.

The scope of health literacy

One of the most widely recognised models of health literacy is that proposed by Nutbeam (2000). Here, the scope of health literacy focuses on three distinct elements: functional, communicative/interactive and an empowerment/critical level (Nutbeam 2000; Kanj and Mitic 2009). The types of health literacy within Nutbeam's (2000) model require different skills to obtain and access information, understand it and use it effectively and are ordered in terms of ascending difficulty, progressively leading to greater empowerment of the individual in relation to participation in decision making and control of health (Heijmans et al. 2014).

Functional health literacy refers to a person's ability to understand their own health status and health concerns, as well as their ability to comprehend information surrounding these, for example, following directions, reading leaflets, reading labels on medication and being able to follow the instructions appropriately (Health Literacy Centre Europe (HLCE) 2015). Rask et al. (2013) refer to functional health literacy as basic health literacy and indicate that at this level individuals tend to know about the basics of maintaining health through hygiene, nutrition, security and support networks as well as certain risks to health such as drug and substance misuse. At this level individuals have some understanding of health services and obtain information through personal and social networks as well as the media. In England it is accepted that levels of functional health literacy are low, and it is thought that much of the health literature in circulation is too complex for 43% of adults between the ages of 16–65 years (Health Literacy UK 2020).

Communicative/interactive health literacy relates to more advanced skills, whereby the individual is better able to identify relevant information about health from a range of sources, understand and derive meaning from that information as well as apply it to different and sometimes changing circumstances (Heijmans et al. 2014). Poor interactive health literacy limits the individual's ability to identify gaps in their health knowledge and also to ask questions about their health (HLCE 2015). This is often compounded by being unable to explain their health concerns, but also to process and remember health related information. Alternatively, those who possess high levels of communicative/interactive health literacy are easily able to communicate their health issues, discuss them and ask questions about them in order to better understand and discuss health with professionals (HLCE 2015).

Critical health literacy refers to more advanced cognitive skills which, together with social skills, can be applied to critically analyse information, and to use this information to exert greater control over life events and situations (Nutbeam 2015). So this is very much about being able to make informed decisions in relation to health, being accountable for one's own health, and also having a sense of control over health (HLCE 2015). Those with high levels of critical health literacy will actively engage with health and seek out information, appraising the quality and reliability of this in order to make decisions (HLCE 2015).

Nutbeam's classification indicates that the different categories of health literacy progressively allow for greater autonomy in decision making and personal empowerment. Progression between categories is not only dependent upon cognitive development but also exposure to different forms of information (content and media). It is also dependent upon a person's confidence to respond effectively to health communications, a process which is usually described as self-efficacy (Rowlands and Nutbeam 2013). Those with the lowest levels of health literacy have the least access to health information – the 'inverse information law' (Rowlands and Nutbeam 2013) – and consequently it is not surprising that a survey for the King's Fund (Buck and Frosini 2012) found the messages conveyed via health promotion campaigns had little effect on the health behaviours of those with lower levels of literacy. Whilst this is concerning, it is important to acknowledge that information about health, particularly that relating to clinical conditions and choices for treatment, is inherently complex. It is likely that there is a mismatch between the existing literacy skills of the population and the health literacy required to understand

and use health information to become and stay healthy and manage illness (Rowlands and Nutbeam 2013). Health literacy is also content- and context-specific, and therefore it is important to concede that even those with good literacy and numeracy skills may find understanding health care information challenging, depending on the specific and individual circumstances they experience (Cornett 2018).

The World Health Organization refers to health literacy as having a central role in determining inequities in health and therefore should be considered a shared responsibility between individuals and governments and health systems (WHO 2016). Indeed, the social dimension features prominently in the WHO (2016) definition of health literacy as the personal characteristics and social resources required for individuals and communities to be able to access, understand and critically evaluate health information in order to make and be involved in decisions about their health. The emphasis here moves beyond understanding health literacy as an individual skill, to pay attention to the role of social support systems as well as policy makers (Heijmans et al. 2015).

As outlined earlier in this chapter, levels of health literacy impact on both access to and utilisation of health and social care services (NHS Scotland 2017), and therefore health literacy can be considered as both a risk and an asset. When viewed in the context of risk, this usually links to clinical care where low levels of health literacy are considered a risk to health in that individuals are less likely to comply with health care advice (Nutbeam 2015). Alternatively, if we view health literacy as an asset, this positions the concept as a goal that offers individuals greater autonomy and control over their health (Nutbeam 2015). Equally, this combines both the individual and the social responsibility associated with improving health, and emphasises that health literacy can be developed through working with individuals as well as by modifying the social environment in order to make it easier for those with lower levels of health literacy to obtain, make sense of and use information in ways that can help to promote and maintain health (Nutbeam 2015).

The policy response

All four nations across the UK recognise the importance of addressing poor health literacy as part of a wider commitment to tackle the determinants of health and wellbeing. The Scottish Government initially recognised the evidence outlining the impact of health literacy on individuals in 2009, initiating an overarching health literacy strategy 'Making it Easy' in 2014, with the ethos of enabling all to have sufficient confidence, knowledge, understanding and skills to live well and do this in the presence of any health conditions (NHS Scotland 2017). This has been followed by the more recent *Making it Easier. A Health Literacy Plan for Scotland* (NHS Scotland 2017). In Wales, there is emphasis on providing the right circumstances for individuals, families and communities to have the resources to live fulfilled and healthy lives, and this includes supporting individuals to develop numeracy and literacy skills as well as increasing awareness and opportunities for individuals to understand, improve and manage their health (Welsh Government

2016). General approaches to addressing the inequalities associated with health literacy in England and Northern Ireland include training for frontline staff, as well as providing environmental change (Protheroe et al. 2015, Health and Social Care Board 2019).

Measuring health literacy

The evidential links between health literacy and health outcomes has meant that health literacy has become a national and international priority. In recent years there has been a growing emphasis on the need for continued efforts to improve health literacy, underlining it as a strategic priority area in order to promote population health and individual empowerment across both the US and Europe (Koh et al. 2012; European Office of the World Health Organization Regional Committee for Europe, 2019). However, in order to produce positive outcomes from such initiatives, health literacy needs to emerge from the side-lines to the forefront of policy and practice. The introduction of an accurate measurement tool is a critical element within the process of improving the identification of those populations most in need of support (Haun et al. 2013). The last 20 years has seen the prolific development of tools designed to measure health literacy in a range of contexts and variations from screening tests to comprehensive assessments. Likewise, the range of procedures to test the validity of the tools is equally as vast (Markwardt and Service 1989, Slosson 2008, Wilkinson 1993). The aim of developing a 'universal' tool to measure health literacy that can be successfully applied to diverse populations is proving a challenge (Jordan et al. 2011; Haun et al. 2013).

The overarching aim of any health literacy measurement tool needs to encompass the assessment of 'relative differences in relevant cognitive and social skills, and the ability of individuals to apply those skills to achieve health outcomes in different circumstances' (Nutbeam 2015, p. 17). Remembering that the skill differences are also categorised in different ways – functional, interactive and critical health literacy – this enables progression for more autonomy in their personal decision making capabilities and level of empowerment (Nutbeam, 2000). The short screening tools adopted by clinicians for use in everyday practice across a varying range of populations are deemed sufficient for clinical practice screening tools, however, they fail to measure in any depth the differences in cognitive and social skill referred to by Nutbeam (2000). What now presides is a diverse range of health literacy instruments. Such diversity is problematic when attempting to choose the appropriate tool due to the range of measurement inconsistencies and complications in interpreting findings across the multitude of studies (Haun et al. 2013). In more recent years there has been development across several countries to create or adapt pre-existing measurement tools into much more complex assessment tools (Chinn and McCarthy 2013, Jordan et al. 2013, Osborne et al. 2013, Sorensen et al. 2013). Such tools aim to assess an individual's capacity to access health information from a range of sources and differentiate between them, understand and personalise the health information and be able to express confidence in using the health information in their decision making and action to benefit their health.

Several direct measures of functional health literacy are recognised and used in the UK. These include the Short Test of Functional Health Literacy in Adults (STOFHL-UK) and the Newest Vital Sign (NVS-UK) measure (Public Health England 2015). In addition, there are some valid and reliable instruments identified within the UK for self-reported measuring; these are the Health Literacy Management Scale (HeLMs) and the Health Literacy Questionnaire (HLQ) (Public Health England 2015).

Whilst there is a predominant focus on the individual, there is also an identified need to consider health literacy from an organisational stance. The Institute of Medicine identified the ten attributes of health literate healthcare organisations, and in response the Health Literate Healthcare Organisation 10-Item Questionnaire (HLHO-10) was developed with satisfactory reliability and validity awarded (Kowalski et al. 2015). The HLHO-10 enables the assessment of the extent to which healthcare organisations enable people to navigate, understand and use their health and social care services and information.

Addressing health literacy

The location and utilisation of a valid and reliable health literacy measurement tool is only one element in addressing health literacy need to enable the reduction of health inequalities. Likewise, only focusing on individuals or the most vulnerable and disadvantaged groups will equally not have the desired extent of impact. Broader action is required to promote the reduction in the steepness of the social gradient in health. Health literacy initiatives and interventions need to be wide ranging, but also have the ability to be scaled up or intensified to be proportionate for the level of disadvantage and those populations most at risk also known as 'proportionate universalism' (NHS Scotland 2014). Practically, an overall strategic stance to improve the health literacy in health and social care systems and address the conditions for individuals across the life continuum is emphasised, however, on a local level this may incorporate targeted approaches to increase the level of health literacy amongst more vulnerable and disadvantaged groups (WHO 2019a).

It is already known that health literacy levels are associated with the social determinants of health, however, equal consideration to the differing needs of individuals across the life continuum is required. So, when addressing strategies some thought is needed to think about age and stage of life (Protheroe et al. 2015). For example, how younger people/older people access information and make decisions about health and what stage an individual or group are at, such as aiming to give the best start in life; encourage education and lifelong learning; employment and working conditions; and ageing well. In order to have the greatest impact, initiatives and interventions need to consider the social conditions of a particular group in tandem with the life stage of the individual or the community demographic.

Five strategic directions identified by the WHO (2019a) aim to develop health literacy over the life course. They identify the need for increased capacity building, involving a range of stakeholders such as policy makers, health and social care practitioners and researchers to name but a few. This will ensure that health literacy is at the forefront and is included by all. Facilitation of cross-sectoral integration and advocacy are fundamental in ensuring that health literacy is promoted in all stages of the life course and that initiatives should aim to link with present skill development opportunities and motivations within each stage. Equally, the implementation of initiatives and interventions from the emerging evidence base is to be promoted and encouraged both with individuals and within communities.

In order to address health literacy and the strategic direction, consideration to the 'how' is required. In the first instance, thought is needed about how health literacy in different settings may be embedded or encouraged, as this will aid the potential direction of interventions and initiatives. When health literacy is dispersed throughout a group (e.g. a family or social group) and that collective knowledge is then used as a resource for understanding health information and making and managing health choices, this is known as 'distributed health literacy' (Edwards et al. 2015). From an organisational aspect the way that they, through their services and systems, make health information and resources accessible and available to their given population is referred to as 'health literacy responsiveness' or 'organisational health literacy'. Community health literacy encompasses the capacities and the assets within communities, such as towns or neighbourhoods, so that the health of all its members is promoted. Increasing health literacy through the life course requires the involvement of all. The support from family and social networks, education and life-long learning, health promotion and health programmes across a range of settings, targeted approaches for the more vulnerable and disadvantaged groups and enabling individuals to locate, access and understand health information is critical to the successful improvement in health literacy and overall health (WHO 2019b).

At a national and regional level, the acknowledgement of health literacy within policy and decision making is paramount. Likewise, regionally and locally the emphasis is on capacity building. Promoting positive health literacy is everyone's responsibility. Capacity building requires those working in health and social care to identify areas of vulnerability and disadvantage and/or capacity gaps and create initiatives. Similarly, this includes building capacity amongst other health and social care practitioners by improving service quality and increasing responsiveness through education, training and research. The ability to communicate effectively with service users who have low levels of health literacy is very much dependent on the ability of the health and social care professional first to identify the issue and second to support a culture of person-centred non-stigmatising service delivery (Cornett 2018). Opportunities arise in a variety of ways, through routine interactions and existing initiatives as well as targeted health literacy interventions. Teachable moments and Making Every Contact Count (MECC, Public Health England 2015), within health and social care practice, such as antenatal/postnatal care, or disease-induced interactions, including newly diagnosed diabetes or heart failure, present openings to explore health literacy on an individual level (Nutbeam 2015, WHO 2019a). Utilising a health literacy toolkit to enable such opportunities can increase levels of health literacy; it takes the form of training, which helps to embed some of the key principles outlined. Teach-back is one of many methods used to improve health literacy, whereby health professionals confirm that service users understand information they have been given by asking them to either demonstrate or repeat back what they have been told. Other simple techniques include chunk and check, using pictures and simple language to improve how individuals communicate and check understanding with others (NHS Scotland 2017). These methods prominently use verbal communication. It is also important that consideration is given to wider communication, especially regarding written information (e.g. public notices, signposts, leaflets and information boards). The use of language, style, design, print, pictures and symbols all need consideration. Health literacy responsiveness requires active assessment and evaluation of the resources used, readability tests such as the Simple Measure of Gobbledygook (SMOG) test, and calculator are useful tools in such assessments (Health Education England 2018).

Health literacy toolkits are also useful resources for community-based peer-support programmes, which also have the potential to address health inequality. Such groups have an overall aim of working with and changing the perceptions of vulnerable or disadvantaged individuals by nurturing common bonds. The equity and commonality shared between the peer-support workers and the participants encourage discussions and involvement in wider social networks. This in turn encourages positive engagement and the sharing of concerns, problems and resolutions, which have been linked to improved health literacy and health outcomes (Harris et al. 2015).

Technology is a central feature of modern life and since health literacy requires the processing of information, digital solutions and endeavours to enhance digital health literacy are fundamental. Responsive health literacy requires organisations to ensure their digital technologies create health information that is accessible and manageable to the whole population, enabling individuals to search and acquire appropriate up-to-date information (WHO 2019b). However, the digital society we now inhabit presents both opportunities and threats. The increase in social networking sites has produced opportunities for international connection with others, and as such a plethora of powerful health communication platforms have emerged (Moorhead et al. 2013). However, these platforms enable the merging of sources into one feed, and therefore create difficulties in extracting the correct information from the fake. Fake, misleading and over-interpreted health information shared on social media poses a potential threat for public health and can in turn hinder health improvement and disease prevention efforts (Sommariva et al. 2018).

It is noted that those with greater levels of digital literacy can access health-related information and use this to manage personal health and care (EurohealthNet 2019), however, as with literacy and health literacy generally, there is a social gradient, and those from more deprived socio-economic groups, as well as those at particular stages of the life-course i.e. older/younger individuals may be less able to navigate the digital world safely and effectively (EurohealthNet 2019). Recent figures indicate that 87% of households across the UK have access to the Internet, however, over one in ten households remain without access and there is great variation in terms of how and the frequency of its use, with those over 55 and above accessing the Internet less frequently and use declining with age (Ofcom 2017).

There is an association between lack of internet use and lower levels of health literacy. Indeed, Protheroe et al. (2015) found that those who had no access to the internet were more than three times as likely to have limited health literacy than those who did have internet access. Strategies at both UK and local level focus on the expansion of and increased access to the Internet; however, given the complexities described, once access is gained equal consideration must be given to helping individuals to understand and use digital health information appropriately and to critically think about the digital information they receive and whether they feel empowered to make decisions about which sources they trust and share. Furthermore, digital health intervention should complement rather than replace existing health systems in a guided and supported manner (WHO 2019b).

Conclusion

The purpose of this chapter was to introduce some of the key concepts and features of health literacy, as well as to highlight the policy and practical response to dealing with health literacy across the UK. Statistical data highlights that significant numbers of the population have low levels of numeracy and literacy and this, along with other wider implications, impacts on health literacy. As such, it is paramount that all in the health and social care arena sustain and expand efforts to address health literacy within their own practice, but also at the wider organisational level. In turn, this needs continued prioritisation within health and social care policy to enable individuals to access, understand and use health information to inform, enhance and maintain their own health, as well as tackle inequalities in health and social care.

Consider the following questions

Having read the chapter, take time to think about the following:
1. What is my understanding of health literacy?
2. What else do I need to know/do?
3. How will I assess health literacy within the context of my role?

Key terms

Health literacy: The degree to which individuals are able to obtain, process and understand health information and services in order to make appropriate decisions about their health.
Literacy: The ability to read, write, speak and listen to communicate effectively and make sense of the world.
Numeracy: An understanding of the role of maths and being able to apply this to make decisions.

Further reading

Health Literacy UK. 2021. *Making Healthcare Easy*. Available at: www.healthliteracy.org. uk [Accessed 11.10.2021].

References

Berry, J. 2016. *Does health literacy matter?* Available at: www.healthliteracyplace.org.uk/ resource-library/article/t/the-test-of-functional-health-literacy-in-adults/ [Accessed 20.03.2020].

Buck, D., Frosini, F. 2012. *Clustering of Unhealthy Behaviours Over Time. Implications for Policy and Practice.* London: The King's Fund.

Chinn, D., McCarthy, C. 2013. All Aspects of Health Literacy Scale (AAHLS): developing a tool to measure functional, communicative and critical health literacy in primary healthcare settings. *Patient Education and Counselling*; 90, 247–253.

Cornett, S. 2018. *Assessing and addressing health literacy.* Available at: www.who.int/ global-coordination-mechanism/activities/working-groups/Assessing-and-Adressing-Health-Literacy.pdf [Accessed 17.04.2020].

Crossley, J. 2015. *Impacts of low health literacy.* Available at: https://epale.ec.europa.eu/en/ blog/impacts-low-health-literacy [Accessed 17.04.2020].

Department for Business, Innovation and Skills 2012. *The 2011 Skills for Life Survey: a survey of literacy, numeracy and ICT levels in England.* Available at: https://assets. publishing.service.gov.uk/government/uploads/system/uploads/attachment_data/ file/36000/12-p168-2011-skills-for-life-survey.pdf [Accessed 16.04.2020].

Edwards, M., Wood, F., Davies, M., Edwards, A. 2015. 'Distributed health literacy': longitudinal qualitative analysis of the roles of health literacy mediators and social networks of people living with a long-term health condition. *Health Expect*; 18(5), 1180–1193.

EuroHealthNet 2019. *Digital health literacy: how new skills can help improve health, equity and sustainability.* Available at: https://eurohealthnet.eu/publication/digital-health-literacy-how-new-skills-can-help-improve-health-equity-and-sustainability/ [Accessed 16.04.2020].

European Office of the World Health Organization Regional Committee for Europe 2019. *Resolution towards the implementation of health literacy initiatives through the life course.* Available at: https://www.euro.who.int/en/about-us/governance/regional-committee-for-europe/past-sessions/69th-session/documentation/resolutions/ eurrc69r9-resolution-towards-the-implementation-of-health-literacy-initiatives-through-the-life-course [Accessed 20.04.2020].

Harris, J., Springett, J., Croot, L., Booth, A., Campbell, F., Thompson, J., Goyder, E., Van Cleemput, P., Wilkins, E., Yang, Y. 2015. Can community-based peer support promote health literacy and reduce inequalities? A realist review. *Public Health Research*, 3(3).

Haun, J. O, Valerio, M. A., McCormack, L. A., Sorensen, K., Paasche-Orlow, M. K. 2013. Health literacy measurement: an inventory and descriptive summary of 51 instruments. *Journal of Health Communication*, 19, 302–333.

Health and Social Care Board 2019. *Health literacy training.* Available at: http://www.hscboard.hscni.net/sessions/ [Accessed 20.04.2020].

Health Education England 2018. *Health Literacy 'How to' Guide.* Available at: www.hee.nhs.uk/our-work/population-health/training-educational-resources [Accessed 01.05.2020].

Health Literacy Centre Europe 2015. *Understanding Health Literacy.* Available at: http://healthliteracycentre.eu/understanding-health-literacy/ [Accessed 16.04.2020].

Health Literacy UK 2020. *Why is health literacy important?* Available at: www.healthliteracy.org.uk/why-is-health-literacy-important [Accessed 19.03.2020].

Heijmans, M., Uiters, E., Rose, T., Hofstede, J., Deville, W., van der Heide, I., Boshuisen, H., Rademakers, J. 2015. *Study on sound evidence for a better understanding of health literacy in the European Union.* Available at: https://ec.europa.eu/health/sites/health/files/health_policies/docs/2015_health_literacy_en.pdf [Accessed 21.04.2020].

Heijmans, M., Waverijn, G., Rademakers, J., van der Vaart, R., Rijken, M. 2014. Functional, communicative and critical health literacy of chronic disease patients and their importance for self-management. *Patient Education and Counselling*, 98(1), 41–48.

Ipsos Mori 2019. *Numerate Nation? What the UK thinks about numbers.* Available at: https://www.ipsos.com/en-uk/numerate-nation-what-uk-thinks-about-numbers [Accessed 16.04.2020].

Jordan, J. E., Buchbinder R., Briggs, A. M. 2013. The Health Literacy Management Scale (HeLMS): a measure of an individual's capacity to seek, understand and use health information within the healthcare setting. *Patient Education and Counselling;* 91(2), 228–235.

Jordan, J. E., Osborne, R. H., Buchbinder, R. 2011. Critical appraisal of health literacy indices revealed variable underlying constructs, narrow content and psychometric weaknesses. *Journal of Clinical Epidemiology;* 64(4), 366–379.

Kanj, M., Mitic, W. 2009. *Promoting Health and Development: Closing the Implementation Gap.* Available at: www.who.int/healthpromotion/conferences/7gchp/Track1_Inner.pdf [Accessed 20.03.2020].

Koh, H. K., Berwick, D. M., Clancy, C. M., Baur, C., Brach, C., Harris, L. M., Zerhusen, E. G. 2012. New federal policy initiatives to boost health literacy can help the nation move beyond the cycle of costly 'crisis care'. *Health Affairs;* 31, 434–443.

Kowalski, C., Lee, S., Schmidt, A. 2015. The Health Literate Health Care Organization 10 Item Questionnaire (HLHO-10): development and validation. *BMC Health Services Research;* 15, 47.

Literacy Trust 2020. *What is Literacy?* Available at: https://literacytrust.org.uk/information/what-is-literacy/ [Accessed 16.04.2020].

Markwardt, F. C., Service, A. G. 1989. *Peabody Individual Achievement Test—Revised: PIAT-R.* American Guidance Service: Circle Pines, MN.

Moorhead, S. A., Hazlett, D. E., Harrison, L., Carroll, J. K., Irwin, A., Hoving C. 2013. A new dimension of health care: systematic review of the uses, benefits, and limitations of social media for health communication. *Journal of Medical Internet Research*; 15(4), 85.

National Numeracy Organisation 2019. *National Numeracy 2019 Impact Report.* Available at: www.nationalnumeracy.org.uk/sites/default/files/nn180_2019_impact_report.pdf [Accessed 12.03.2022].

National Numeracy Organisation 2020. *What is Numeracy?* Available at: www.national numeracy.org.uk/what-numeracy [Accessed 17.04.2020].

NHS Scotland 2014. *Proportionate Universalism and Health Inequalities.* Available at: www. healthscotland.com/uploads/documents/24296-ProportionateUniversalismBriefing. pdf [Accessed 30.04.2020].

NHS Scotland 2017. *Making it Easier. A Health Literacy Action Plan for Scotland.* Available at: www.gov.scot/binaries/content/documents/govscot/publications/strategy-plan/ 2017/11/making-easier-health-literacy-action-plan-scotland-2017-2025/documents/ 00528139-pdf/00528139-pdf/govscot%3Adocument/00528139.pdf   [Accessed 16.03.2020].

Nutbeam, D. 2000. Health literacy as a public health goal: a challenge for contemporary health education and communication strategies into the 21st century. *Health Promotion International*; 15(3), 259–267. https://doi.org/10.1093/heapro/15.3.259

Nutbeam, D. 2008. The evolving concept of health literacy. *Social Science and Medicine*; 67, 2072–2078.

Nutbeam, D. 2015. Defining, measuring and improving health literacy. *HEP*; 42(4), 16–21.

Ofcom (2017) *Internet and Online Content.* Available at: www.ofcom.org.uk/__data/assets/ pdf_file/0010/105004/wales-internet-online.pdf [Accessed 04.05.2020].

Osborne, R. H., Batterham, R. W., Elsworth, G. R. 2013. The grounded psychometric development and initial validation of the Health Literacy Questionnaire (HLQ). *BMC Public Health*; 13, 658.

Protheroe, J., Whittle, R., Bartlam, B., Estacio, E. V., Clark, L., Kurth, J. 2015. Health Literacy, Associated Lifestyle and Demographic Factors in the Adult Population of an English City: A Cross-sectional Survey. *Health Expectations*. pp. 108. Wiley: Chichester.

Public Health England 2015. *Local Action on Health Inequalities. Improving Health Literacy to Reduce Health Inequalities.* Available at: https://assets.publishing.service.gov.uk/ government/uploads/system/uploads/attachment_data/file/460709/4a_Health_Literacy-Full.pdf [Accessed 16.03.2020].

Rask, M., Uusiautti, S., Määttä, K. 2013. The fourth level of health literacy. *International Quarterly of Community Health Education*; 34(1), 51–71.

Roberts, J. 2015. *Local Action on Health Inequalities. Improving Health Literacy to Reduce Health Inequalities.* Practice Resource: September 2015. Public Health England: London.

Rowlands, G., Nutbeam, D. 2013. Health literacy and the 'inverse information law'. *British Journal of General Practice*; 63(608), 120–121.

Rowlands, G., Tabassum, B., Campbell, P., Harvey, S., Vaittinen, A., Stobbart, L., Thomson, R., Wardle-McLeish, M., Protheroe, J. 2020. The evidence-based development of an intervention to improve clinical health literacy practice. *International Journal of Environmental Research and Public Health*; 17(5), 1513. https://doi.org/10.3390/ijerph17051513

Scottish Government 2020. *Adult Literacies in Scotland 2020: Strategic Guidance*. Available at: www.gov.scot/publications/adult-literacies-scotland-2020-strategic-guidance/pages/3/ [Accessed 16.04.2020].

Slosson, R.L. 2008. *Slosson Oral Reading Test – Revised (Sort-R3)*. East Aurora, New York: Slosson Educational Publications.

Smith, S. G., Curtis, L. M., O'Connor, R., Federman, A. D., Wolf, M. S. 2015. ABCs or 123s? The independent contribution of literacy and numeracy skills on health task performance among older adults. *Patient Education and Counselling*; 98(8), 991–997.

Sommariva, S., Vamos, C., Mantzarlis, A., Uyên-Loan Đào, L., Tyson, D. M. 2018. Spreading the (fake) news: exploring health messages on social media and the implications for health professionals using a case study. *Journal of Health Education*; 49(4), 246–255.

Sorensen, K,. van den Broucke, S., Pelikan, J. M. 2013. Measuring health literacy in populations: illuminating the design and development process of the European Health Literacy Survey Questionnaire (HLS-EU-Q). *BMC Public Health*; 13, 948.

Welsh Government 2016. *Measuring the health and well-being of a nation. Public Health Outcomes Framework for Wales*. Available at: https://gov.wales/sites/default/files/publications/2019-06/measuring-the-health-and-well-being-of-a-nation.pdf [Accessed 23.04.2020].

Wilkinson, G. S. 1993. *Wide Range Achievement Test. WRAT3*. Lutz, FL: Wide Range, Incorporated.

World Health Organization 2016. *The mandate for health literacy*. Available at: www.who.int/healthpromotion/conferences/9gchp/health-literacy/en/ [Accessed 18.03.2020].

World Health Organization 2019a. *Draft WHO European roadmap for implementation of health literacy initiatives through the life course*. Available at: www.euro.who.int/__data/assets/pdf_file/0003/409125/69wd14e_Rev1_RoadmapOnHealthLiteracy_190323.pdf?ua=1 [Accessed 30.04.2020].

World Health Organization 2019b. *WHO guildeline: recommendations on digital interventions for health system strengthening*. Available at: www.who.int/reproductivehealth/publications/digital-interventions-health-system-strengthening/en/ [Accessed 01.05.2020].

Section 2:

EARLY INTERVENTION

5

HEALTHY CHILD DEVELOPMENT

AMANDA HOLLAND

LEARNING OUTCOMES

By the end of this chapter you will be able to:

- Gain a brief understanding of some well-known theories of child development.
- Consider the role of epigenetics on child development.
- Make links between the sustainable development goals and child health.
- Compare child health programmes offered in the UK.

Introduction

Child development is a dynamic process that begins from conception and continues gradually throughout childhood. During this time children experience physical, emotional, social and cognitive changes, developing skills and abilities to use in the world around them. Positive relationships and loving nurturing environments facilitate secure attachments where healthy child development can occur in a planned, organised way as children gradually progress from dependency on their parents or carers to increasing independence. Child development is determined by genetic inheritance and is highly influenced by experiences, particularly during the first years of life. During the early years, the foundations for all future learning, behaviour, health and successes in school and later life are laid down.

This chapter will provide a brief introduction to some of the most well-known theories of child development and aid an understanding of the nature of human growth and healthy development. It will briefly consider child morbidity and mortality from a global perspective and provide an overview of international growth standards and child health programmes within the UK. It is recommended that this chapter is read in conjunction with Chapter 6, The Influence of Early Relationships on Child Development and Long-term Health and Wellbeing and Chapter 16 Safeguarding Children and Young People.

Key legislation and government policy aimed at promoting and protecting child health

> Every child has the right to life. Governments must do all they can to ensure that children survive and develop to their full potential. (United Nations 1989, Art. 6).

Article 6 of the *United Nations Convention on the Rights of a Child* (UNCRC) (UN 1989) explains how every child has the right to thrive and survive and how adults and governments must work together to protect and promote child health and ensure children enjoy their rights. Legislation aimed at promoting and protecting child health sets out duties and responsibilities of those who must by law take action to make sure the rights of infants, children and young people to life and achievement of their full potential is ensured. Table 5.1 briefly lists some key legislation that underpins the direction of government health policy and strategies committed to supporting and enabling child health and wellbeing. For legislation relating specifically to safeguarding children, see Chapter 16.

Child development theories

The nature of child development is viewed as a continuous process covering a wide variety of competencies that manifest across childhood. Behaviours, skills and knowledge emerge as healthy children grow and attain developmental milestones. Child

Table 5.1 Key legislation that underpins the direction of government health policy and strategies committed to supporting and enabling child health and wellbeing

United Nations Convention on the Rights of a Child (1989)	• The most widely ratified international human rights treaty in history • 54 articles setting out children's rights, covering all aspects of a child's life, all with equal importance • The convention came into force in the UK in 1992, since forming the basis of further legislation and policy aimed at protecting and promoting child health There are four general principles; 1. Non-discrimination (article 2) 2. Best interest of the child (article 3) 3. Right to life survival and development (article 6) 4. Right to be heard (article 12)
The Children's Act 1989 and 2004	Focuses on the well-being of children in the UK. The main principles of the act are; • Allow children to be healthy • Help children to be happy and enjoy life • Allowing children to remain safe in their environments • Help children to succeed • Help achieve economic stability for the future of children • Help make a positive contribution to children's lives
The Equality Act 2010	The Act protects people from discrimination and guarantees the rights of children and young people. It sets out legal requirements to ensure children are treated without discrimination irrespective of their race, colour, sex, language, religion, ethnic or social origin, disability, birth or other status.
Children and Young People (Scotland) Act 2014	The Act sets out to shift public services towards the early years of a child's life, and towards early intervention encouraging preventative measures, rather than crises' responses. The Act establishes a legal framework within which services are to work together in support of children, young people and families.
Well-being of Future Generations (Wales) Act 2015	The Act is unique to Wales. It requires public bodies to consider the impact of their decisions, to work better with people, communities, and each other, and to prevent persistent problems such as poverty, health inequalities and climate change. The law sets 7 goals; • A globally responsible Wales • A prosperous Wales • A resilient Wales • A healthier Wales • A Wales of cohesive communities • A Wales of vibrant culture and thriving Welsh Language • A more equal Wales
Children's Services and Co-operation Act (Northern Ireland) 2015	The Act aims to improve co-operation amongst departments and agencies and places a duty on Children's Authorities to co-operate where appropriate and deliver services aimed at improving the well-being of children and young people. It sets the strategic direction to achieving improvements in the well-being of children and young people in NI.

development is commonly grouped into different domains such as biological (changes in physical growth, e.g. fine and gross motor development), emotional (changes in attention, emotional regulation, understanding and experiences), social (changes in social communication and relationships) and cognitive (changes in thought processes, speech, language and communication) (Keenan et al. 2016, Sharma and Cockerill 2014). Age periods for the study of child development typically focus on:

- The first thousand days – conception to age 2
- Early childhood – 2 to 6 years
- Middle childhood – 6 to 11 years
- Adolescence – 11 to 18 years
- Early adulthood – 18 to 25 years

Theories of child development provide a framework to aid an understanding about the nature of child development and human growth at various ages and stages. A very brief introduction to some of the most well-known theories can be seen in Table 5.2.

Erickson's (1963) developmental theory centres on psychosocial development. He believed that the development of personality is impacted by relationships and social experiences across the lifespan. His work focused on eight psychosocial stages of development and growth from birth through to adulthood and older age, (see Table 5.2). The skills and capabilities accomplished at each stage support the acquisition of new skills towards progressing through the next stage of development. At each stage Erickson believed individuals experience conflict, and that if dealt with successfully this enables psychological strength and growth paving the way for healthier developmental outcomes. However, failing to resolve conflict can lead to less optimal outcomes and delays in the continued development of essential skills required to master future challenges and conflicts (Erickson 1963). A criticism of Erickson's theory is that it does not explain what needs to happen to support individuals to complete each stage or how development occurs. Bowlby's (1988) theory of attachment, on the other hand, indicates that secure attachments enable children to develop the skills required to manage and

Table 5.2 Theories of Child Development

Developmental theory	Stages of development
Erikson's Psychosocial Developmental Theory (Erikson 1963)	• Stage 1: basic trust versus mistrust - birth to 1 year • Stage 2: autonomy versus shame and doubt - 1 to 3 years • Stage 3: initiative versus guilt - 3 to 6 years • Stage 4: industry versus inferiority - 6 to 11 years • Stage 5: identity versus identity diffusion - adolescence • Stage 6: intimacy verses isolation - young adulthood • Stage 7: generativity versus stagnation - middle adulthood • Stage 8: ego integrity versus despair - old age
Freud's Psychosexual Developmental Theory (Freud 2001)	• Oral stage: birth to 1 year • Anal stage: 1 to 3 years • Phallic stage: 3 to 6 years • Latency stage: 6 years to puberty • Genital stage: puberty to adulthood
Piaget's Cognitive Developmental Theory (Piaget 1971)	• Sensorimotor stage: birth to 2 years • Preoperational stage: 2 years to 7 years • Concrete operational stage: 7 to 12 years • Formal operational stage: age 12 and up

overcome challenging conflicts. Secure attachment between parents and their children develops where caregiving is loving, responsive, nurturing and consistent. This creates an optimum environment for children to gain confidence that their needs will be met, physically, socially and emotionally. Sensitive and responsive care is essential, particularly during the early years, to enable children to develop empathy, trust and the ability to problem solve and manage their feelings and emotions (Bowlby 1988). See Chapter 6 for further discussion of Bowlby's attachment theory.

Freud's psychosexual developmental theory proposed that personality development occurs through five psychosexual stages from birth to puberty and beyond (see Table 5.2). Each stage of development represents different areas of the body that become important sources of frustrations and pleasure as a person grows. Each stage revolves around psychosexual energy (libido) expressed through different parts of the body and is described as the driving force of behaviours at different stages of growth. For example, during the oral stage (from birth to approximately 18 months) infants gain pleasure through their mouth by sucking, chewing and biting. As with Erickson's theory, a person must overcome conflict at each stage to successfully develop a healthy personality. Where conflict remains unresolved, Freud (2001) believes fixations can occur and an individual may remain stuck in a stage. A potential source of conflict during the anal stage may be a child's desire to immediately open their bowels verses the parents attempt to train them to wait and use the toilet. In this example, unresolved conflict can result in delays to becoming fully toilet trained in readiness for school. While Freud's theory enables an understanding of development, it has been heavily criticised as it largely focused on males and neglected to examine important aspects of female development; furthermore, his significant claims have not been scientifically validated.

Bandura's (1977) social learning theory suggests that learning and behaviour are influenced by the environment and cognitive factors. Development is said to occur through observing, modelling and imitating behaviours and emotions of others. In one of Bandura's best known experiments, children were observed to model acts of aggression towards a doll known as a 'bobo doll'. The experiment involved children observing an adult behaving physically and verbally aggressive towards the doll. When left alone with the doll children were observed to repeat similar acts of aggression towards the doll, thereby demonstrating the role of modelling in the development of aggressive behaviour (Bandura et al. 1961). Bandura's theory emphasises the importance of children being exposed to positive role models; however, a criticism is that his theory lacks exploration of wider contextual environmental variables such as socioeconomic factors, race, sex and education (Keenan et al. 2016).

Piaget's (1971) cognitive development theory focuses on understanding how children acquire knowledge and explains how intelligence changes as children grow and adapt their knowledge to the world around them. Piaget believed that children's cognitive development progresses through a series of four stages (see Table 5.2). As a child moves through the four different stages they acquire increased sophistication of thought. For example, in the sensorimotor stage a child lives in the present and has not yet developed a mental picture of the world, then as they move to the preoperational stage they develop the ability to think using symbolic representations such as language and mental imagery.

During the concrete operational stage children begin to think logically, with the ability to think abstractly developing in the formal operation stage. Piaget's work considers how children develop at different rates and progress through stages at their own pace; however, it has been criticised for its conception of development occurring in stages rather than a continuum of development. Furthermore, is lacks consideration of environment factors such as cultural and social differences, proposing universality. Bronfenbrenner (1977), on the other hand, views the environment as a dynamic entity, constantly changing, with a significant impact on child development.

Bronfenbrenner (1977) proposed a bioecological model of human development where environmental influences on child development extend beyond the immediate surroundings, taking into account wider social and cultural aspects (see Figure 5.1). The model places the child at the centre of four layers that represent different aspects of the environment, the inner most layer being the microsystem, followed by the second layer, the mesosystem, then the third layer, the exosystem, and the fourth layer, the macrosystem, with the chronosystem, a fifth layer, added at a later date. The microsystem refers to immediate relationships with family, peers, neighbours, church and school, and considers the influence of close relationships on child development. At this level Bronfenbrenner believed relationships can be bidirectional, with parents directly influencing the child's behaviours and beliefs and the child influencing parenting behaviours. Bronfenbrenner acknowledged that these influences could occur at any level, however, he suggested that this was strongest in the microsystem.

The mesosystem refers to quality and frequency of relationships between those within the microsystem. For example, educational attainment such as learning to read can be optimised with positive relationships between parents and teachers, where learning in school extends to learning within the home. Where parents lack the desire to form positive relationships with teachers, perhaps due to their own negative experiences as school children, conflict between learning in school and learning in the home can occur, adversely impacting on an optimum environment for child growth.

The exosystem refers to social structures that indirectly impact on child development and interact with various aspects within the mesosystem, such as parental employment, mass media, community services, social support networks and government agencies. These structures can provide important support for families and enhance child development, such as child-friendly employment with flexible working hours, low-cost childcare, and paid maternity and paternity leave. Children can either benefit from their parents' income to meet their needs or experience negative effects from their parents' busy work schedules. However, parental unemployment, financial insecurity, overcrowding and poor social networks have been linked with increasing the risk of child maltreatment (Sidebotham et al. 2002).

The macrosystem considers how wider influences such as graphical locations, ethnicity, cultural ideologies and laws directly impact on the upbringing and development of a child. This layer recognises how wider cultural patterns, values, beliefs and political decisions have a powerful influence on child development. The fifth and final layer of Bronfenbrenner's bioecological model, the chronosystem (not shown in Figure 5.1), considers

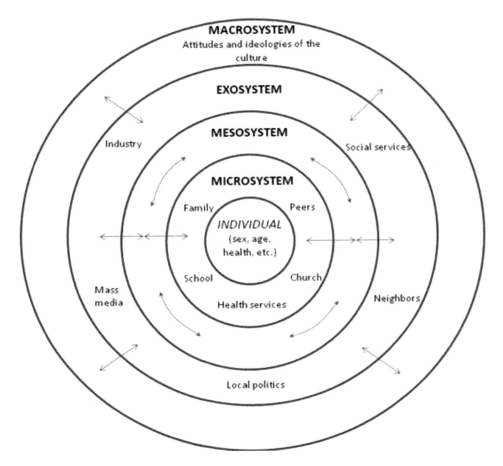

Figure 5.1 Bronfenbrenner's bioecological model of development
(Keenan et al. 2016, p.38)

environmental changes that occur over a lifetime which impact on development such as change in family structures and societal changes such as economic changes and wars. Bronfenbrenner's theory demonstrates how parents and carers can positively influence the microsystem and mesosystem, however, the direct influences from within the other systems can adversely impact child development, perhaps thereby demonstrating how it really does take a village to raise a child.

Knowledge of various theories of child development can support practitioners in understanding the nature of child growth and development, and how wider influences can either support or hinder developmental outcomes.

The role of epigenetics

An emerging area of scientific research known as 'epigenetics' reveals how early experiences, behaviours and the environment can negatively impact on healthy child development, temporarily or permanently. Epigenetics can cause changes that affect the way genes are expressed. Epigenetic changes do not change DNA, but they can change how the body reads DNA sequences by changing gene expression, turning genes 'on' or 'off'. One of the most well-known epigenetic changes is DNA Methylation; this works by adding a chemical group to DNA where it blocks the proteins that attach to DNA to 'read' the gene, turning the gene 'off'. Demethylation, on the other hand, removes the group of chemicals, turning the gene 'on'. Body cells have the same genes but they function differently, and epigenetics help to determine which function a cell will have, for example a muscle cell or nerve cell. Epigenetics allows a muscle or nerve cell to turn on genes to make proteins important to specific muscles or nerve cells; however, experiences and the environment can affect how these genes are expressed (Centre for Disease Control and Prevention 2021).

Consider the developing brain. The construction of brain architecture begins before birth, with the most rapid period of growth occurring before the age of two. During this time specialised brain cells known as 'neurons' that enable basic brain functions construct at an estimated rate of one million new neural connections every second, stimulating lightning-fast communications between different parts of the brain. Through a process of pruning, less stimulated neural connections reduce and brain circuits become more efficient, enabling the development of the first sensory pathways of vision and hearing, with language skills and higher cognitive function following (Centre on the Developing Child 2007). Although brain development is strongly influenced by genetic factors, experiences dictate the growth of neurons and the neural connections that are kept and those which are lost through the pruning process. Neural pathways that are used more frequently become more strongly wired, whether in response to positive or negative stimuli. At birth the brain is approximately 25% of an adult brain weight, by the age of two the brain will grow to 75% of an adult brain weight (Shaffer 2002). It is most flexible and adaptable in the early years and most sensitive to epigenetic changes. Traumatic experiences particularly during pregnancy and the first years of life such as war, famine, slavery, domestic abuse, can severely compromise the chemistry that encodes genes in brain cells, changing gene expressions as described above. This results in epigenetic modifications which increase the risk of developmental delay, and poor physical and mental health outcomes in the long term (Centre for Disease Control and Prevention 2021, Centre on the Developing Child 2021). High-quality health care for pregnant women, infants, children and young people together with support for parents and carers can influence positive epigenetic expressions and healthy gene potential.

A brief global perspective of child mortality and morbidity

Enabling children to thrive and survive and to reach their full potential is a human right and essential for sustainable development (United Nations 1989), yet many children face significant challenges to survive past infancy. In 2019, 6.1 million children and young adolescents died worldwide, mostly from preventable and treatable causes (UNICEF 2019). Children under the age of five accounted for 5.2 million of these deaths, with 2.4 million deaths occurring in infants under the age of 28 days, 1.5 million in infants aged one month to eleven months, and 1.3 million deaths occurring in children aged between one to four years (WHO 2020). The leading cause of deaths in children under five years are from preterm birth complications, birth asphyxia/trauma, pneumonia, congenital anomalies, diarrhoea, malaria and non-communicable diseases such as heart disease, stroke, cancer and diabetes. Older children and adolescents are more exposed to accidents and injuries, such as drowning or road traffic accidents, and unintended pregnancies. The risk of mortality and morbidity increases for children and adolescents living within areas of humanitarian crises. Worldwide, progress has been made to reduce the rates of child mortality with deaths in the under-fives dropping by 59% since 1990, from 93 deaths per 1,000 live births to 38 deaths per 1,000 live births in 2019. However, differences across regions and countries continue to exist with 80% of deaths in the under-fives occurring in Sub-Saharan Africa and Southern Asia (WHO 2020).

The Sustainable Development Goals and child health

Global childhood mortality remains unacceptably high, particularly as most deaths are preventable or treatable. The Sustainable Development Goals (SDGs) aim to address continued child deaths, health inequalities and emerging child health priorities. The SDGs were adopted by the United Nations in 2015, setting out 17 goals to achieve better health and a more sustainable future for all through a global partnership involving 193 developed and non-developed countries (United Nations 2021). Goals range from tackling poverty and hunger to promoting health, quality education, sustainable cities, communities, forests and life below water. Goal 3: *Ensure healthy lives and promote wellbeing for all ages*, specifically sets out targets to end preventable deaths of newborns and children under 5 years by 2030 through two targets:

- Reduce newborn mortality to at least as low as 12 per 1,000 live births in every country.
- Reduce under-five mortality to at least as low as 25 per 1,000 live births in every country.

Other targets include reducing premature mortality from non-communicable diseases, halving the number of global deaths and injuries from road traffic accidents, and strengthening prevention and treatment services for substance misuse (WHO 2020). A priority is placed on strengthening healthcare systems to promote health and prevent ill health across the lifespan through universal health coverage with access to good quality services and affordable medicines and vaccines. To ensure targets are met, governments are encouraged to:

- *Strengthen primary healthcare systems to reach every child.*
- *Focus on maternal, newborn and child survival.*

- *Prioritise child and adolescent health and wellbeing, including mental health.*
- *Support responses to reduce the impact on children and families of natural disasters, complex emergencies and demographic shifts*

(UNICEF 2021)

All 193 countries signed up to the SDGs agreement are expected to contribute to all goals and deliver them domestically. The COVID-19 pandemic has resulted in challenges to achieving goals, with the most urgently shared agenda focusing on globally accessible vaccination. Much action is needed over the next decade to achieve the SDGs and reduce global child mortality and morbidity, securing improved health outcomes for all children and a more sustainable future. For a brief discussion on how nature plays an important role in the achievement of SDGs and child health, refer to the text box below.

Nature and child development

Over the past decade, there has been a growing body of research to understand the relationship between children and nature. The research confirms many significant benefits of spending time in nature on healthy child development, across physical, cognitive, affective and social domains (Beery and Lekies 2021).

A study by the World Health Organization (2019) found that 80% of adolescents were physically inactive due to time spent watching TV, video game playing and other sedentary behaviours. Worldwide, the prevalence of obesity has nearly tripled since 1975 resulting in 39 million children under the age of 5 and 340 million aged 5 to 19 classified as overweight or obese (WHO 2021). A sedentary lifestyle is known to increase the risks of gaining too much weight or becoming obese, whereas children who experience nature are known to be more physically active. The mental health of children who have contact with nature is supported and well developed because time spent in nature helps to develop brain cognition (Bulut and Maraba, 2020). A study by Natural England (2020) found that eight in ten children reported that being in nature made them very happy.

The non-medical term 'Nature Deficit Disorder' describes how children spend less time in nature and how this can result in behavioural changes (Louv 2005). Research has shown that being in contact with nature boosts psychological wellbeing and mood (Harvey et al. 2020), enhances attention span, self-regulation and behavioural development (Lee et al. 2019, Taylor and Butts-Wilmsmeyer 2020), supports stress reduction, resilience and aids motivation for learning (Dettweiler et al. 2015, 2017); furthermore, it can increase positive family interactions (Izenstark et al. 2021).

During the UK COVID-19 lockdown, there was a surge of people spending time in nature (Natural England 2020). A study found that during this period, 66% of parents/guardians reported that their children spent more time in nature than usual, and how they are now more likely to advocate for their children to play outdoors (Lemmey 2020). There are, however, clear inequalities for child access to nature, with Natural England (2020) indicating that 71%

of children from Black and minority ethnic backgrounds reported spending less time outside since COVID-19 compared with 57% of children from other backgrounds. Furthermore, 73% of children from households with a total annual income below £17,000 spent less time outdoors, compared with 57% from households with an annual income above £17,000. The reported health benefits of children spending more time in nature over lockdown include lessened anxiety (Chaudhury and Banerjee 2020) and decreased air pollution (Lemmey 2020).

All parts of society should have access to green spaces to support health and wellbeing, as set out in the Government's 25 Year Environment Plan (GOV UK 2018). This goal has much support from non-profit environmental organisations such as The Wildlife Trust, The National Trust, Friends of the Earth and others.

Nature plays an important role in achieving the Sustainable Development Goal 3 'Good Health and Wellbeing', and indeed no child should be left behind. Health and social care practitioners can promote the significant benefits of nature on healthy child development within their practice.

(Lucy Holland, Environmental Scientist, MRes in Conservation, Trustee and Ambassador for the Gwent Wildlife Trust)

Promoting healthy child development through child health programmes

In 2006, the World Health Organization (WHO) developed international Child Growth Standards for infants and young children based on the understanding that children across the globe have the potential to develop within the same range of height and weight when given the optimum start in life for health, growth and development. The standards assess for physical growth, nutritional status and motor development in all children from birth to age five and allow for early detection of nutritional and health care needs. The standards resulted from an intensive study initiated by the WHO in 1997 in partnership with the United Nations University and involved more than 8,000 children from Brazil, Ghana, India, Norway, Oman and the USA. The children were selected based on optimum environments for growth, that is, breast-fed infants and children receiving recommended feeding practices, good healthcare, mothers who did not smoke and other factors associated with good health outcomes. The study confirmed that although there are individual differences in growth among children, across large populations, regionally and globally, the average growth is similar. According to the WHO the new standards prove that the differences in children's growth to the age of five are more influenced by nutrition, feeding practices, health care and the environment than genetics or ethnicity (WHO 2006).

In the UK, governments across the four nations have varying universal child health programmes to promote and support healthy child development, placing children's rights, needs and resources as central to evidence-based early intervention and prevention services. Programmes are implemented through a multi-professional, multi-agency approach involving practitioners such as midwives, health visitors, school nurses, mental health services, social services and education. Child health programmes are delivered within home settings, community centres, GP surgeries, pre-school and school settings.

The core components of child health programmes are:

- Childhood screening (e.g. newborn screening tests, newborn physical examination) and targeted developmental reviews.
- Health promotion, protection (e.g. safeguarding children from harm) and prevention (e.g. accident and injury prevention, smoking cessation).
- Parenting support (parenting programmes, breast-feeding groups, fathers' groups).
- Immunisation (childhood immunisation programmes).

Child health programmes aim to provide a structured approach through universal contacts and integrated services so that all children and families benefit from evidence-based public health programmes (see Table 5.3). Early intervention and prevention are key to supporting healthy child development, and child health programmes provide a gateway for skilled practitioners to assess child and family needs including physical, emotional, social and environmental needs. Based on assessment of need, more enhanced or intensive services are available to support those identified as in greater need (Department of Health, Social Services and Public Safety 2010, Public Health England 2021, Scottish Government 2015, Scottish Government 2018, Welsh Government 2016).

Child health programmes are mostly led by Specialist Community Public Health Nurses (SCPHNs). In the UK, SCPHNs are nurses or midwives, registered with the Nursing and Midwifery Council (2021), who have undertaken an additional post-registration qualification in SCPHN to gain the award of health visitor or school nurse. Health visitors lead health programmes for children under the age of five whilst school health nurses lead health programmes for children aged five to nineteen years. As highly skilled professionals they follow a biopsychosocial model of health working in partnership with individuals, families, schools and communities to support healthy child development from conception in preparation for school and beyond. Health visitors deliver universal provisions within the home, and this puts them in a unique position to promote and influence positive health outcomes for children and their families. Through a salutogenic (health creating) approach health visitors proactively search for health needs, stimulate awareness of health needs and facilitate appropriate health-enhancing activities (Cowley and Frost 2006).

Child health programmes and commissioning groups for health visiting services vary considerably across the four nations. For example, in Wales seven NHS boards are responsible for the commissioning of health visiting services. Two child health programmes exist, the Healthy Child Wales Programme and the Flying Start programme. The Healthy Child Wales programme offers eight mandatory universal contacts to families and their children, with options for enhanced or intense home visiting based on need. Flying Start is a targeted programme offering 11 home visits with the addition of a further nine face-to-face visits, either in a community setting or in the home. The Flying Start service is targeted towards families with children under four years who live in some of the most deprived areas in Wales. In England, health visiting services are commissioned

Table 5.3 Universal child health programmes in the UK

	Wales	Scotland	England	Northern Ireland
Name of child health programme	Healthy Child Wales Programme (Welsh Government 2016)	Getting it Right for Every Child (Scottish Government 2017)	Healthy Child Programme (Department of Health 2009/2021)	Healthy Child, Healthy Future programme (Department of Health, Social Services and Public Safety 2010)
Age range	Pregnancy to 7 years	Pregnancy to 19	Pregnancy to 19 years	Pregnancy to 19 years
Ages of mandatory and recommended reviews				
Early antenatal	√	√	√	
Late antenatal	√	√	√	√
Birth-72 hours	√	√	√	√
10-14 days	√	√	√	√
3-5 weeks		√		√
6-8 weeks	√	√	√	√
12 weeks	√	√	√	√
4 months	√	√		√
6 months	√		√	√
7-8 months		√		
9-12 months			√	√
13-15 months	√	√		√
24-30 months	√	√	√	√
36 months				√
42 months	√			√
4-4 ½ years Hand over to School Nurse	√	√	√	√
Primary School reviews	√	√	√	√
Post primary school reviews		√	√	√

through local authorities and regulation requires only five mandatory contacts by the health visitors; however, in 2021 a further two contacts at three months and six months were added, although these are only recommended, not mandatory. In Northern Ireland, health visitors are required to make nine home visits to the family home before the child reaches school age. Services are commissioned by the Health and Social Care Board in partnership with the Public Health Agency and five local commissioning groups.

In Scotland, 14 NHS boards are responsible for commissioning services in their regions, with the health visitor pathway offering 11 home visits to all families.

Variations and inequity in child health programmes and investments in services and workforce capacity to deliver programmes across the UK has caused much debate with professional organisations such as the Community Practitioner and Health Visitor Association (CPHVA) (Scott 2019) and the Institute of Health Visiting (iHV) (Adams 2019) calling for action from central and devolved governments to invest in health visiting, particularly in England where the service lags behind other countries.

Conclusion

This chapter briefly discussed several theories of child development that aid an understanding of human growth at various ages and stages while also considering wider environmental influences that impact on child development, child morbidity and mortality. International growth standards and child health promotion programmes in the UK were briefly explored. Variations and inequalities in child health programmes exist throughout the four nations of the UK and across the globe. Every child has equal rights to thrive and survive, an understanding of child development and child health programmes aimed at supporting healthy child development and wellbeing will support practitioners in their roles when working with children and their families.

Consider the following questions

1. What are the 54 articles of the United Nations Convention on the Rights of a Child and how do they support healthy child development?
2. How do the theories of child development support your understanding of human growth?
3. How do the Sustainable Development Goals support child health?
4. How might variations in child health programmes across the four nations impact on inequalities in child health from a UK-wide perspective?

Key terms

Attachment: The enduring connection between the infant and the primary caregiver that develops through a tendency of the infant to naturally seek and maintain closeness particularly during stressful situations.

COVID-19: An infectious disease caused by a newly discovered coronavirus.

Epigenetics: The study of how a person's behaviours and environment can cause changes that affect the way their genes work.

Salutogenisis: Health-creating approach.

Further reading

Centre for Disease Control and Prevention. 2022. *CDC's Developmental Milestones*. Available at: www.cdc.gov/ncbddd/actearly/milestones/index.html [Accessed 12.03.2022].

Emond, A. 2019. *Health for All Children*. (5th edn). Oxford University Press: Oxford.

World Health Organization. 2006. *Child Growth Standards*. Available at: www.who.int/tools/child-growth-standards [Accessed 12.03.2022].

References

Adams, C. 2019. *iHV launches 'Health Visiting England: A Vision for the Future. Institute of Health Visiting*. Available at: https://ihv.org.uk/news-and-views/news/ihv-launches-health-visiting-in-england-a-vision-for-the-future/ [Accessed 10.02.2021].

Bandura, A. 1977. *Social Learning Theory*. Prentice-Hall: Englewood Cliffs, NJ.

Bandura, A., Ross, D., Ross, S. A. 1961. Transmission of aggression through imitation of aggressive models. *Journal of Abnormal Social Psychology*; 63, 575–582.

Beery, T. H., Lekies, K. S. 2021. Nature's services and contributions: the relational value of childhood nature experience and the importance of reciprocity. *Frontiers in Ecology and Evolution*; 9, 251.

Bowlby, J. 1988. *A Secure Base*. Routledge: New York.

Bronfenbrenner, U. 1977. Toward an experimental ecology of human development. *American Psychologist*; 32(7), 515–531.

Bulut, S., Maraba, D. 2020. The effect of nature on child development. *Current Research in Psychology and Behavioral Science (CRPBS)*; 1(2), 1–2.

Centre for Disease Control and Prevention. 2021. *Genomics and Precision Health. What is epigenetics?* Available at: www.cdc.gov/genomics/disease/epigenetics.htm [Accessed 10.07.2021].

Centre on the Developing Child, Harvard University. 2007. *In brief: the science of early childhood development*. Available at: https://developingchild.harvard.edu/resources/inbrief-science-of-ecd/ [Accessed 20.02.2021].

Centre on the Developing Child, Harvard University. 2021. *Epigenetics and child development: how children's experiences affect their genes*. Available at: https://developingchild.harvard.edu/resources/what-is-epigenetics-and-how-does-it-relate-to-child-development/ [Accessed 05.02.2021].

Chaudhury, P., Banerjee, D. 2020. 'Recovering with nature': a review of ecotherapy and implications for the COVID-19 pandemic. *Frontiers in Public Health*, 8.

Cowley, S., Frost, M. 2006. *The Principles of Health Visiting: Opening the Door to Public Health Practice in the 21st Century*. Community Practitioners' and Health Visitors' Association: London.

Department of Education. 2015. *Children's Services Co-operation Act (Northern Ireland) 2015*. Available at: https://www.education-ni.gov.uk/childrens-services-co-operation-act-northern-ireland-2015 [Accessed 21.09.2021].

Department of Health. 2009. *Healthy Child Programme. Pregnancy and the first five years of life*. Available at: https://www.gov.uk/government/publications/healthy-child-programme-pregnancy-and-the-first-5-years-of-life [Accessed 21.09.21].

Department of Health, Social Services and Public Safety. 2010. *Healthy child, healthy future. A framework for the Universal Child Health Promotion Programme in Northern Ireland. Pregnancy to 19 years*. Available at: www.health-ni.gov.uk/sites/default/files/publications/dhssps/healthychildhealthyfuture.pdf [Accessed 15.04.2021].

Dettweiler, U., Becker, C., Auestad, B. H., Simon, P., Kirsch, P. 2017. Stress in school. Some empirical hints on the circadian cortisol rhythm of children in outdoor and indoor classes. *International Journal of Environmental Research and Public Health;* 14(5), 475.

Dettweiler, U., Ünlü, A., Lauterbach, G., Becker, C., Gschrey, B., 2015. Investigating the motivational behavior of pupils during outdoor science teaching within self-determination theory. *Frontiers in Psychology;* 6, 125.

Erickson, E. H. 1963. *Childhood and Society*. (2nd edn). Norton: New York.

Freud, S. 2001. *The Standard Edition of the Complete Psychological Works of Sigmund Freud. Volume 111*. Vintage: London.

GOV.UK. 2018. *25 Year Environment Plan*. Available at: www.gov.uk/government/publications/25-year-environment-plan [Accessed 06.09.2021].

Harvey, D. J., Montgomery, L. N., Harvey, H., Hall, F., Gange, A. C., Watling, D. 2020. Psychological benefits of a biodiversity-focussed outdoor learning program for primary school children. *Journal of Environmental Psychology;* 67, 101381.

Izenstark, D., Ravindran, N., Rodriguez, S., Devine, N., 2021. The affective and conversational benefits of a walk in nature among mother–daughter dyads. *Applied Psychology: Health and Well–Being;* 13(2), 299–316.

Keenan, T., Evans, S., Crowley, K. 2016. *An Introduction to Child Development*. (3rd edn). Sage Publishing: London.

Lee, M., Kim, S., Ha, M. 2019. Community greenness and neurobehavioral health in children and adolescents. *Science of the Total Environment;* 672, 381–388.

Legislation.gov.uk. 1989. *Children Act 1989*. Available at: https://www.legislation.gov.uk/ukpga/1989/41 [Accessed 10.09.2021].

Legislation.gov.uk. 2004. *Children Act 2004*. Available at: https://www.legislation.gov.uk/ukpga/2004/31/contents [Accessed 10.09.2021].

Legislation.gov.uk. 2010. *Equality Act 2010*. Available at: https://www.legislation.gov.uk/ukpga/2010/15/contents [Accessed 10.09.2021].

Legislation.gov.uk. 2014. *Children and Young People (Scotland) Act 2014*. Available at: https://www.legislation.gov.uk/asp/2014/8/contents/enacted [Accessed 10.09.2021].

Lemmey, T. 2020. *Research Report. Connection with Nature in the UK During the COVID-19 Lockdown*. In association with the Centre for national Parks and Protected Areas, University of Cumbria.

Louv, R. 2005. *Last Child in the Woods: Saving our Children from Nature-Deficit Disorder*. Algonquin Books: Chapel Hill, NC.

Natural England. 2020. *The People and Nature Survey for England: Children's Survey*. Available at: www.gov.uk/government/statistics/the-people-and-nature-survey-for-england-child-data-wave-1-experimental-statistics/the-people-and-nature-survey-for-england-childrens-survey-experimental-statistics [Accessed 06.09.2021].

Nursing and Midwifery Council. 2021. Available at: www.nmc.org.uk/ [Accessed 10.05.2021].

Piaget, J. 1971. *Biology and Knowledge: An Essay on the Relations Between Organic Regulations and Cognitive Processes.* University of Chicago Press: Chicago, IL.

Public Health England. 2021. *Best start in life and beyond. Improving public health outcomes for children, young people and families. Guidance to support commissioning of the Health Child Programme 0 to 19. Guide 1: Background information on commissioning and service model.* Available at: https://assets.publishing.service.gov.uk/government/uploads/system/uploads/attachment_data/file/969168/Commissioning_guide_1.pdf [Accessed 10.04.2021].

Scott, A. 2019. Shining the light. *Community Practitioner.* February.

Scottish Government. 2015. *Universal Health Visiting Pathway in Scotland: pre-birth to pre-school.* Available at: www.gov.scot/publications/universal-health-visiting-pathway-scotland-pre-birth-pre-school/pages/2/ [Accessed 15.04.2021].

Scottish Government. 2018. *Transforming nursing, midwifery and health professions roles: the school nursing role in integrated community nursing teams.* Available at: www.gov.scot/publications/school-nursing-role-integrated-community-nursing-teams/ [Accessed 15.04.2021].

Shaffer, D. R. 2002. *Developmental Psychology: Childhood and Adolescence.* (6th edn). Wadsworth: Belmont, CA.

Sharma, A., Cockerill, H. 2014. *Mary Sheridan's from Birth to Five Years. Children's Developmental Progress.* (4th edn). Routledge: New York.

Sidebotham, P., Heron, J., Golding, J. 2002. Child maltreatment in the 'Children of the Nineties': deprivation, class and social networks in a UK sample. *Child Abuse and Neglect*; 26, 1243–1259.

Taylor, A. F., Butts-Wilmsmeyer, C., 2020. Self-regulation gains in kindergarten related to frequency of green schoolyard use. *Journal of Environmental Psychology*; 70, 101440.

Trevelyan, A. M. 2020. *Speech: Achieving the SDGs amidst COVID-19. UK National Statement to the UN High Level Political Forum 2020.* Available at: www.gov.uk/government/speeches/achieving-the-sdgs-amidst-COVID-19 [Accessed 13.04.2021].

UNICEF. 2019. *Health: Every Child Has the Right to Thrive and Survive.* Available at: www.unicef.org/health [Accessed 10.01.2021].

UNICEF. 2021. *Goal 3: Good Health and Well-being. Ensure Healthy Lives and Promote Well-being for All at All Ages.* Available at: https://data.unicef.org/sdgs/goal-3-good-health-wellbeing/ [Accessed 10.07.2021].

United Nations. 1989. *United Nations Convention on the Rights of a Child.* The Office of United Nations High Commissioner for Human Rights: Geneva.

United Nations. 2021. *Sustainable Development Goals.* Available at: www.un.org/sustainabledevelopment/health/ [Accessed 10.01.2021].

Welsh Government. 2015. *Well-being of Future Generations (Wales) Act 2015.* Available at: https://gov.wales/well-being-of-future-generations-wales [Accessed 10.09.2021].

Welsh Government. 2016. *An Overview of the Healthy Child Wales Programme*. Available at: https://gov.wales/sites/default/files/publications/2019-05/an-overview-of-the-healthy-child-wales-programme.pdf [Accessed 10.02.2021].

World Health Organization. 2006. *World Health Organization Releases New Child Growth Standards*. Available at: www.who.int/news/item/27-04-2006-world-health-organization-releases-new-child-growth-standards [Accessed 10.02.2021].

World Health Organization. 2019. *To Grow Up Healthy, Children Need to Sit Less and Play More*. Available at: www.who.int/news/item/24-04-2019-to-grow-up-healthy-children-need-to-sit-less-and-play-more [Accessed 10.02.2021].

World Health Organization. 2020. *Children: Improving Survival and Well-being*. Available at: www.who.int/news-room/fact-sheets/detail/children-reducing-mortality [Accessed 12.01.2021].

World Health Organization. 2021. *Obesity and Overweight*. Available at: www.who.int/news-room/fact-sheets/detail/obesity-and-overweight [Accessed 28.09.2021].

6

THE INFLUENCE OF EARLY RELATIONSHIPS ON CHILD DEVELOPMENT AND LONG-TERM HEALTH AND WELLBEING

AMANDA HOLLAND AND KATE PHILLIPS

LEARNING OUTCOMES

By the end of this chapter you will be able to:

- Gain an understanding of how parent–child relationships influence child development.
- Understand how past parenting experiences and adverse childhood experiences influence both parenting capacity and child development.
- Consider the wider social and environmental factors that influence parenting capacity and positive parenting behaviours.
- Gain a recognition of the diversity of differing family dynamics and parenting roles.

Introduction

The responsibility of raising children to become well-rounded young people and adults primarily rests with parents and families. Whilst wider society and governments also have a crucial role to play, the building blocks for healthy child development are established from conception and are dependent on positive responsive caregiving that nurtures secure relationships and provides the social and emotional foundations required for optimum child development. Most parents want to do the best they can for their children, however, complex factors such as poverty, mental ill health, addiction and violence can cause disruptions that interfere with the development of secure relationships, ultimately impacting on the health and wellbeing of children through adolescence into adulthood. This chapter examines the influence of early relationships on child development and why this is important in terms of short- and long-term outcomes of children. For the purpose of this chapter the term 'parent' is used and refers to mother, father or major biological or non-biological caregiver.

Policy context

The United Nations Convention on the Rights of a Child (CRC) (UN 1989) is the most widely ratified human rights treaty in history containing 54 articles that sets out civil, political, economic, social and cultural rights of children, aged 17 and under, regardless of their race, religion or abilities, and states how adults and governments must work together to protect children's rights. The CRC became ratified in the UK in 1991 and came into force in 1992, underpinning the direction of UK Government legislation and policy initiatives aimed at supporting, promoting and protecting the healthy development and wellbeing of children (Children Act 1989, Children Act 2004, Child Poverty Act 2010).

Much research identifies early childhood as a crucial window of opportunity to support healthy child development particularly in the first 1,000 days, from conception to age two (Center on the Developing Child 2007). Evidence clearly indicates the importance of positive parent–child relationships in influencing long-term outcomes for children, for better or for worse (National Scientific Council on the Developing Child 2004).

Policy initiatives across the devolved four nations in the UK have taken different approaches to incorporate legislation into public health programmes placing children's rights, needs and resources at the centre of health care activities (Welsh Government 2016, Public Health Scotland 2015, Department of Health, Social Services and Public Safety 2010, Department of Health 2009). Child health programmes place importance of investment in the early years to enable every child a healthy start in all aspects of their life and to realise their full potential. Key priorities include screening, immunisation and surveillance, that is, monitoring and supporting child development. The promotion of positive parent–child relationships and secure bonding and attachment is a fundamental aspect to improving health outcomes. Professional teams including health visitors, family nurses, nursery nurses and school nurses deliver child health programmes; however, midwives, social care workers, allied health professionals, teachers and anyone who has contact with children all have a key role to play and must work together to identify parents and families that need support and children who may be at risk of poor outcomes.

Attachment and bonding

Positive parent–child relationships and secure attachment and bonding is associated with positive developmental outcomes and is the single most important factor in reducing child abuse (National Society for the Protection of Cruelty to Children 2015). Bonding and attachment are often used interchangeably, however 'attachment' refers to the enduring connection between the infant and the primary care giver that develops through a tendency of the infant to naturally seek and maintain closeness particularly during stressful situations. Bonding, on the other hand, refers to the primary caregiver's relationship with their new infant where they come to know, love and accept their new baby (Bowlby 1988).

Babies are born into the word totally dependent on their parents and carers for survival. It is most often the mother who initially provides food and comfort for the newborn and to whom the infant develops a primary attachment. However, a primary adult with an intimate connection who can predict and respond to the infant's needs with sensitivity and consistency will provide a sense of security where the infant comes to realise their needs will be met, giving them a feeling of safety in which they can begin to explore the world from a secure base (Bowlby 1988). Children experience their world through an environment of human relationships. The child's first relationships, that with parents, will have a profound impact on their future health and wellbeing. Experiences in the first years of life, particularly the first 1,000 days, have a profound impact on the ongoing development and wellbeing of children. Where parenting is loving, responsive, consistent and predictable children grow to feel safe and develop secure attachment relationships with their parents, and this provides an optimum environment in which they develop trust, empathy and flourish, physically, socially and emotionally. On the other hand, where parenting is repeatedly unavailable, neglectful or intrusive, unresponsive or unpredictable, insecure relationships may develop where children adapt to their environment and learn to avoid closeness and emotional connections as they come to realise they cannot depend upon the parent to meet their needs. Secure relationships enable children a secure base to learn about themselves and others, to develop confidence, empathy, social skills and trust; however, insecure relationships can create feelings of uncertainty and confusion where children are less likely to learn how to regulate their emotions or develop social skills as they learn to live without the love and support of others. Poor attachment in the early years is highly correlated with poor cognitive, emotional and behavioural outcomes and chronic physical illness such as obesity, asthma and heart disease (Gold 2017).

Most parents naturally develop loving and responsive relationships with their children and want to do the best they can. Indeed, human ethology assumes that parenting behaviours are pre-programmed and develop in response to their baby's natural

Table 6.1 Attachment categorisations (Holland 2021, adapted from Bowlby 1979, Ainsworth et al. 1978)

Attachment Style	Caregiver Response	Infant/Child Behaviour
Secure Attachment	Sensitive, responsive, consistent, attuned, reliable. For example, prompt comforting when child is distressed, warm interested response to infant's wish to communicate or play.	Able to regulate emotions, seek help from others when distressed, adaptable to changing circumstances and able to explore the world.
Insecure (Avoidant)	Connected enough to protect the infant; minimises the importance of attachment issues; can be dismissive of infant's attachment cues; insensitive to infant's signals and emotional needs. Distant, irritated, anxious.	Shows little distress on separation and minimal joy when reunited with caregiver; avoidance of emotional intimacy and defensive focus on exploration. Does not seek out physical contact. Indiscriminate about who they interact with.
Insecure (Ambivalent/Resistant)	Inconsistent or unpredictable emotional availability and responses to infant's emotional needs. For example, at times overprotective or overstimulating and at other times rejecting or ignoring.	Overly engaged with attachment figure and may feel too anxious about caregiver's emotional availability to freely explore the environment.
Disorganised insecure attachment	Unresponsive, intrusive, hostile or violent. These parents may have experienced trauma themselves.	Chaotic and confusing behaviour e.g. hypervigilant, freeze or fear when parent appears.

behaviours and needs. For example, the need to be soothed when frightened, in pain or crying, to be fed, kept warm and protected. However, not all parenting behaviours manifest themselves completely but are learnt through examples from others, education, and parents' own experiences of being parented (Bowlby 1988).

The pioneering work of psychologists John Bowlby (1979) and Mary Ainsworth (Ainsworth et al. 1978) on attachment theory defined and categorised secure and insecure attachment. It is helpful for those working with children and families to understand attachment styles in relation to caregiver responses and infant/child behaviours to guide observations and discussions about the nature of parent–child relationships (see Table 6.1). Where concerns arise partnership working with parents, their children and multidisciplinary/multiagency child development services would enable timely assessment, diagnosis and agreed plans of care to support parents and their children.

Bioecological influences

Bronfenbrenner's (1974) bioecological model of human development describes how the effects of the environment have a profound impact on child development and their relationship with their parents, as discussed in Chapter 5. The model describes four layers of systems, each representing different aspects of the environment, from the innermost layer, the micro system which refers to the immediate setting in which the child lives and experiences close relationships, to the outermost level, the macrosystem which considers the overarching ideology of attitudes and cultural influences, such as values, laws, regulations and customs. With the child as central to the model, all systems will interact with each other and ultimately influence the development of relationships with an enduring effect on overall child development. This model enables understanding of the breadth of influences on the development of parent–child relationships, and how children are raised and parented.

Parenting styles

Child development is influenced by parenting approaches and the style of parenting. In the 1960s, Baumrind's (1967) pioneering research focused on the classification of parenting styles. Through exploring child behaviour and parenting practices Baumrind identified three common parenting styles: authoritative, authoritarian and permissive. **Authoritative** parenting describes warm, loving and responsive parenting, where limitations and boundaries are clearly set and fairness and consistency provides reasons and explanation rather than coercion to help guide future behaviour. This style of parenting is associated with positive child outcomes, for example, emotional stability, the development of empathy and good social skills, adaptive patterns of coping, self-esteem and self-confidence. On the other hand, **authoritarian** parenting is described as demanding and controlling, rather than nurturing or supporting, little warmth or positive attention is given, rather instructions and rules with no explanation for orders. Children may react with obedience, hostility or avoidance, and even imitate harsh parenting with other children. This style of parenting leads to the poorest outcomes for children and can result in low academic attainment and depressive symptoms. **Permissive** parenting describes warm and emotionally responsive parenting but lacks consistency and authority with little demands and expectation on the child. As a result, children may lack control, self-esteem, feel insecure, lack academic motivation, take less responsibility, and may show aggression due to the lack of boundaries and discipline (Power 2013). Maccoby and Martin (1983) later identified a neglecting, uninvolved style of parenting. This describes a parent who is psychologically unavailable and overwhelmed by their own problems, they may feel little or no emotional bond with their child. This style of parenting may result in insecure attachment as described in Table 6.1. Authoritative parenting results in the best outcomes for children, however, Baumrind's research dates back 50–60 years yet Power (2013) argues that these styles of parenting still have the strongest empirical basis. Indeed, Baumrind's authoritative parenting is supported and encouraged in many countries around the world (Carson et al. 1999, Mayseless et al. 2003, Martínez et al. 2007), however, further research is needed to examine cultural differences as children from some cultures are known to perform well with authoritarian parenting, where strict parenting behaviours are related to training (Chao 1994).

Parenting capacity

Parenting capacity refers to the parents' ability to appropriately protect their child from the risk of harm and to nurture their physical, social, emotional and educational developmental needs. Exploring parental capacity involves considering whether parenting is *good enough* to fulfil a child's needs. Winnicott (1953) refers to *good enough* as parenting that adequately meets the child's needs including love, care, responsiveness and commitment which is adaptive to the experiences and development of the child. In contrast to *perfect* parenting, Winnicott described the term 'good enough' as parenting that is responsive, appropriate and sensitive to the child's needs, temperament and developmental stages, supporting the child's transition over time from a dependent position to an increasingly more autonomous one. Winnicott recognised that it is impossible for parents to be empathetic and available all the time; however, he refers to the process of *good enough* parenting as adequately responding to the child's changing needs over time without a detrimental impact on the child's long-term health and development.

The Framework for the Assessment of Children in Need and their Families (Department of Health 2000) is commonly used today to support assessment and identify parental strengths and difficulties in adequately meeting their child's needs. The framework reflects the principles of the United Nations Convention on the Rights of a Child (1989) and is informed by the Children Act (1989). With the child at the centre of the assessment, the framework takes an ecological approach to enable an understanding of how wider environmental factors impact on healthy child development. It consists of three domains: 1. the child's developmental needs; 2. the parents' or caregivers' capacities to respond appropriately; 3. the wider family and environmental factors. The dimensions of parenting capacity explore parents' ability to provide basic care, ensure safety, emotional warmth and stimulation, guidance and boundaries, and stability (see Table 6.2). However, a multitude of factors can impact on a parent's capacity to provide *good enough* parenting such as poverty, mental illness, domestic abuse and parents' own experiences of being parented, some of which are discussed further in this and other chapters.

The influences of parents' own childhood experiences

The way parents feel about their children and their behaviour towards them will likely be influenced by their own experiences during childhood (Siegel and Hartzell 2014). Many parents can describe experiences of positive and enjoyable childhoods. On the other hand, studies have identified how many adults have experienced adversity in childhood (Hughes et al. 2017). Research into the harmful effects of adverse childhood experiences (ACEs), such as child maltreatment or exposure to parental mental illness or domestic violence, indicates an increased risk of long-term negative effects on health and wellbeing. This can range from physical health conditions, cancer, obesity, heart disease, to mental ill health conditions, problematic alcohol and drug use, interpersonal and self-directed violence (Hughes et al. 2017). Repeated exposure to ACEs during childhood can result in increased risk of disruptions in parental capacity to protect their child from risk of harm and to nurture their development and wellbeing. Where a parent's own childhood trauma remains unresolved they may likely find it difficult to reflect on their relationships with their own children (Gold 2017). Their capacity to mentalise, that is, to think about their own feelings and the feelings of their child, may be disrupted and negatively impact on the development of a positive parent–child relationship (Fonagy et al. 1991). Early childhood experiences do not, however, always determine fate. Where parents have had a difficult childhood, they may not necessarily recreate the same negative interactions with their own children. Where parents come to understand and make sense of their own experiences it can help them to build a positive enjoyable relationship with their own children; however, without such understanding history may likely repeat itself as negative interactions are passed down through the generations (Siegel and Hartzell 2014).

The Department of Education (2013) have explored how ACEs can compromise parenting practices in accordance with the key dimensions of parenting capacity outlined in the Common Assessment Framework (Department of Health 2000); these have been explored in Table 6.2.

Negative parenting behaviours associated with ACEs, as described in Table 6.2, can have a detrimental influence on the development of a secure attachment between the child and parent. This will compromise the development of a child's confidence to interact and understand the world around them, including an inability to form healthy social relationships and respond and overcome stress and adversity in their future life situations (Hardcastle & Bellis 2019). The causes of these parental difficulties can be complex and have social and environmental influences, which may include socio-economic deprivation, social isolation or previous exposure to ACEs in childhood creating a generational cycle of adversity. Those working with families have a professional responsibility to assess potential social and environmental challenges and identify the individual parenting behaviours that may put a child at risk of poor outcomes. Supportive interventions can then be implemented to strengthen parenting capacity to protect future child health and developmental outcomes. This will be explored further within Chapter 16 Safeguarding Children and Young People.

Working closely with families and developing trusting relationships where parents feel safe to discuss their experiences of being parented offers a crucial opportunity for practitioners to understand parenting behaviours and support parents through a non-judgemental strengths-based approach.

Fathers' influence on child development

Fathers who are responsive to their infant's needs and seek to provide a caring environment that fosters opportunities for learning can provide unique and nurturing experiences that build a firm foundation for long-term positive outcomes (Fatherhood Institute 2010). This includes the promotion of a child's emotional and social wellbeing and cognitive capabilities in preparation for school. It is important to highlight the paternal role of the father and the diversity this parenting role has on child development. The unique

Table 6.2 Dimensions of parenting capacity and parenting behaviours associated with ACEs

Dimensions of Parenting Capacity	Examples	Parenting behaviours associated with ACEs – Substance Misuse, Mental Illness or Domestic Violence
Basic Care	Providing for the child's physical needs, medical and dental care, provision of food, drink, shelter, clean and appropriate clothing and adequate personal hygiene.	• Parents may have difficulties perceiving and prioritising their children's basic care needs over their own. • Parents may prioritise the need to purchase substances over purchasing essential resources to meet their child's needs, including food, clothing and basic home necessities.
Ensuring Safety	Protection from harm or danger, from unsafe adults or self-harm. Protection from danger in the home and elsewhere.	• Parents may have difficulties managing their emotions and their perceptions may be distorted creating an inability to perceive potential dangers and inadvertently expose their children to unsafe environments. • This could include exposure to drug taking paraphernalia or exposure to unsafe adults. • Exposure to domestic violence poses significant physical risk to children and a fear for their own safety.
Emotional Warmth	Providing emotional warmth, love and affection, promoting a sense of self and being valued, a positive sense of racial and cultural identity.	• Parents can experience excessive stress which causes them to become emotionally unavailable with an inability to be warm and responsive to their child's needs. • Parents are more likely to use harsh or coercive behaviour management styles. • This hinders the development of a secure attachment and facilitation of an authoritative parenting style.
Stimulation	Promoting the child's learning and intellectual development through interaction, communication, talking and responding to the child's language and questions, encouraging and joining the child's play and promoting educational opportunities.	• These stressful circumstances can cause parents to have a low self-esteem and depressive symptoms. This can compromise their self-efficacy to provide a stimulating environment and interact with their child in an educationally stimulating way.
Guidance and Boundaries	Enabling the child to regulate their emotions and behaviour, which involves setting boundaries, so that the child is able to develop an internal model of moral values and conscience.	• Parents exposure to ACEs is correlated with inconsistent and unpredictable parenting behaviours. This can include harsh or coercive discipline, inappropriate boundaries and inconsistent guidance and supervision. • These difficulties are heightened if a parent's perceptions are distorted due to the influence of substance misuse.

(Continued)

Table 6.2 (Continued)

Dimensions of Parenting Capacity	Examples	Parenting behaviours associated with ACEs – Substance Misuse, Mental Illness or Domestic Violence
Stability	Providing an environment to enable a child to develop a secure attachment to the primary caregiver(s).	• These potential risks and compromised parenting capacity can create an unpredictable and unstable environment for a child and influence their sense of stability. • A child will lack confidence that their needs will be met within a warm and responsive environment due to inconsistent parenting behaviours. • Frequent address changes may be necessary to manage home circumstances and risk factors which creates further instability. (Department of Education 2000, 2013)

contribution from fathers differs to a mother's contribution (Rollè et al. 2019), and this is strongly correlated to how fathers communicate with their children and encourage them to manipulate and interact with their environment (Russell 2012).

Fathers appear to donate a considerable quantity of their paternal involvement to facilitating play activities with their children and develop the father–child relationship through the facilitation of these activities (Asmussen and Weizel 2010). Playtime often incorporates physical, dynamic pursuits that help to build a child's autonomy and curiosity to investigate their environment (Rollè et al. 2019). This curiosity is enhanced because fathers provide play situations that are often unpredictable and give children the opportunity to exercise their independence, allowing freedom for explorations and the development of problem-solving capabilities (Hogg 2014). This is often referred to as 'rough and tumble play', which provides essential challenges for children through the facilitation of tasks that encourage risk-taking and the achievement of goals (e.g. climbing, piggy-back/shoulder rides, play fighting). These challenging experiences empower children to develop the ability to regulate their emotions and control negative feelings or impulses, which is fundamental in learning the ability to communicate in a socially acceptable manner in the future (Rosenberg and Bradford-Wilcox 2006), equipping them with the skills to develop positive future social relationships with their peers which will promote optimum emotional and social wellbeing (Flanders et al. 2009).

Fathers have been complemented to possess a strong commitment to promote and encourage their child's achievements, whereas research suggests mothers are more committed to protect and nurture (Rosenberg and Bradford-Wilcox 2006). Stevenson and Crnic (2013) suggest fathers are more demanding and less sensitive when interacting with their child, which promotes speech and language skills and confidence in social communication. Although both parents positively contribute to their child's literacy and language development through the facilitation of reading activities, mothers are more likely to communicate through emotions and fathers are reported to use more abstract and exploratory language which enhances a child's conceptualisation of knowledge (Fatherhood Institute 2014a). Overall, fathers' involvement can support and promote child development by adding diversity to the learning environment.

Healthy child development can be influenced by a positive father–child relationship, where fathers are able to take an active role and are highly involved in their child's development. A structured definition of parental involvement was developed by Lamb et al. (1987), known as the Three Part Model of Paternal Involvement. It describes how fathers become highly involved and categorises a father's involvement into three dimensions:

Engagement: The direct contact a father has with his child, engaging in mutual activities. This can include reading, playing or physical care.

Availability: The time a father donates to the child to create opportunities for engagement.

Responsibility: Providing the necessary resources that are required to fulfil the child's developmental needs, including the responsibility to make choices regarding the child's care and wellbeing.

The relationship between both parents has a direct effect on the three dimensions of a father's involvement as highlighted above. A positive parental relationship is important to the overall effectiveness of a father's involvement and will collectively motivate both parenting behaviours (Rosenberg and Bradford-Wilcox 2006). For example, if fathers experience affection and support from the parental relationship they may likely feel valued within the family network, and this can encourage more sensitive and responsive interactions (Coleman and Garfield 2004). The Fatherhood Institute (2014b) suggest that involved fathers can be highly influential in supporting infant feeding choices following birth and advocating healthy maternal lifestyle choices in pregnancy such as alcohol and smoking cessation. They also suggest that increased father involvement in parenting is correlated with reduced parental stress and offers a protective barrier against maternal postnatal depression.

Certain circumstances such as parental separation or care orders may mean that fathers cannot always be involved in raising their children, but where they can be involved unique barriers exist that can impact on the level of involvement fathers have in family life and childcare activities, as described in Table 6.3.

Legislative paternal leave entitlement varies across the globe with many countries treating fathers differently to mothers in this respect. Where equal choice is offered this can promote fathers' involvement, supporting and enabling the paternal bond. The provision of flexible working arrangements also helps to accommodate work–life balance commitments, especially in the current economic climate whereby caring responsibilities may need to be shared when both parents are in employment. Those working with families should champion the role of both parents within health and social care provision. If both parents are aware of the valuable impact a loving father can have on their child's development, it may empower mothers to support the involvement of fathers, enabling

Table 6.3 Barriers to father involvement

Barrier	Description
Gender Roles	Traditional gender stereotypes have created inequality between the parenting roles of both mother and father. Traditionally fathers have taken on the role of provider or breadwinner, whilst mothers have dominated the responsibility of running the family home and caring for the children (Hauari and Hollingworth 2009).
Employment	Employment can restrict the time a father has available for his involvement in child-nurturing activities (Russell 2012).
Maternal Gatekeeping	Mothers can have a strong influential power over a father's participation in his child's care. This maternal force is recognised as 'Maternal Gatekeeping', it is described as a mother's action or behaviour that directly or indirectly reduces the father's ability to actively contribute to the family and its functioning, arbitrating the roles a father can pursue within the home. This can impact on the quality of the father-child relationship as it limits the time and activities shared between the father and child (Hauari and Hollingworth 2009).
Gendered Services	Parent is often misinterpreted to signify 'Mother'. Fathers can therefore misinterpret the value and importance of their role and feel excluded from services offering parenting support (Morgan et al. 2009).

them to appreciate that their children will benefit from both parents' contribution to their care (Hauari and Hollingworth 2009). It may also motivate fathers to challenge their potential gender stereotypes and empower their overall involvement.

Same-sex parenting

Contemporary family dynamics in the 21st century are diverse and includes co-parenting in same-sex relationships. In these circumstances same-sex parents are more likely to adopt children or require the use of reproductive support (Gates 2015). The planning and emotional challenges these routes to parenthood may bring has been identified to positively influence the parental motivation to provide a warm and nurturing environment for a child (Tasker 2010). Same-sex couples are also viewed to have a potential advantage as Short et al. (2007, p.9) believes they are not guided by gender role stereotypes and *'organise family life and caring for children far more equitably than heterosexual couples do'*. This could promote less parental conflict and stress, empowering parental responsiveness and further supporting the emotional and behavioural development of children. Ultimately, within any family life setting the important ingredient, irrespective of parental gender composition, is the stability, warmth and stimulating environment the parental relationship provides that will have the most impact on a child's development (Bos et al. 2016). As with all families, the quality of parenting and the responsive environment facilitated is also influenced by both social and environmental systems as depicted in Bronfenbrenner's (1974) model, as this chapter and chapter 5 briefly explores. It is important to be aware also that same-sex parents may have experienced prejudice and discrimination in relation to their sexual orientation, so may fear how their family will be accepted within society and this may influence how they access or integrate with parenting support services and practitioners. It is fundamental that practitioners working with parents and families are sensitive to these unique needs and facilitate the social integration of differing family dynamics within health and social care provision. This is further explored within Chapter 22.

The impact of COVID-19 on parent–child relationships

The COVID-19 pandemic and lockdown restrictions have had a detrimental effect on the parenting journey due to isolation from loved ones and lack of support from face-to-face early years services. At the time of writing this chapter it has been a year since the first lockdown restrictions were enforced across the UK. Research exploring the implications of lockdown on child development and parent–infant relationships is only now beginning to emerge, indicating severe and long-lasting negative consequences. This was evident in a recent UK-wide report detailing findings from a survey seeking parental views of pregnancy, birth and life at home with a new baby during this unique time. Nearly 5,500 parents responded to the survey revealing wide regional variation and inequalities between different communities. The full data-set and analysis will be made public in August 2021, however, from the report early indications revealed 25% of parents reported concern about their relationship with their baby and 35% wanted help with this, 26% reported their baby crying more than usual and 68% felt the changes brought about by COVID-19 were affecting their unborn baby, baby or young child (Saunders and Hogg 2020). During this time Ofsted reported an increase in serious incidents involving babies, over one-fifth more than in the same period the previous year, before the pandemic, resulting in eight deaths that could have been avoided or mitigated through the delivery of adequate supportive early years services (Spielman 2020).

Conclusion

This chapter has discussed the influence of early relationships and parenting on child development and wellbeing. The building blocks for healthy child development are established in the early years and are dependent on positive responsive caregiving that nurtures secure relationships and provides the social and emotional foundations required to enable and support optimum child development and positive long-term outcomes. Gaining an understanding of complex factors and wider influences that can affect parenting capacity to form positive relationships and nurture infant and child development is important for those working with children and families. This should include ACE awareness, recognition of diverse family dynamics, the influence of differing parental roles and the potential challenges parents encounter within their parenting journey.

CONSIDER THE FOLLOWING QUESTIONS

1. How does the development of secure attachment and bonding support child development?
2. What social and environmental systems influence parenting capacity?
3. What is authoritative parenting and how does this style of parenting affect child development?

Key terms

Adverse Childhood Experiences (ACEs): Stressful, traumatic experiences occurring in childhood such as being a victim of abuse or neglect (physical, sexual, emotional, psychological), witnessing domestic violence, parental ill mental health, abandonment through parental separation or divorce, growing up in a household where adults are experiencing alcohol or drug use problems, or a member of the household is incarcerated.

Attachment: The enduring connection between the infant and the primary care giver that develops through a tendency of the infant to naturally seek and maintain closeness particularly during stressful situations.

Bonding: The primary caregiver's relationship with their new infant where they come to know, love and accept their new baby.

COVID-19: An infectious disease caused by a newly discovered coronavirus.

Parenting capacity: The parents' ability to appropriately protect their child from the risk of harm and to nurture their physical, social, emotional and educational developmental needs.

Further reading

Centre on the Developing Child. Available at: https://developingchild.harvard.edu/ [Accessed 12.03.2022].

Parent–Infant Foundation. Available at: https://parentinfantfoundation.org.uk/ [Accessed 12.03.2022].

Zero to Three. Available at: www.zerotothree.org/ [Accessed 12.03.2022].

References

Ainsworth, M. S., Blehar, M. C., Waters, E., Wall, S. N. 1978. *Patterns of Attachment: A Psychological Study of the Strange Situation.* Erlbaum: Hillsdale, NJ.

Asmussen, K., Weizel, K. 2010. *Evaluating the Evidence: Fathers, Families and Children.* National Academy for Parenting Practitioners: London.

Baumrind, D. 1967. Child care practices anteceding three patterns of preschool behavior. *Genetic Psychology Monographs;* 75(1), 43–88.

Bos, H. W., Knox, J., Rijn-van-Gelderen, L., Gartrell, N. K. 2016. Same-sex and different-sex parent households and child health outcomes: findings from the National Survey of Children's Health. *Journal of Developmental and Behavioural Paediatrics*; 37(3), 179–187.

Bowlby, J. 1979. *The Making and Breaking of Affectional Bonds*. Tavistock: London.

Bowlby, J. 1988. *A Secure Base*. Routledge: New York.

Bronfenbrenner, U. 1974. Developmental research, public policy, and the ecology of childhood. *Child Development*; 45, 1–5.

Carson, D., Chowdhury, A., Perry, C. K., Pati, C. 1999. Family characteristics and adolescent competence in India: investigation of youth in southern Orissa. *Journal of Youth and Adolescence*; 28, 211–233.

Center on the Developing Child. 2007. *The Science of Early Childhood Development* (InBrief). Available at: https://developingchild.harvard.edu/resources/inbrief-science-of-ecd/ [Accessed 10.01.2021].

Chao, R. K. 1994. Beyond parental control and authoritarian parenting style: understanding Chinese parenting through the cultural notion of training. *Child Development*; 65, 1111–1119.

Coleman, W. L., Garfield, C. 2004. Fathers and paediatricians: enhancing men's roles in the care and development of their children. *Pediatrics*; 113(5), 1406–1411.

Department of Education. 2013. *Assessing Parental Capacity to Change When Children Are On the Edge of Care: An Overview of Current Research Evidence*. Available at: https://assets.publishing.service.gov.uk/government/uploads/system/uploads/attachment_data/file/330332/RR369_Assessing_parental_capacity_to_change_Final.pdf [Accessed 15.02.2021].

Department of Health. 2000. *The Framework for the Assessment of Children in Need and their Families*. The Stationery Office: London.

Department of Health. 2009. *Healthy Child Programme: Pregnancy and the First Five years of Life*. Available at: www.gov.uk/government/publications/healthy-child-programme-pregnancy-and-the-first-5-years-of-life [Accessed 12.01.2021].

Department of Health, Social Services and Public Safety. 2010. *Healthy Child, Healthy Future. A Framework for the Universal Child Health Promotion Programme in Northern Ireland. Pregnancy to 19 years*. Available at: www.health-ni.gov.uk/publications/healthy-child-healthy-future [Accessed 13.02.2021].

Fatherhood Institute. 2010. *FI Research Summary: Father's Impact on their Child's Learning & Achievement*. Fatherhood Institute: Marlborough.

Fatherhood Institute. 2014a. *FI Research Summary: Fathers' Impact on Young Children's Language and Literacy*. Fatherhood Institute: Marlborough.

Fatherhood Institute. 2014b. *FI Research Summary: Supportive Fathers – Healthy Mothers*. Fatherhood Institute: Malborough.

Flanders, J. L., Leo, V., Paquette, D., O'Pihl, R., Séguin, J. R. 2009. Rough-and-tumble play and the regulation of aggression: an observational study of father–child play dyads. *Aggressive Behavior*; 35, 285–295.

Fonagy, P., Steele, M., Steele, H., Moran, G. S., Higgitt, A. C. 1991. The capacity for understanding mental states: the reflective self in parent and child and its significance for security of attachment. *Infant Mental Health Journal*; 12, 201–218.

Gates, G. 2015. Marriage and family: LGBT individuals and same-sex couples. *The Future of Children*; 25(2), 67–87. Available at: www.jstor.org/stable/43581973 [Accessed 08.01.2021].

Gold, C. M. 2017. *The Developmental Science of Early Childhood. Clinical Applications of Infant Mental Health Concepts from Infancy Through Adolescence*. W. W. Norton: New York.

Hardcastle, K., Bellis, M. A. 2019. *Asking about ACEs in Health Visiting*. Public Health Wales NHS Trust: Wrexham.

Hauari, H., Hollingworth, K. 2009. *Understanding Fathering, Masculinity, Diversity and Change*. Joseph Rowntree Foundation: York.

Hogg, S. 2014. *NSPCC: All Babies Count: The Dad Project*. NSPCC: London.

Hughes, K., Bellis, M. A., Hardcastle, K. A., et al. 2017. The effects of multiple adverse childhood experiences on health: a systematic review and meta-analysis. *Lancet Public Health*; 2(8), e356–e366.

Lamb, M. E., Pleck, J. H., Charnov, E. L., Levine, J. A. 1987. A biosocial perspective on paternal behavior and involvement. In J. Lancaster (Ed.), *Parenting Across the Life Span: Biosocial Dimensions* (pp. 111–142). Aldine Publishing: New York.

Maccoby E., Martin J. 1983. Socialization in the context of the family: parent–child interaction. In P. H. Mussen (Ed.), *Handbook of Child Psychology*. Wiley: New York.

Martínez, I., García, J. F., Yubero, S. 2007. Parenting styles and adolescents' self-esteem in Brazil. *Psychol. Rep.*; 100(3 Pt 1), 731–745.

Mayseless, O., Scharf, M., Sholt, M. 2003. From authoritative parenting practices to an authoritarian context: exploring the person-environment fit. *Journal of Research on Adolescence*, 17, 23–50.

National Scientific Council on the Developing Child 2004. *Young children develop in an environment of relationships: Working Paper No. 1*. Available at: https://developingchild.harvard.edu/resources/wp1/ [Accessed 20.01.2021].

National Society for the Protection of Cruelty to Children. 2015. *Serious Case Reviews. Case Reviews Published in 2015*. Available at: www.nspcc.org.uk/preventing-abuse/child-protection-system/case-reviews/2015/ [Accessed 19.02.2021].

Power, T. 2013. Parenting dimensions and styles: a brief history and recommendation for future research. *Child Obesity*; 9(1), 14–21.

Public Health Scotland. 2015. *Child Health Programme – Pre-school*. Available at: https://beta.isdscotland.org/topics/child-health/child-health-programme/child-health-systems-programme-pre-school/ [Accessed 10.02.2021].

Rollè, L., Gullotta, G., Trombetta, T., et al. 2019. Father involvement and cognitive development in early and middle childhood: a systematic review. *Front. Psychol.*; 10, 2405. doi: 10.3389/fpsyg.2019.02405

Rosenberg, J., Bradford-Wilcox, W. 2006. *The Importance of Fathers in Healthy Development of Children.* National Clearing on Child Abuse & Neglect Information. Washington, DC.

Russell, B. 2012. *Step by Step: Engaging Fathers in Programs for Families.* Best Start Resource Centre/Health Nexus: Toronto.

Saunders, B., Hogg, S. 2020. *Babies in Lockdown. Listening to Parents to Build Back Better.* Available at: https://babiesinlockdown.info/download-our-report/ [Accessed 10.03.2021].

Short, E., Riggs, D. W., Perlesz, A., Brown, R., Kane, G. 2007. *Lesbian, Gay, Bisexual and Transgender (LGBT) Parented Families.* The Australian Psychological Society: Melbourne.

Siegel, D. J., Hartzell, M. 2014. *Parenting from the Inside Out: How a Deeper Self-understanding Can Help You Raise Children Who Thrive.* Scribe Publications: London.

Spielman, A. 2020. *Speech at the Online National Children and Adult Services Conference.* Available at: www.gov.uk/government/speeches/amanda-spielman-at-ncasc-2020 [Accessed 24.02.2021].

Stevenson, M., Crnic, K. 2013. Intrusive fathering, children's self-regulation and social skills. A mediation analysis. *Journal of Intellectual Disability Research*; 57(6), 500–512.

Tasker, F. 2010. Same-sex parenting and child development: reviewing the contribution of parental gender. *Journal of Marriage and Family*; 72(1), 35–40.

The Child Poverty Act. 2010. Available at www.legislation.gov.uk/ukpga/2010/9/contents [Accessed 28.03.2021].

The Children Act. 1989. Available at: www.legislation.gov.uk/ukpga/1989/41/contents [Accessed 28.03.2021].

The Children Act. 2004. Available at: www.legislation.gov.uk/ukpga/2004/31/contents [Accessed 28.03.2021].

United Nations. 1989. *United Nations Convention on the Rights of a Child.* The Office of United Nations High Commissioner for Human Rights: Geneva.

Welsh Government. 2016. *An Overview of the Healthy Child Wales Programme.* Available at: https://gov.wales/healthy-child-wales-programme-0 [Accessed 20.12.2020].

Winnicott, D. 1953. Transitional objects and transitional phenomena. *International Journal of Psychoanalysis*; 34, 89–97.

7

PERINATAL MENTAL HEALTH

JANE HANLEY

LEARNING OUTCOMES

By the end of this chapter you will be able to:

- Understand the importance of good perinatal mental health.
- Be aware of the signs and symptoms of perinatal mental health and illness.
- Understand the impact on the family.
- Gain knowledge of the assessment process.
- Understand the different management options.

Introduction

The term 'perinatal mental health' is well established and is defined as the period from conception until two years following the birth. It was, however, only introduced into common usage during the 2000s. Prior to that, 'postnatal depression' was the more popular label for the mother who suffered from mood disorders following childbirth. There were vague references to puerperal psychosis, but as psychosis was a rare event, midwives were more likely to be in contact with mothers who experienced it, and the condition was only occasionally encountered by health visitors. Bipolar disorder was hardly mentioned, and any other stress-related disorders or illnesses were consigned to institutions and asylums.

Often, the depressed mother consulted her General Practitioner (GP) because she felt tired. However, her 'sick note' had *backpain* written on it as the excuse for her not to return to work following the birth of her infant. In some instances, this malady lasted for over a year. In truth, it was shameful to admit to feeling anxious or depressed, for to do so would make the mother a bad person and question the reasoning for her depression when she had a beautiful baby and loving husband. That was, and still is in some cases, the attitude of the society in which she lived.

In reality, a sea change occurred throughout the globe when individuals decided that something had to be done to ensure that postnatal depression was understood to be an illness to be taken seriously and not denied by mothers. A combination of factors highlighted its importance: the scientific exploration for mothers' distress, the indignancy of the inequality of health services for depressed mothers, the insight that perinatal mental illness was real, and the acknowledgement of the significant impact on infants, fathers and families.

The expression 'perinatal mental health', has been expanded and covers from conception to one year following the birth of the infant. It encapsulates a wide range of conditions, some of which will be discussed. There are various accounts of the number of women who might be affected, and this ranges from one in ten in the UK (Shorey et al. 2018), one in seven in the USA (Wisner et al. 2013) to 20% of new mothers in developing countries (WHO 2020). These numbers pose a significant public health problem, compared with perhaps the 16% of mothers who develop gestational diabetes (Diabetes UK 2020). It has also been accepted that relationships between couples can be fraught and that fathers too can be affected by and suffer from anxiety and depression. From that perspective, rather than refer to 'mothers', the term 'parents' is used throughout this chapter.

No one really knows why high anxiety levels and depressive mood states occur and why some are or not affected by adverse life events. It is not uncommon for mothers to feel elements of anxiety or mild depressive symptoms during and after their pregnancy, and with support and understanding these symptoms can be allayed. If they are not, and risk factors are present, then it is possible that the signs and symptoms may intensify and the mother's anxious state or low mood may increase. However, identifying these risk factors can play a significant role to enable the practitioner to understand when difficulties are more likely to occur.

Risk factors

Risk factors during pregnancy are not always evident; however, it is within the remit of practitioners to determine them. There are several obvious risk factors, which include poverty and poor social support, but others may be less clear and therefore need to be elucidated by sensitive enquiry. There is value in obtaining a family history, particularly in the light of transgenerational mental health and illness (Gutierrez-Galve et al. 2019).

Those mothers with complex social needs are less likely to access and maintain contact with perinatal mental health services (NICE 2016). The exposure to violence, which might be domestic, sexual, gender or race-based, can cause persistent anxiety, from which there may be little respite for the pregnant mother. There is evidence to suggest a depressed father sometimes has a less positive attitude towards both the pregnancy and the infant (Noergaard et al. 2017). Parents who have been subjected to extreme environmental conditions can be isolated from their normal social support systems which, in turn, can exacerbate their symptoms of anxiety and/or depression. Societal changes have radically altered the role of parents; more women are working well into their pregnancies and returning to work shortly after the infant is born. High stress levels within the workplace are not conducive to a stress-free pregnancy, whilst a change of working patterns might ameliorate this.

The importance of social connections is well established, yet for some, parenthood can be an isolating experience. It has been suggested that approximately one in five fathers appear to lose contact with close friends, thus missing out on the vital protective support which acts as a buffer during this key transition stage of their life. The diverse changes in the family structure now include single fathers who may have sole care of the infant, with little or no support from the mother. Stay-at-home fathers can suffer the same loneliness or social isolation as the new mother, and their mental health is equally liable to be affected (Caperton et al. 2019). Whilst there are same gender parents, the research on their mental health is sparse; however, one study found that stable and happy same gender relationships can promote psychological wellbeing (Whitton and Kuryluk 2014).

As the UK becomes increasingly multicultural, there needs to be considerations around diversity and equality. Mothers whose native language is not English, who have sought refuge fleeing from conflict, persecution or war, have some of the risk factors for anxiety and depressive states. The use of translators may not always be feasible, therefore the practitioner should seek the communicative skills and knowledge of local spiritual and health leaders to develop the rapport necessary to gain the mother's confidence and, in, turn understand their background history and cultural identity.

Stress, particularly during the antenatal period, is taken seriously. Epigenetics explain how environmental influences affect the expressions of genes. The mother's mental health, particularly having anxiety during pregnancy, can exert specific effects on the developing foetus through neurobiological foetal programming. This may have a long-term effect on the infant's development and health. Infants whose mothers were stressed during their pregnancy are more likely to be anxious themselves and are at greater risk of poor development and behavioural disorders (Talge et al. 2007).

Presentation of anxiety disorders during the perinatal period

It is important to understand that anxiety disorder is a strong predictor of postnatal depression at all points of time after delivery (Nakić Radoš et al. 2018) and should not be dismissed as a transient mood state. Some of the symptoms may be obscure and when divided into physical, emotional and behavioural signs it is often the behaviours that provide a clearer indication of the parent's mood state.

Physical signs and symptoms

It is sometimes difficult to determine what is a physical or emotional consequence of pregnancy, and the postnatal period has some organic causes. For example, the headaches, sweating and nausea could be a result of eclampsia, or the sensations of the palpitations and shortness of breath triggered by a pulmonary embolism, yet these are some of the symptoms that can be an indication of anxiety. Other symptoms of anxiety include restlessness, aches and pains, dizziness and dry mouth.

These may remain largely unnoticed unless the practitioner questions the parent about how they are feeling.

Emotional signs and symptoms

These may be easier to determine, particularly if the parent has expressed feelings of anxiousness, with their mind racing, worrying unnecessarily, complaining of decreased concentration and confusion, thus making it difficult to make decisions. Their sleep may be disrupted, not because of the needs of the infant but because they are unable to relax. Statements of anxiety and concern may be in relation to the infant, with excessive questions about feeding regimes, exaggeration or perceived problems with the infant's physical ailments and the need for constant reassurance. However, for a parent to admit to this takes significant trust, which may not have fully developed between the parent and the practitioner. Therefore, there is value in administering an assessment tool which can help the practitioner to determine how and what the parent is experiencing.

Behavioural signs and symptoms

There may be a crossover between the way the parents behave and the emotions which are driving this. In the more extreme cases the parent may make excuses not to attend clinics or become over anxious about home visits. There may be a tendency to be more fussy than relaxed, but at the same time appearing exhausted with the intensity of their actions. They may ruminate excessively over what they perceive as problems, and feel impotent at the fact that they are unable to control situations.

Obsessive compulsive disorder (OCD) is one manifestation of stress and can be evidenced by compulsive behaviours of avoidance, which are in response to intrusive, irrational negative thoughts. In such instances, the parent may feel the need to perform ritualistic behaviours to avoid situations which could create further anxiety. The actions are often compelling and the severity of the illness can seriously interfere with daily life.

The astute practitioner will question the reasons for the parent's unease and with subtle enquiry may prompt the parent to confess the actual reasons for their distress, and be able to focus on solutions. If these concerns are not addressed, then it is likely that the severe anxiety will develop or co-exist with depression and may result in future safeguarding issues.

Presentation of depressive disorders during the perinatal period

A depressive disorder can occur at any time during the perinatal period and is a debilitating illness. It has been defined in three parts: mild, moderate, severe.

However, it can be difficult to differentiate between the mood states. What are the distinct differences between mild and moderate? In reality, it is the intensity of the presentation and duration of the symptoms. There is no clinical diagnosis for perinatal depression but instead the diagnostic criterium is for 'depression'. There must be five or more symptoms during the same two-week period and at least one of the symptoms should be either depressed mood or loss of interest or pleasure (APA 2013).

Science has provided significant weight to the fact that depression is not a lifestyle choice or sign of weakness, but a neurological condition whereby alterations within the activities of the brain structure influences its functions and has implications for the origins of depressive disorders (El-Sayed et al. 2012).

Physical signs and symptoms

As with signs and symptoms of anxiety, there will be a cross-over in the signs of depression. There tends to be a lack of energy, with tasks appearing to take longer than usual to perform. This loss of drive can cause a slowing down of all motor functions, in particular movement and speech, which may be more sluggish than usual. In the more severe forms of depression, the parent may find it difficult to form sentences, which can cause frustration and irritability. Overall vigour may be absent, and efforts to go to the gym or carry out routine exercises or daily activities become tedious chores. As a result of changes in the dietary habits, there may be changes in bowel movements, with constipation being a common feature. Complaints about vague aches and pains, imagined or real, become almost a preoccupation and can be an excuse to avoid intimate or sexual behaviours. Depressive symptoms often cause changes to the libido, which is either lowered or in some cases lost.

Emotional signs and symptoms

The loss of their previous self and the confusion and anguish this provokes can lead to a myriad of mood states which can escalate or diminish over a period of time. There may be feelings of worthlessness, which can cause guilt and anger. The parent no longer has enjoyment from the activities they once had pleasure in doing. Interest is lost and nega-tive thoughts pervade their mind. This can be overpowering and the parent has little control over the way they feel or would like to feel. Sometimes this can cause resentment and the parent may be cautious about sharing these thoughts with a practitioner.

Behavioural signs and symptoms

An observation of the deterioration of their personal appearances and home environ-ment can provide significant clues about the parents' state of mind. The parent may be distressed and make excuses about themselves, but at the same time feel that they are unable to remedy the way they are. When managing their infant, depressed parents sometimes tend to focus on themselves and their own negative perceptions about their abilities. They are more likely to self-blame if they unable to control or solve a situation involving their infant (Singley and Edwards 2015).

However, it is not always easy to determine if something is wrong simply by paying attention to the parent's appearance, as sometimes the parent is well aware of the timing of the practitioner's visit or the impact their visit to the practitioner may make on any judgements about them or their home. The myth about the practitioner taking the infant into care if the mother is depressed still perpetuates. Each parent may collude with the other to ensure there are few clues that either is not coping.

Another symptom is the parent's manner: they can show apathy and indifference to either the pregnancy in the antenatal period, or towards the infant postpartum. There may be signs of their inability to concentrate or to be preoccupied with minor inci-dents. Conversely, the parent may be so frustrated and overwhelmed that they may both look and feel sad. They may be unable to control their emotions and either implode or explode, by shouting, crying or becoming exasperated with themselves and/or the infant (Edhborg et al. 2005).

Sleep patterns, unrelated to the pregnancy or the infant, may be disrupted. There may be periods when it is difficult to fall asleep at night or get out of bed in the morning, often with diurnal variations of rest. This behaviour may be evidenced by the parent looking and admitting to feeling tired all the time and being unable to rest, despite no external interruptions (Hanley and Williams 2019).

Equally, appetite may be affected, with either an over- or under-consumption of food during mealtimes. Normal eating patterns may be substituted with erratic dietary habits or by consuming very little. This might be observed by the lack of weight gain in the pregnant mother, or the mother quickly loses her 'baby weight' postpartum. Questions about the types and timings of food intake can clarify the parent's attitude to food and why their behaviour towards it has changed.

However, it is crucial to note that the impact of a new infant on their lifestyle has to be taken into account, and no rash conclusions should be made without careful consideration.

In some cases, the parent may feel so overwhelmed by their feelings of hopelessness and helplessness that they contemplate suicide (Sit et al. 2015). They may be unable to reconcile their overall feelings of despair and exhaustion and crave release from their situation. They may feel they are a bad parent and that their infant and partner would have a better life without them. It is not uncommon for a parent to act on these thoughts and feelings. Therefore, it is imperative that any signs or suggestions of suicide intent are taken seriously and the parent is referred for immediate medical help. In the UK, calling the emergency services should be the first reaction and then remaining with the parent until help is available.

Puerperal psychosis

Puerperal psychosis is a severe mental illness and is an emergency situation. It usually occurs a few days following childbirth. Paternal psychosis is very rare, with very few reported cases (Shahani 2012). One or two in a thousand new mothers may require hospital admission to a Mother and Baby Unit following an episode of puerperal psychosis or a recurrent affective psychosis disorder. It is more common in the first-time mother with the added risk that about one-quarter of mothers will suffer from a reoccurrence in subsequent pregnancies. Postpartum psychosis is considered to be on the bipolar spectrum and a history of depression and/or anxiety is a strong risk factor. Women with bipolar disorder, where their mood can significantly fluctuate between manic and depressive states, are therefore at increased risk of postpartum psychosis (Lewis et al. 2018).

If untreated, it is possible psychosis will last for more than 6 to 8 months, but with early intervention the mother may feel completely well within 1 to 3 months. The evidence suggests that the triggers for the condition are pregnancy related, which makes vulnerable women more susceptible to episodes that may occur during the third trimester of the pregnancy. However, the most powerful determinant appears to be during the first 10 days following delivery (Boyce and Barriball 2010).

The first indication that the mother is unwell is bizarre behaviour; however, this may not always be the case and the odd way in which the mother behaves can be associated with the normality of childbirth, therefore is sometimes overlooked.

In puerperal psychosis, florid, nihilistic, bizarre delusions are often present. A common example is that the mother truly believes her baby is not her own and she has no idea to whom the infant belongs. This causes her great distress and anxiety. The more eccentric and pervading the belief, the more the mother is likely to respond. Her anguish causes her irrational behaviour and she may rapidly become a danger to herself and her infant.

Hallucinations can affect all of her senses; auditory hallucination may cause her to hear incoherent, distorted, sometimes aggressive voices at unpredictable times, confusing the mother about what is real and what is not. Often the voices are accompanied by vivid, violent visions, smells and touch, which confirm the mother's perception of herself and feels that her internal world is more real than the external world. The mother is profoundly ill and disabled by her illness, therefore she needs to be managed by a specialist team and treated with antipsychotic drugs.

Assessment

It has long been argued that the Edinburgh Postnatal Depression Scale (EPDS) is one of the more useful assessment tools to use in the postnatal period. It has also been validated for use in the antenatal period and with fathers (Cox et al. 1987, Massoudi et al. 2013). However, there remains reticence to use it, and many policies include its use only after negative answers to the three brief and focused Whooley et al. (1997) questions that address both the mood and interest of the parent. There is a case for assessing all parents in the perinatal period, which would not only ascertain any hidden histories of mental illnesses or disorders but also normalise the process of asking questions about mental health (Austin 2013). Clinical judgement can determine whether the parent needs any treatment and if so, what the most appropriate route should be.

Management options

There are a number of ways in which perinatal mental health may be managed, and these are discussed below.

Listening visits

The answers given on the EPDS can act as a precursor to the Listening Visit which is a skilled therapeutic intervention that can be implemented by appropriately trained practitioners. It is based on a person-centred approach and is a therapeutic arrangement between the parent and practitioner. The sessions concentrate on the non-directive, non-judgemental attitude of the practitioner with the ability to offer empathetic responses without being prescriptive. The important factors are to allow the parent the space, trust and confidence to be able to talk about their innermost thoughts and feelings and to know that they will be empowered to remedy or rectify situations which will help them to get better (Hanley 2015).

Therapeutic techniques

Other therapies that include problem solving and cognitive behavioural techniques can be introduced to help to resolve issues which may be more challenging. Rather than suggest a solution, the practitioner encourages the parent to identify their needs and generate their own problem and solution on their terms. The 'want' is determined by sieving through what is important or unimportant. The parent is encouraged to think of their own answers and decide which is the more suitable, thereby solving their own problems.

Cognitive behavioural techniques can also help when exploring the parent's negative thoughts. The principle is to examine life situations, problems and difficulties. It explores the reasons for the negative thinking and behaviours, and attempts to alter them to more positive responses. The therapy focuses on the challenging and changing behaviours that limit the parent's ability to function because their thinking is mostly in negative terms. When altered this influences their belief system and ultimately the way they behave.

The use of relaxation techniques can help to destress the parent who may find it difficult to be calm before a therapeutic session. The technique can also help them relax before they sleep or when they are aware that they are becoming anxious. Exercise techniques and regimes also have merit in reducing stress and depression, whilst baby massage classes can provide peer support and a relaxing atmosphere. The successful bonding between the parent and infant can improve both the parent and infant mood states.

Mindfulness

This is becoming increasingly popular as a way of focusing the mind to be aware of the surrounding sensations, what is happening both inside and outside the body. It is easy for thoughts to ruminate and be all consuming. Mindfulness quiets the mind and allows the parent to think of what is happening in the here and now. It includes being aware of the sense of touch, the sense of sounds, with an awareness of both noise and silence and being conscious of the differing smells and odours. Concentrating and being focused on just one object helps to clear any thoughts, and in that moment there is little opportunity to regret the past or worry about the future. The awareness of the present sensations and perceptions allows the mind to filter out more intrusive thoughts and feelings. To perfect this takes practice, and it is sometimes recommended to try the technique for at least 15 minutes per day (Kabat-Zinn 2015). Mindfulness is as effective as antidepressants and can reduce the occurrence of depression by 40–50% compared with other methods of treatment (NICE 2009).

However, some solutions are not always appropriate and the parent may need to be referred on to a specialist perinatal mental health service for further treatment.

Medication for anxiety

The medications of choice for anxiety are either anxiolytics or sedatives. Anxiolytics, or antianxiety drugs such as the benzodiazepines, release gamma aminobutyric acid, which helps the muscles to relax, slows the breathing and has a calming effect. Its actions inhibit the receptors and neurotransmitters and slows down the depressive actions in the brain. It helps to blunt the feelings of anxiety, control the emotions and can aid sleep. However, prolonged use should be avoided because of the possibility of dependence (BNF 2015).

Medication for depression

There may be reticence to take any form of medication but in some instances, particularly the more severe forms of depression, this may be the only recourse to ensure the parent's mental state improves. However, often a combination of medication and a therapeutic intervention can have positive results. What has to be weighed is the length of time it takes for both types of treatment to be effective. Talking therapies often take up to four weeks to be effective, and so does medication; however, whereas the prescription can be picked up from the chemist almost straight away, the talking therapy might take weeks to arrange. With this in mind, some parents would prefer the former, whereas if the Listening Visits were tailored to an immediate response, then the waiting times would be negligible.

It is important that the practitioner has some knowledge of the type of medication that may be prescribed, the possible side effects and the efficacy of the drug. Some will argue that this is the remit of the doctor, yet most practitioners will be familiar with the actions of the medicines that are dispensed during the ward drug round.

There are differing effects of the variety of antidepressants, with some being more effective and better tolerated than others. Escitalopram and Sertraline enhance the levels of the neurotransmitter serotonin, whilst other drugs, mirtazapine for instance, alters the serotonin and noradrenaline activity. For the best results, some may require a combination or differing types of medication. Prozac, or fluoxetine, is one of the only antidepressants which is significantly more effective at reducing major depression after eight weeks (Halle et al. 2015).

Some parents may be reluctant to take any form of psychopharmaceutical medication because it makes them drowsy and can induce long periods of sleep. This makes it difficult to respond to the 24-hour demands of an infant and has consequences for timing of feeds and so on. Sometimes parents admit to discontinuing the drug because they found the effects difficult to cope with or they were persuaded by relatives to prevent them becoming 'addicted'.

The most commonly used antidepressants are relatively safe for breastfeeding babies. The dose that is received from the milk is generally small and is far less than the known safe doses of the same drug which is given directly to neonates and infants (Hotham and Hotham 2015).

Antidepressants on the whole are usually well tolerated, have fewer side effects and are less likely to be harmful if an overdose is taken. Studies on the efficacy of antidepressants in the treatment of minor depression have found clinically relevant benefits over placebos (Naber and Bullinger 2018). Under half of those treated with a placebo improved compared with over 60% who took an antidepressant. The number of prescribed antidepressants has doubled over the past ten years, making them one of the more popular treatments (Lacobucci 2019).

The possible side effects can include a dry mouth, difficulty in swallowing and sometimes feeling nauseous. There is often an increase in appetite and subsequent weight gain, which can be distressing for mothers in particular who are already attempting to lose their 'baby weight' (Gafoor et al. 2018). The parent can also be predisposed to constipation and problems with micturition. Eye problems usually subside within a few weeks, and fatigue is also common but this usually resolves.

Loss or lack of libido can be challenging as there is a lack of desire for sex, getting aroused, suffering from discomfort or decreased orgasms. For the man it can cause erectile dysfunction. These side effects may be minor, and for the majority once the body adjusts to the medication the normal libido resumes. If it becomes problematic, introducing Sildenafil or Viagra may re-establish a normal sex life.

Within four weeks the medication should start to work, but it is recommended that it is continued for at least nine months from the first signs of improvement in mood. It is sometimes easy to discontinue the treatment once the parent feels better, but if the medication is not taken regularly, then it is likely that the cycle of depression will continue.

Self-help groups and other interventions

There is significant evidence to suggest that support groups, also on social media, are effective in relieving perinatal mental disorders and are also cost efficient. The discussions generated within the safe group situation are felt to be valuable and appreciated. The relationships that form can lead to social interactions to help satisfy the basic need to affiliate with others. If the group programme has educational as well as cognitive behavioural components, this further helps to reduce the parent's depressive mood state. The intervention of human contact appears to have a beneficial effect on most if not all parents.

The importance of the third and voluntary sector should always be considered, as peer support has considerable merit. Support principles are based on values which are designed to help the peer supporters create and deliver a service that is safe, inclusive and meets the needs of parents and their families, but which remains distinct from clinical services (MMHA 2019). The basic premise is that all the support services offer help to parents and a time when the impact of poor mental health can be greater than at any other time, particularly if left untreated.

Conclusion

As we enter an enlightened and engaging age of promoting perinatal mental health, it is essential that practitioners take the opportunity to develop services that recognise the importance of parent–baby relationships and relationships within the wider family (NICE 2018). The promotion of a healthy lifestyles for both parents encourages a healthy pregnancy and relationship, which in turn creates a healthy infant. However, early identification and the provision of quality services for any mental health disorder is paramount in order for parents to experience the real joy of being a parent. It is the responsibility of front-line workers to ensure that this happens.

CONSIDER THE FOLLOWING QUESTIONS

1. What are the risk factors for perinatal mental health and illness?
2. What are the possible physical signs of anxiety?
3. What are the possible behavioural signs of depression?
4. What assessment tools are recommended?
5. What is a Listening Visit?

Key terms

Eclampsia: This is a rare but serious condition where high blood pressure results in seizures during pregnancy.
Listening Visit: This is a form of non-directive counselling that is client focused.
Puerperal psychosis: This is a rare, but serious mental illness which usually occurs in the days following childbirth.
Pulmonary embolism: This is a *blood clot* in the lungs, which can damage the lung and decreases the levels of oxygen in the blood.

Further reading

Hanley, J. 2009. *Perinatal Mental Health: A Guide for Health Professionals and Users*. Wiley-Blackwell: Chichester.

Hanley, J. 2015. *Listening Visits in Perinatal Mental Health*. Routledge: Oxford.

Hanley, J., Williams, M. 2019. *Fathers and Perinatal Mental Health*. Routledge: Oxford.

Williams, M. 2018. *Daddy Blues: Postnatal Depression and Fatherhood*. The Foundation Centre: Newark.

References

American Psychiatric Association. 2013. *Diagnostic and Statistical Manual of Mental Disorders*. (5th edn). https://doi.org/10.1176/appi.books.978089042559

Austin, M.-P. 2013. *Marcé International Society Position Statement on Psychosocial Assessment and Depression Screening in Perinatal Women*. Marcé International Society for Perinatal Mental Health: Brentwood, TN.

BNF. 2015. *NICE Guidelines for Benzodiazepines*. Royal Pharmaceutical Society of Great Britain, British Medical Association: London.

Boyce, P., Barriball, E. 2010. Puerperal psychosis. *Archives of Women's Mental Health*; 13(1), 45–47.

Caperton, W., Butler, M., Kaiser, D., Connelly, J., Knox, S. 2019. Stay-at-home fathers, depression, and help-seeking: a consensual qualitative research study. *Psychology of Men & Masculinities*; 21(2), 235–250.

Cox, J., Holden, J., Sarkovsky, R. 1987. Detection of postnatal depression. *Development of the 10-item Edinburgh Postnatal Depression Scale Br J Psychiatry*, 150: pp. 782–6.

Diabetes UK. 2020. www.diabetes.org.uk

Edhborg, M., Friberg, M., Lundh, W., Widström, A.-M. 2005. 'Struggling with life': narratives from women with signs of postpartum depression. *Scandinavian Journal of Public Health*; 33(4), 261–267.

El-Sayed, A. M., Haloossim, M. R., Galea, S., Koenen, K. C. 2012. Epigenetic modifications associated with suicide and common mood and anxiety disorders: a systematic review of the literature. *Biol. Mood Anxiety Disord.*; 14: 10. doi: 10.1186/2045-5380-2-10

Gafoor, R., Booth, H. P., Gulliford, M. C. 2018. Antidepressant utilisation and incidence of weight gain during 10 years follow up population-based cohort study. *BMJ*; 361: k1951.

Gutierrez-Galve, L., Stein, A., Hanington, L., Heron, J., Lewis, G., O'Farrelly, C., Ramchandani, P. G. 2019. Association of maternal and paternal depression in the postnatal period with offspring depression at age 18 years. *JAMA Psychiatry*; 76(3), 290–296.

Halle, R. A., Gartlehner, G., Gaynes, B. N., Forneris, C., Asher, G. N., Morgan, L. C., Coker-Schwimmer, E. C., Boland, E., Lux, J. L., Gaylord, S., Bann, C., Pierl, C. B., Lohr, K. N. 2015. Comparative benefits and harms of second-generation antidepressants and cognitive behavioral therapies in initial treatment of major depressive disorder: systematic review and meta-analysis. *BMJ*; 351, h6019.

Hanley, J. 2015. *Listening Visits in Perinatal Mental Health*. Routledge: Oxford.

Hanley, J., Williams, M. 2019. *Fathers and Perinatal Mental Health*. Routledge: Oxford.

Hotham, N., Hotham, E. 2015. Drugs in breastfeeding. *Australian Prescriber*; 38(5), 156–159.

Kabat-Zinn, J. 2015. Mindfulness. *Mindfulness*; 6(6), 1481–1483.

Lacobucci, G. 2019. NHS prescribed record number of antidepressants last year. *BMJ*; 364: l1508.

Lewis, K. J., DiFlorio, A., Gordon-Smith, K., Perry, A., Craddock, N., Jones, L., Jones, I. 2018. Mania triggered by sleep loss and risk of postpartum psychosis in women with bipolar disorder. *Journal of Affective Disorders*; 225(1), 624–629.

Massoudi, P., Hwang, C. P., Wickberg, B. 2013. How well does the Edinburgh Postnatal Depression Scale identify depression and anxiety in fathers? A validation study in a population based Swedish sample. *J. Affective Disord.*; 149(1–3), 67–74.

MMHA. 2019. www.maternalmentalhealthalliance.org

Naber, D., Bullinger, M. 2018. Should antidepressants be used in minor depression? *Dialogues in Clinical Neuroscience*; 20(3), 223–228.

Nakić Radoš, S., Tadinac, M., Herman, R. 2018. Anxiety during pregnancy and postpartum: course, predictors and comorbidity with postpartum depression. *Acta. Clin. Croat.*; 57(1), 39–51.

National Institute for Health and Clinical Excellence (NICE) 2009. *The Management of depression in adults: recognition and management*. Clinical guideline [CG90].

National Institute for Health and Clinical Excellence (NICE) 2016. Antenatal and postnatal mental health. *Quality Standard QS115*.

National Institute for Health and Clinical Excellence (NICE) 2018. Antenatal and postnatal mental health: clinical management and service guidance. *Clinical guideline CG192*.

Noergaard, B., Ammentorp, J., Fenger-Gron, J., Kofoed, P. E., Johannessen, H., Thibeau, S. 2017. Fathers' needs and masculinity dilemmas in a neonatal intensive care unit in Denmark. *Adv. Neonatal Care*; 17(4), E13–E22.

Shahani, L. A. 2012. Father with postpartum psychosis. Case Reports. *BMJ*: bcr1120115176.

Shorey, S., Cheeb, C. Y. I., Nga, E. D., Chanc, Y. H., et al. 2018. Prevalence and incidence of postpartum depression among healthy mothers: a systematic review and meta-analysis. *Journal of Psychiatric Research*; 104(9), 235–248.

Singley, D., Edwards, L. 2015. Men's perinatal mental health in the transition to fatherhood. *Prof. Psychology: Research and Practice*; 46(5), 309–316.

Sit, D., Luther, J., Buysse, D., et al. 2015. Suicidal ideation in depressed postpartum women: associations with childhood trauma, sleep disturbance and anxiety. *J. Psychiatr. Res.*; 66–67: 95–104. doi:10.1016/j.jpsychires.2015.04.021

Talge, N., Neal, N., Glover, V. 2007. Antenatal maternal stress and long-term effects on child neurodevelopment: how and why? *Journal of Child Psychology and Psychiatry*; 48(3/4), 245–261.

Whitton, S. W., Kuryluk, A. D. 2014. Associations between relationship quality and depressive symptoms in same-sex couples. *Journal of Family Psychology*; 28(4), 571–576.

Whooley, M. A., Avins, A. L, Miranda, J., Browner, W. S. 1997. Case-finding instruments for depression. Two questions are as good as many. *J. Gen. Intern. Med.*; 12(7), 439–445.

Wisner, K., Sit, D., McShea, M. S., et al. 2013. Onset timing, thoughts of self-harm, and diagnoses in postpartum women with screen-positive depression findings. *JAMA Psychiatry*; 70(5), 490–498.

World Health Organization. 2020. *Maternal Mental Health.* www.who.int.org

Section 3:

INEQUALITIES IN PUBLIC HEALTH

8

INEQUALITIES IN HEALTH

LINDA MAGES

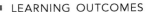

LEARNING OUTCOMES

By the end of this chapter you will be able to:

- Define health inequalities and describe their link with global and UK health conditions, identifying examples that have implications for your practice.
- Identify the determinants of health inequalities, know how they are measured, use theoretical models to examine their impact, and consider what implications they have for your practice.
- Understand health inequalities between populations defined by age, gender, ethnicity, socio-economic status and geography and explain how the inverse care-law impacts these populations, identifying examples that are relevant to your practice.
- Describe equality and human rights legislation relevant to health inequalities and debate the challenges presented by concepts of *inequality*, *equality* and *equity* for your practice and in developing public health programmes to address health inequalities.
- Discuss strategies to tackle health inequalities including your role in advocacy. Consider the challenges and benefits of using a multidisciplinary asset-based approach and examine why actions cannot be confined to a healthcare system, such as the NHS.

Introduction

The Universal Declaration of Human Rights (UN 1948) assert that everyone should have the opportunity to live a healthy life. On addressing health inequalities the UK has been a world leader, but in the last decade the Institute of Equity (2020a) spotlight increasing time spent in ill health by people who are poor. These differences in health status are unfair and occur between people within a country and between countries. They are often deeply rooted and complex, with health services continuing to be inversely related to need (Tudor 1971). Emphatically, the COVID-19 pandemic has underlined the issue of health inequalities, most particularly in the BAME population (NHS Confederation 2020).

This chapter explores the environmental, societal and social determinants that create health inequalities. It will outline key public health challenges, behavioural risk factors, and discuss the use of theoretical models. Relevant policy is integrated throughout this chapter with key terms and an exploative exercise at the end.

Health inequalities defined

A clear understanding of health inequalities is paramount for development of policies and interventions that support making services, treatment and care relevant, accessible and proportionate to need (Institute of Equity 2020a). Whitehead (2007) defined health inequalities as differences in health status between people or communities that are potentially preventable because they are socially and systematically produced. Hunter (2009) asserted that such complex issues cannot be tackled by individual action but require a multi-faceted, multi-disciplinary societal approach. Evidence demonstrates a 'socioeconomic gradient' for lifestyle behaviours, which are now regarded as symptoms and causes of health inequalities. It is therefore pertinent that health be considered within a political context so that ill health can be identified as generated by political socioeconomic decision making.

Health inequalities are important because they describe unjust and avoidable differences in health status, access to services, experience of care, and opportunities people have to live healthy lives (see Table 8.1) (King's Fund 2020).

The human right to make healthy choices and enjoy good health is not experienced equally across populations (UN 1948). Since the publication of the *Black Report* (Black et al. 1988), there is no doubt on the unequal distribution of ill health and premature death between affluent and poor populations (Acheson 1998, Marmot et al. 2010, OPHI 2018, Wanless 2004, WHO 2019).

Overview of global and UK health inequalities

The Sustainable Development Goals (SDGs) (UN 2020) recognise the socio-political injustice that causes inequalities in health and premature death. Climate change has created direct and indirect risks to health and life which disproportionately impact on those who are vulnerable and less able to adapt (Institute of Equity 2020b). Health inequalities across the lifespan present a global priority and their elimination is a major public health goal (European Parliamentary Research Service 2020). Ruckert et al. (2017) argue that implementation of a Universal Basic Income could significantly reduce health inequalities. Other strategies include global and local level Public Private Partnerships (World Bank Group 2020) along with Universal Health Coverage, considered most important to reducing the financial impact of healthcare on poor people (WHO 2020b).

Post Acheson (1998) Britain was regarded as a global leader in reducing health inequalities but more recently UK health inequalities continue to widen, in particular due to long-term conditions and complex co-morbidity (Department of Health Northern Ireland 2019, Public Health Wales Observatory 2020, Scottish Government 2020). This trend is attributed to policy focused on behaviour change rather than the wider determinants of lifestyle. There are also notable health inequalities between children from high- and low-income families (Collishaw et al. 2019, Royal College of Paediatrics and Child Health 2020). The British Medical Association (2017) report that poverty has cost the NHS £29 billion a year and excess hospitalisations £4.8 billion (Asaria et al. 2016). Marmot et al. (2010) estimate that health inequalities have the cost the UK around £31 billion in lost production.

Models to explore causes of inequalities in health

'Determinants' are characteristics that influence health and life expectancy. They may be biogenetic, such as sex, age and gender, or societal, referred to as 'social determinants'. The latter include demographic, behaviour, sociocultural, educational, healthcare, economic, ecology and climate elements (Cesta 2020). Determinants also affect the way people choose to look after their own health and utilise healthcare (Equality and Health Inequalities Unit 2015). Behaviours that impact negatively or positively on health are driven by complex interactions between determinants throughout an individual's life and are mostly beyond the control of individual and family agency (Marmot 2017).

Individual health can be explored using the Dimensions of Health (see Figure 8.1) (Naidoo and Wills 2016).

The inner circle encompasses six dimensions, each representing a continuum of wellbeing from optimal to extremely poor. They are enclosed by social and environmental determinants that include planet sustainability, peace, governance, transport, housing, water, sanitation, food and income. Changes in one dimension can directly or indirectly affect another, resulting in positive or negative impacts on risk factors and health status.

Using Bronfenbrenner's (1974) reconceptualized Bioecological Model (Bronfenbrenner and Ceci 1994), the processes that transform genetic 'phenotypes' and 'genotypes' (Figure 8.2) can be examined to gain insight into the influence of context on parents and children at five interrelated levels from 'micro' to 'chrono' (Khanom et al. 2020).

The 'micro' level explores direct contact on the child by people and settings recognised as crucial to nurturing development (Guy-Evans 2020). A 'meso' focus considers

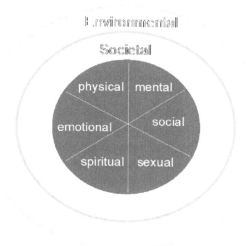

Figure 8.1 Dimensions of health (adapted from Naidoo and Wills 2016)

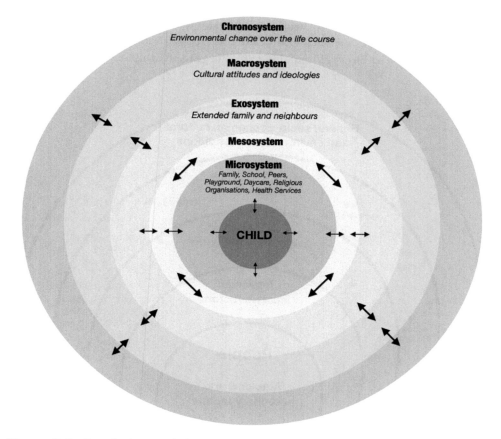

Figure 8.2 Bronfenbrenner's (1974) socio-ecological model of interrelated influences on child development (adapted from Guy-Evans 2020)

neighbourhood settings in which the family are actively involved. The 'exo' level examines environments that are not directly experienced by the child such as a parent's work place (Khanom et al. 2020). At a societal level the 'macro' view examines ideological, cultural, socioeconomic and ethnic influences. The 'chrono' level examines changes in wellbeing produced by key life transitions such as starting school or work, having children and retiring (Guy-Evans 2020).

Barton and Grant's (2006) Health Map (Figure 8.4) and its antecedent by Dahlgren and Whitehead (1991) (Figure 8.3) locate people at the centre of their models, enclosed by and interacting with the social, economic, political, built, natural and global environments. This enables practitioners to articulate negative and positive relationships between the physical and socioeconomic environment and health inequalities supporting identification of enablers and constraints on health. Barton and Grant (2006, p. 252) designed the Health Map to challenge the building of 'unhealthy conditions' and to support the Healthy Cities Movement (WHO, 2020c).

How are health inequalities measured?

When health inequalities are discussed it is important to identify and measure the influences, quantify health outcomes, and describe the population groups impacted. 'Life expectancy', 'healthy life years' and 'disability life years' harshly reflect the impact on

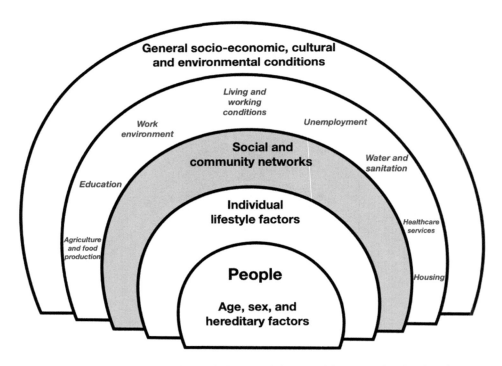

Figure 8.3 Determinants of health (adapted from Dahlgren and Whitehead 1991)

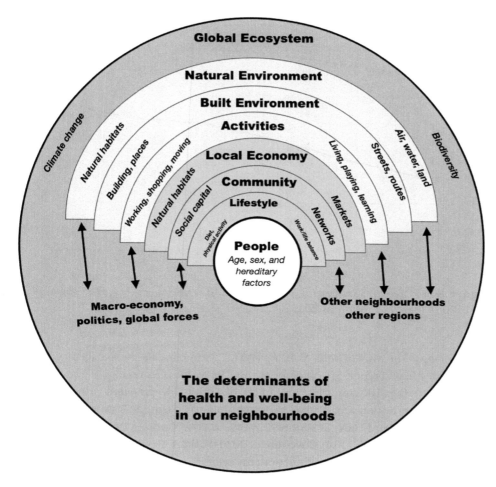

Figure 8.4 Health map of the local human habitat (adapted from Barton and Grant 2006)

health of the unjust distribution of social determinants. Marmot (2017) refers to this 'socioeconomic gradient' of health and ill health as the 'health gap' which he powerfully illustrates using 'life expectancy' and 'disability-free life expectancy' data (Figure 8.5). That health inequalities do not occur randomly or by chance provides a powerful argument for their reduction.

Data is central to prioritisation of health inequities (WHO, World Bank and USAID 2015). The World Health Data Platform (WHO 2020a) provides databases across a multitude of issues that make health inequalities visible and strengthen global capacity to address them. The progress of countries in tackling the SDGs is evaluated using the Multidimensional Poverty Index (MPI) which measures three dimensions of poverty using 10 indicators across health, education and standard of living (Figure 8.6) (OPHI 2018). It identifies who is poor and how they are poor, and supports comparison of countries and

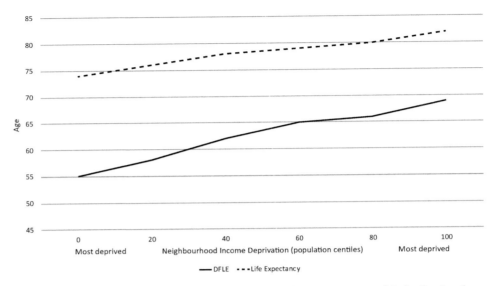

Figure 8.5 Life expectancy and disability-free life expectancy at birth: England 1999–2003 (based on Marmot 2017)

world regions. The *World Health Statistics* (WHO 2019) compile life expectancy trends, causes of death, and report SDG progress across 194 Member States.

Within the four UK countries the Indices of Multiple Deprivation provide relative measures of deprivation across small geographical areas (Figure 8.7) (Ministry of Housing, Communities and Local Government 2020a, 2020b, Northern Ireland Statistics and Research Agency 2017, Scottish Government 2020, Social Value Portal 2020, Welsh Government 2020a, 2020b). 'Deprivation' not only refers to income poverty, it also includes reduced opportunities, resources and services.

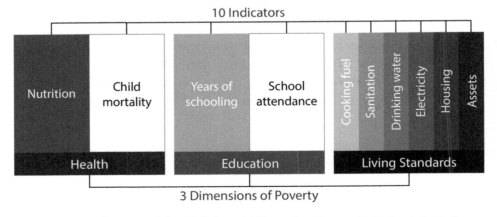

Figure 8.6 Indicators of the global multidimensional poverty index (adapted from OPHI 2018)

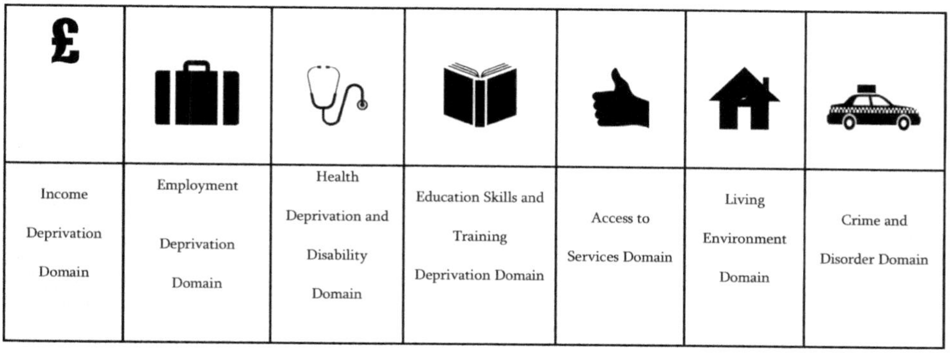

£						
Income Deprivation Domain	Employment Deprivation Domain	Health Deprivation and Disability Domain	Education Skills and Training Deprivation Domain	Access to Services Domain	Living Environment Domain	Crime and Disorder Domain

Figure 8.7 Domains of deprivation (adapted from Northern Ireland Statistics and Research Agency 2017)

Healthcare system determinants

The design, funding and delivery of healthcare systems supported by sustained political support can benefit populations beyond preventing ill health and treating illness. It is asserted that health systems should improve health by contributing to achieving the SDGs (UN Department of Economic Affairs, 2020), add years of life and reduce disability life years. Healthcare systems can not only contribute to protecting vulnerable populations from disease, they can also invest a sense of common purpose, inclusiveness and life security. However, the Inverse Care Law persists (Tudor, 1971). This is illustrated in the UK by comparison of General Practices in high- and low-socioeconomic areas (Fisher et al. 2020). Across the globe, it is exemplified in disproportionate levels of blindness in low- and middle-income countries (Buchan et al. 2019).

Across the globe people grapple with healthcare insecurity to immediate or future healthcare (Gama 2016). Poor access to *essential* quality healthcare affects around half the world's population, with 12% spending at least 10% of their household income on healthcare with unexpected illness necessitating borrowing and depletion of assets, often impacting most on children (WHO 2020b). Access is further exacerbated by a lack of healthcare infrastructure, a trained labour force, poor health literacy and a lack of service user voice (Gama 2016). This issue is not limited to low- and middle-income countries. In the USA, 10% of the population (33 million people) are without health insurance and rely on 'safety-net' providers that offer limited access to services while millions are 'underinsured' (Freeman et al. 2020).

The Universal Health Coverage (UHC) movement regards people as a county's greatest asset and on this premise advocates population health improvement as a means to strengthen human capital and national economies (WHO, World Bank and USAID 2015). As with all health inequalities, UHC should be supported by multisectoral action and human resource development (Figure 8.8) (World Bank 2019). Because primary health care is vital to socially and geographically disadvantaged people it is considered the most appropriate and cost-efficient way forward to UHC (WHO 2020b). Sacks et al. (2020)

emphasise the need for effective community leadership and community participation in improving access and quality of health services. Governments are supported towards achieving UHC through The Universal Health Coverage Partnership (UHC-P), which focuses on noncommunicable disease and health security (WHO 2020a).

Impact of health inequalities

Most modern drivers of population health, and of inequalities in health, lie outside healthcare systems. It is necessary to look beyond the direct biological and lifestyle causes of disease to sources that are less visible and referred to as the 'causes of the causes' (Marmot 2010). The concept of 'intersectionality' enables examination of the impact the interplay of power relations and the social determinants have on inequalities in health (Gkiouleka et al. 2018). Exploration of lay perspectives can be harnessed but Smith and

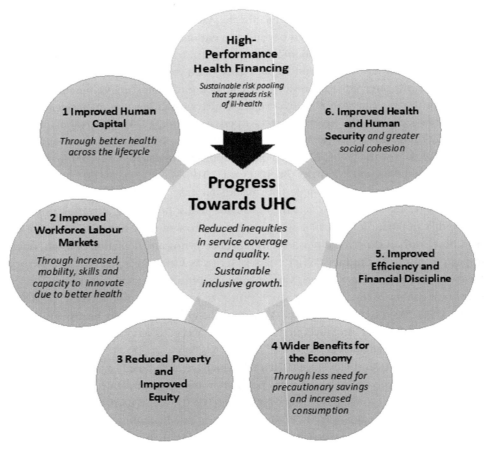

Figure 8.8 Health financing for Universal Health Coverage (adapted from World Bank 2019, p.19)

Anderson (2018) expose a reluctance by disadvantaged people to recognise health inequalities which they attribute to stigma and shame.

A key demographic factor of health inequality is age, but findings are complicated by the known association of age with increased risk of illness (Acciai, 2018). Ethnicity is a diverse determinant, where the prevalence of racism also needs to be understood and addressed (Otu et al. 2020). Health inequalities attributed to gender have to consider differences in ascribed roles and life opportunities within their societal context (Heinz et al. 2020). Education has been shown to protect individuals from later-life disadvantage. The continued participation of educated older people through paid work and social activities may sustain good health (Arpino 2019). Education is an important modifiable social determinant of health across the lifespan (The Health Foundation 2017).

Wilkinson and Pickett (2009) highlight the 'pernicious' effect of income inequality on health and social outcomes in more socioeconomically unequal societies.

Economic stability, or lack of it, encompasses housing quality and homelessness, access to healthy food, crime and violence, transportation facility and cost, green open spaces; exposure to pollutants; and social and community cohesion, inclusion and participation (Cesta, 2020). Healthcare determinants include access, intervention concordance, use of primary care and health literacy. Achieving improvements in health literacy is important to achieving increased rates of services use. Overall, people who have multiple disadvantages often need to exert excessive effort to access health services, and social exclusion is recognised as an important driver of inequalities in health (van Bergen et al. 2017).

Health is remarkably sensitive to the social environment within which people grow, learn, live, work and age. This manifests starkly by the least advantaged groups having shorter lives and more ill health (Marmot et al. 2010). A lifespan examination reveals the socioeconomic and genetic influences on child health and development starting at conception, or earlier. Maternal and foetal health is particularly susceptible to the socioeconomic environment (Larranaga et al. 2018). Different socioeconomic and environmental maternal circumstances have positive or negative influences on the risk of severe disease and also result in differing health outcomes from similar severe disease occurrences. Evidence shows that perinatal health, intrauterine growth and preterm birth are strong reflections of poverty during pregnancy. They are considered to underpin the transmission of health inequalities throughout childhood and indicate higher risk of long-term conditions and premature death during adulthood (Larranaga et al. 2018).

The impact on individuals of living in deprivation during pregnancy and throughout childhood accumulate and 'cast a long shadow' over subsequent social development, health behaviours and adult wellbeing (Marmot 2010, p.40). Adolescence is also a critical period, where risk behaviours adversely affect academic attainment and future adult health. Affluent socioeconomic conditions protect the health of individuals supporting high self-esteem, resilience and healthy behaviour choices, while impoverished circumstances undermine self-esteem, social skills and educational attainment creating conditions for the development of physical and mental ill health (Fisher et al. 2020).

COVID-19, health inequalities and ethnicity

In the UK, late presentation of COVID-19 for treatment is associated with poverty, and the mortality rate in the most deprived areas is reported to be twice that of affluent areas (Otu et al. 2020). Evidence across diverse BAME populations highlight influence by different determinants, which is further complicated by racism and discrimination (Launer 2020). In addition, some health professionals can feel uncomfortable engaging with issues concerning ethnic inequalities (Salway et al. 2016). An investigation by Public Health England (2020a) confirmed disparities of 10% to 50% in the risk of death from COVID-19 among varied BAME populations compared to white British people. Further research on the systemic inequities that drive BAME health inequalities in the UK is urgently needed (Mulholland and Sinha, 2020).

Equality and equity in relation to health inequalities

Reducing health inequalities cuts to the heart of the NHS values and 'Constitution' which upholds a comprehensive service available to all, free at the point of need and declares a duty to improve access and health outcomes of vulnerable 'groups and sections of society' (Department of Health and Social Care 2015). The Equality Act 2010 requires all public sector bodies to advance equality (GOV.UK 2020). It was not until the Health and Social Care Act 2012 (Legislation.gov.uk 2012) that NHS and Clinical Commissioning Groups were legally required to 'properly and seriously' consider how to reduce health inequalities (Equality and Health Inequalities Unit 2015). This focus was strengthened by the Social Value Act 2012 that required public sector commissioners to consider how to improve the local socioeconomic environment (NHS England 2020).

It is important to differentiate the concept of 'equality' from 'equity'. Turner (1986) described equality as a modern and progressive value. In the context of health, equality is about equal rights to the same standard of treatment or care to achieve equal outcomes. Ideologically, Tawney (1931, p.47) considered equality unattainable, but asserted that it should be 'sincerely sought', while Dahrendorf (1969, p.21) saw inequality as an impetus 'towards liberty' and described equality as 'terrible'. Within health, achieving equality requires differences to be considered (Lister 1997). Sometimes 'sameness' of intervention does not result in a fair or 'equitable' outcome. Equity is an ethical principle and in health refers to ensuring everyone has the opportunity and is provided with what they need to achieve health (Braveman and Gruskin, 2003). Equity can therefore realise equality of outcome by treating people differently depending on their need.

Action on health inequalities

Actions to reduce health inequalities have the potential to save money across the lifespan even though longevity may increase (Asaria et al. 2016). Addressing inequalities in health requires a lifespan multidisciplinary approach that aims to achieve more equal and equitable health outcomes across diverse populations using universal and targeted interventions (NHS England 2017, Public Health England 2017). Dahlgren and Whitehead (1991) identified prioritisation of structural interventions to tackle the causes of ill health, such as redistributive tax policies, workforce regulation, welfare benefits and improved access to healthcare provision (Addison et al. 2020). The dynamic complexity and persistence of health inequalities led Hunter (2009) to frame them as 'wicked issues' requiring multifaceted, multi-professional interventions. Generally, it is asserted that strategies to address health inequalities pay insufficient attention to obtaining and understanding concerns conveyed by community voices.

The *Marmot Review* (Marmot et al. 2010, p.177) identified nine policy areas for intervention across the wider determinants of health using a life course approach (Table 8.1).

Many of these interventions are 'service based', and adopt a systematic, scaled-up approach that is outcome focused (Public Health England, 2017). The *NHS Long Term Plan* (NHS 2019) commits to tackling wider threats to health through socioeconomic policy and action on preventable or modifiable lifestyle determinants. Assessment and management of conditions associated with health inequalities are the focus of the NHS Health Check Programme in England (NHS 2020b). Key behavioural risk factors including obesity, physical inactivity, smoking and alcohol, and physiological factors comprising high blood pressure, blood glucose and cholesterol, are targeted by all UK countries (Public Health Agency (Northern Ireland) 2019, Public Health Scotland 2020b, Public Heath Wales 2013). Diabetes Type 2 is a leading preventable cause of vision loss, kidney failure, heart disease and stroke. The NHS Diabetes Prevention Programme (NHS 2020a) identifies those at high risk of developing Type 2 diabetes.

Community development is 'place-based' and referred to as Community Capacity Building (CCB), an asset-based approach that strengthens communities towards achieving changes that improve their facilities and environment, subsequently impacting positively on health (Scottish Community Development Centre, 2020). A community's capacity is enhanced by its social networks, including intergenerational dialogue (Murayama et al. 2019) which contribute to improved community resilience, sustainable change and better outcomes through successful 'co-production' (Morris and McDaid, 2017). Smith and Anderson (2018) advise sensitive planning to avoid unintentional exacerbation of shame and stigma regarding their socioeconomic situation (Figure 8.9).

Table 8.1 Policy areas for wider determinant interventions (Marmot et al. 2010, p.177)

Early child development and education	Employment arrangements and working conditions	Social protection
Built environment	Sustainable development	Economic analysis
Delivery systems and mechanisms	Priority public health conditions	Social inclusion and social mobility

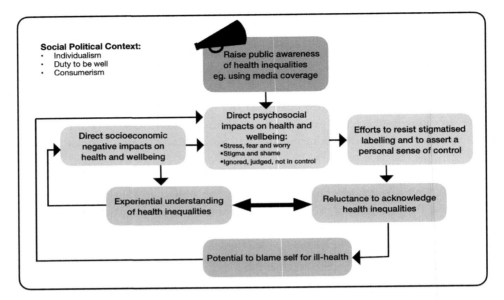

Figure 8.9 Impact of raising public awareness on health inequalities (adapted from Smith and Anderson 2018, Fig. 2)

Core values include recognition by services that communities already have assets and social capital (Scottish Community Development Centre 2020) contrasting with the deficit-based approach that focuses on needs (Steiner 2016). The process of developing co-production is referred to as 'community engagement', the nature of which can be described by using Arnstein's (1969) Ladder of Participation (Figure 8.10).

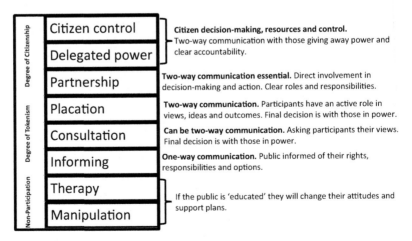

Figure 8.10 The 'ladder of participation' showing community engagement (adapted from Arnstein 1969)

Characteristics of successful interventions

Although considerable effort and research has been directed at tackling inequalities of health, it is asserted that their evaluations are often over short-term timeframes, making it difficult to attribute health outcomes to an intervention. Tools have been developed to help professionals and commissioning bodies, such as Local Authorities and CCGs, to measure any reduction in health inequalities (NHS, 2020c). Monitoring and evaluation provide insight into the change process enabling more effective use of resources and understanding of impact. Characteristics that are associated with successful interventions include:

- Reporting on implementation and impact (Public Health England 2017).
- Use of specific measures to improve health of the most disadvantaged groups (Public Health Wales 2013).
- High levels of individual, parent, family or community engagement (Matwiejczyk et al. 2018).
- Priorities owned by key stakeholders (Public Health England 2017).
- Enabling the most disadvantaged to have a voice without shame or stigma (Smith and Anderson 2018).
- An inclusive approach that ensures access, empowers and develops health literacy (Public Health England 2015).
- An asset-based approach (Public Health England 2017).
- Co-produced improved life-span health (Scottish Community Development Centre 2020).
- Integrated multi-professional working using shared budgets (Public Health Agency Northern Ireland 2019).
- Multifaceted preventative measures not relying on single interventions (Hunter 2009).
- Sustainable resource availability (Marmot et al. 2010).
- Clear timescales, monitoring and evaluation from the start (Public Health England 2017).

Conclusion

Across the globe, the relationship between health inequalities, disadvantaged groups, and biogenetic, socioeconomic and ecological determinants have been demonstrated. The unequal impact of COVID-19 on the mortality and health of vulnerable individuals, households and communities is unequivocal (Health & Equity in Recovery Plans Working Group 2020). It is strongly established that health inequalities result from complex interactions between multiple influences that are cumulative over our lifespan and include power relationships, racism and discrimination. They can be unchangeable (genetic, ethnicity and age), accumulative (family, lifestyle, abuse and poverty), direct (family, friends, participation, isolation, income, housing, air pollution, food security, culture, violence, lifestyle, access to healthcare, climate change), indirect (education, transport, climate change), modifiable (diet, exercise, income, housing), and preventable (smoking, alcohol, income, housing, access to healthcare). Examination of power relationships and lay perspectives are limited with policy focusing on lifestyle change and healthcare access, but all health and social care professionals can act as advocates for individuals, families and communities in order to tackle health inequalities.

Consider the following questions

1. Explore national statistics for one UK country using the data sources below to identify:
    a. determinants and consider how the they impact on health and life expectancy;
    b. where the highest concentrations of different types of deprivation are and reflect on the implications for communities.
    Compare statistics for the UK with those for other countries.

Northern Ireland
Northern Ireland Statistics and Research Agency (2020a, 2020b).

Wales
Public Health Wales Observatory (2020).
Welsh Government (2020a, 2020b).

Scotland
Public Health Scotland (2020a).
Scottish Government (2020).
Scottish Index of Multiple Deprivation (2020)

England
GOV.UK (2020a).
Ministry of Housing, Communities and Local Government (2020b).
Public Health England (2020b, 2020c).

World Health Statistics
Oxford Poverty and Human Development Initiative (2018).
World Health Organization (2020a, 2019).

2. How can you integrate health literacy support into your practice?
3. Identify lifestyle challenges in children that have implications for adult health.
4. When considering inequality, equality and equity, does health and healthcare have special importance?
5. Justice has been described as 'an account of permissible inequalities', at what point do health inequalities become unjust?

Key terms

BAME: People who are Black, Asian and Minority Ethnicity.

CCGs: Clinical Commissioning Groups led by elected GPs, nurses and secondary care consultants who decide local services needed and ensure their provision.

Community capacity building: Support community groups access to address issues which are important to them.

Community resilience: Ability of communities to harness local resources to help themselves.

Co-production: A reciprocal relationship between service providers and service users.

Dahrendorf, R. G: German-British sociologist, philosopher and liberal politician.

Disability life years (DALY): Expressed as the number of years lost due to ill health, disability or early death.

Disability-free life expectancy (DFLE): Average number of years a person would live disability-free with no limiting long-term illness.

Fuel poverty: A household has above average fuel costs and if they spent that amount would have an income below the poverty line.

Genotype: Set of heritable genes that can be passed from parents to children.

Health literacy: A person's ability to acquire, understand and use information about health and health services.

Health security: Protects national populations from health threats such as pandemics.

Healthy life years (HLY): The number of years a person is expected to continue to live in a healthy condition.

Intergenerational practice: Builds support between older and younger members of communities to tackle fear, prejudice and build respect.

Intersectionality: A theoretical framework that practitioners can use to gain insight into how interaction across socially constructed categories – such as race, class, gender, sexual orientation and disability – create inequality, disadvantage and oppression.

Perinatal period: From the 28th week of pregnancy to the end of the 1st week after birth.

Phenotype: Genetic observable characteristics or traits of an individual.

Proportionate universalism: Universal services that are proportionate to degree of need.

Social capital: Trust and reciprocity among families, groups and communities.

Tawney, R. H.: English economic historian, ethical socialist.

Universal basic income: Unconditional income granted irrespective of work or a means test.

Universal health coverage: Improve accessibility of essential health services for poor people and ensure financial protection of healthcare provision.

Further reading

Institute of Equity. 2020. *Health Equity in England. The Marmot Review 10 Years On.* University College London, Institute of Equity: London.

PHE. 2020. *Wider Determinants of Health*. Office for Health Improvement & Disparities: London. Available at: https://fingertips.phe.org.uk/profile/wider-determinants [Accessed 21.03.2022].

Wilkinson, R., Pickett, K. 2009. *The Spirit Level: Why More Equal Societies Almost Always Do Better.* Allen Lane: London.

References

Acciai, F. 2018. The age pattern of social inequalities in health at older ages: are common measures of socio-economic status interchangeable? *Public Health*; 157, 135e141.

Acheson, D. 1998. *Independent Inquiry into Inequalities in Health: Report.* HMSO: London. Available at: https://assets.publishing.service.gov.uk/government/uploads/system/uploads/attachment_data/file/265503/ih.pdf [Accessed 11.03.2022].

Addison, M., Kaner, E., Johnstone, P., Hillier-Brown, F., Moffatt, S., Russell, S., Barr, B., Holland, P., Salway, S., Whitehead, M., Bambra, C. 2020. Equal North: how can we reduce health inequalities in the North of England? A prioritization exercise with researchers, policymakers and practitioners. *Journal of Public Health*; 41(4), 652–664.

Arnstein, S. 1969. A ladder of citizen participation. *Journal of the American Institute of Planners*; 35(4), 216–224.

Arpino, B. 2019. Education inequalities in health among older European men and women: the role of active aging. *Journal of Aging and Health*; 31(1), 185–208.

Asaria, M., Doran, T., Cookson, R. 2016. The costs of inequality: whole-population modelling study of lifetime inpatient hospital costs in the English National Health Service by level of neighbourhood deprivation. *Journal of Epidemiology and Community Health*; 70(10), 990–996.

Barton, H., Grant, M. 2006. A health map for the local human habitat. *The Journal of the Royal Society for the Promotion of Health*; 126(6), 252–253.

Black, D., Morris, J. N., Smith, C., Townsend, P. 1988. *Inequalities in Health: The Black Report.* (Eds. Townsend, P. and Davidson, N.). Penguin: Harmondsworth.

Braveman, P., Gruskin, D. 2003. Defining equity in health. *Journal of Epidemiology and Community Health*; 57, 254–258.

British Medical Association. 2017. *Health at a Price. Reducing the Impact of Poverty.* BMA: London. Available at: www.bma.org.uk/media/2084/health-at-a-price-2017.pdf [Accessed 11/03/2022].

Bronfenbrenner, U. 1974. Developmental research, public policy, and the ecology of childhood. *Child Development*; 45(1), 1–5.

Bronfenbrenner, U., Ceci, S. J. 1994. Nature–nurture reconceptualised: a bio-ecological model. *Psychological Review*; 10(4), 568–586.

Buchan, J. C., Dean, W. H., Ramke, J., Burton, M. J. 2019. The inverse-research law of eye health. *Eye*; 33, 1976–1977.

Cesta, T. 2020. *Understanding the Social Determinants of Health.* AHC Media LLC.

Collishaw, S., Furzer, E., Thapur, A.K., Sellers, R. 2019. Brief report: a comparison of child mental health inequalities in three UK population cohorts. *European Child & Adolescent Psychiatry*; 28, 1547–1549.

Dahlgren, G., Whitehead, M. 1991. *Policies and Strategies to Promote Social Equity in Health*. Institute for Future Studies: Stockholm.

Dahrendorf, R. G. 1969. The nature and types of social inequality. In A. Beteille (Ed.), *Social Inequality*. Penguin: London.

Department of Health (Northern Ireland). 2019. *Health Inequalities. Annual Report 2019*. Public Health Information & Research Branch, Information Analysis Directorate: Belfast.

Department of Health and Social Care. 2015. *The NHS Constitution for England*. Available at: www.gov.uk/government/publications/the-nhs-constitution-for-england/the-nhs-constitution-for-england [Accessed 01.12.2020].

Equality and Health Inequalities Unit. 2015. *This Guidance is to Support Clinical Commissioning Groups and NHS England to Meet their Legal Duties with Regard to Equality and Health Inequalities*.

European Parliamentary Research Service. 2020. *Addressing Health Inequalities in the European Union*. Available at: www.europarl.europa.eu/RegData/etudes/IDAN/2020/646182/EPRS_IDA(2020)646182_EN.pdf [Accessed 11.03.2000].

Fisher, R., Dunn, P., Asaria, M., Thorlby, R. 2020. *Briefing: Level or Not? Comparing General Practice in Areas of High and Low Socioeconomic Deprivation in England*. The Health Foundation: London.

Freeman, T., Gesesew, H. A., Bambra, C., Giugliani, E. R. J., Popay, J., Sanders, D., Macinko, J., Musolino, C., Baum, F. 2020. Why do some countries do better or worse in life expectancy relative to income? An analysis of Brazil, Ethiopia, and the United States of America. *International Journal of Equity in Health*; 19, 202.

Gama, E. 2016. Health insecurity and social protection: pathways, gaps, and their implications on health outcomes and poverty. *International Journal of Health Policy and Management*; 5(3), 183–187.

Gkiouleka, A., Huijts, T., Beckfield, J., Bambrac, C. 2018. Understanding the micro and macro politics of health: inequalities, T intersectionality and institutions – a research agenda. *Social Science and Medicine*; 200, 92–98.

GOV.UK. 2020b. *The Equality Act 2010*. Available at: www.gov.uk/guidance/equality-act-2010-guidance [Accessed 01.12.2020].

Guy-Evans, O. 2020. *Simply psychology. Bronfenbrenner's ecological systems theory*. Available at: www.simplypsychology.org/Bronfenbrenner.html [Accessed 01.12.2020].

Health & Equity in Recovery Plans Working Group. 2020. *Direct and Indirect Impacts of COVID-19 on Health and Wellbeing*. Champs Public Health Collaborative, Public Health Institute. John Moores University: Liverpool. Available at: www.ljmu.ac.uk/~/media/phi-reports/2020-07-direct-and-indirect-impacts-of-COVID19-on-health-and-wellbeing.pdf [Accessed 11.03.2022].

Heinz, A., Catunda, C., van Duin, C., Torsheim, T., Willems, H. 2020. Patterns of health-related gender inequalities. A cluster analysis of 45 countries. *Journal of Adolescent Health*; 66, S29eS39.

Hunter, D. 2009. Leading for health and wellbeing: the need for a new paradigm. *Journal of Public Health*; 31(2), 202–204.

Institute of Equity. 2020a. *Health Equity in England. The Marmot Review 10 Years On.* University College London, Institute of Equity: London. Available at: www.health. org.uk/publications/reports/the-marmot-review-10-years-on [Accessed 11.03.2022].

Institute of Equity. 2020b. *Sustainable Health Equity: Achieving a Net-zero UK.* Available at: www.instituteofhealthequity.org/resources-reports/sustainable-health-equity-achieving-a-net-zero-uk/main-report.pdf [Accessed 11.03.2022].

Khanom, A., Evans, B. A., Lynch, R., Marchant, E., Hill, R. A., Morgan, K., Rapport, F., Lyons, R. A., Brophy, S. 2020. Parent recommendations to support physical activity for families with young children: results of interviews in deprived and affluent communities in South Wales (United Kingdom). *Health Expectations*; 23, 284–295.

King's Fund. 2020. *What are Health Inequalities?* Available at: www.kingsfund.org.uk/publications/what-are-health-inequalities#what [Accessed 01.12.2020].

Larranaga, I., Santa-Marina, L., Molinuevo, A., Alvarez-Pedrerol, M., Fernandez-Somoano, A., Jimenez-Zabala, A., Rebagliato, M. 2018. Poor mothers, unhealthy children: the transmission of health inequalities in the INMA study, Spain. *The European Journal of Public Health*; 29(3), 568–574.

Launer, J. 2020. Ethnic inequalities in health: should we talk about implicit white supremacism? *Postgraduate Medical Journal*; 96, 1132.

Legislation.gov.uk. 2012. *Health and Social Care Act 2012.* Available at: www.legislation. gov.uk/ukpga/2012/7/contents/enacted [Accessed 01.12.2020].

Lister, R. 1997. *Citizenship: Feminist Perspectives.* Palgrave Macmillan: Basingstoke.

Marmot, M. 2010. Inclusion health: addressing the causes of the causes. *Lancet*; 391(10117), 186–188.

Marmot, M. 2017. The health gap: the challenge of an unequal world: the argument. *International Journal of Epidemiology*; 1312–1318.

Marmot, M., Allen, J., Goldblatt, P., Boyce, T., McNeish, D., Grady, M., Geddes, I. 2010. *Fair Society, Healthy Lives. The Marmot Review.* University College: London. Available at: www.parliament.uk/globalassets/documents/fair-society-healthy-lives-full-report. pdf [Accessed 11.03.2022].

Matwiejczyk, L., Mehta, K., Scott, J., Tonkin, E., Coveney, J. 2018. Characteristics of effective interventions promoting healthy eating for pre-schoolers in childcare settings: an umbrella review. *Nutrients*; 10, 293. Available at: www.mdpi.com/2072-6643/10/3/293/htm [Accessed 11.03.2022].

Ministry of Housing, Communities and Local Government. 2020a. *The English Indices of Deprivation 2019.* Available at: www.gov.uk/government/statistics/english-indices-of-deprivation-2019 [Accessed 01.12.2020].

Ministry of Housing, Communities and Local Government. 2020b. *The English Indices of Deprivation 2019.* Available at: http://imd-by-postcode.opendatacommunities.org/imd/2019 [Accessed 01.12.2020].

Morris, L., McDaid, M. 2017. Compassionate communities – from frailty to community resilience – making a public health approach to end of life care a reality. *International Journal of Integrated Care*; 17(5), 1–8.

Mulholland, R. H., Sinha, I. P. 2020. Ethnicity and COVID-19 infection: are the pieces of the puzzle falling into place? *BMC Medicine*; 18, 206.

Murayama, Y., Murayama, H., Hasebe, M., Yamaguchi, J., Fujiwara, Y. 2019. The impact of intergenerational programs on social capital in Japan: a randomized population-based cross-sectional study. *BMC Public Health*; 19, 156.

Naidoo, J., Wills, J. 2016. *Foundations for Health Promotion*. Elsevier: London.

NHS. 2019. *NHS Long-term Plan*. Available at: www.longtermplan.nhs.uk [Accessed 01.12.2020].

NHS. 2020a. *NHS Diabetes Prevention Programme (NHS DPP)*. Available at: www.england.nhs.uk/diabetes/diabetes-prevention/ [Accessed 01.12.2020].

NHS. 2020b. *NHS Health Check Helping you Prevent Diabetes, Heart Disease, Kidney Disease, Stroke and Dementia*. Available at: www.healthcheck.nhs.uk/ [Accessed 01.12.2020].

NHS. 2020c. *Tools and Resources to Help Measure Reduction on Health Inequalities*. Available at: www.england.nhs.uk/ltphimenu/right-care-tools-and-resources/ [Accessed 01.12.2020].

NHS Confederation. 2020. *Tackling Health Inequalities. Learning from Each Other to Make Rapid Progress*.

NHS England. 2017. *Next Steps on the NHS Five-year Forward View*.

NHS England. 2020. *Key Legislation. Equality, Diversity and Health Inequalities*. Available at: www.england.nhs.uk/about/equality/equality-hub/resources/legislation/ [Accessed 01.12.2020].

Northern Ireland Statistics and Research Agency. 2017. *Northern Ireland Multiple Deprivation Measure 2017*. Available at: www.nisra.gov.uk/sites/nisra.gov.uk/files/publications/NIMDM17-%20with%20ns.pdf [Accessed 11.03.2020].

Northern Ireland Statistics and Research Agency. 2020a. *COVER Pre-release Access List*. Available at: www.nisra.gov.uk/statistics [Accessed 01.12.2020].

Northern Ireland Statistics and Research Agency. 2020b. *Northern Ireland Multiple Deprivation Measure 2017*. Available at: www.ninis2.nisra.gov.uk/InteractiveMaps/Deprivation/Deprivation%202017/SA_Deprivation_Map/atlas.html [Accessed 01.12.2020].

Otu, A., Ahinkorah, B. O., Ameyaw, E. K., Seidu, A., Yaya, S. 2020. One country, two crises: what COVID-19 reveals about health inequalities among BAME communities in the United Kingdom and the sustainability of its health system. *International Journal for Equity in Health*; 19, 189.

Oxford Poverty and Human Development Initiative (OPHI). 2018. *Global Multidimensional Poverty Index 2018: The Most Detailed Picture to Date of the World's Poorest People*. Oxford Poverty and Human Development Initiative, University of Oxford: Oxford.

Public Health Agency (Northern Ireland). 2019. *Strong Partnerships Required to Tackle Health Inequalities*. Available at: www.publichealth.hscni.net/news/strong-partnerships-required-tackle-health-inequalities [Accessed 01.12.2020].

Public Health England. 2015. *Local Action on Health Inequalities. Improving Health Literacy to Reduce Health Inequalities*. PHE: London. Available at: https://assets.publishing.service.gov.uk/government/uploads/system/uploads/attachment_data/file/460709/4a_Health_Literacy-Full.pdf [Accessed 11.03.2022].

Public Health England. 2017. *Reducing Health Inequalities: System, Scale and Sustainability*. Available at: https://assets.publishing.service.gov.uk/government/uploads/system/uploads/attachment_data/file/731682/Reducing_health_inequalities_system_scale_and_sustainability.pdf [Accessed 11.03.2022].

Public Health England. 2020a. *Disparities in the Risk and Outcomes of COVID-19*. Available at: https://assets.publishing.service.gov.uk/government/uploads/system/uploads/attachment_data/file/908434/Disparities_in_the_risk_and_outcomes_of_COVID_August_2020_update.pdf [Accessed 11.03.2022].

Public Health England. 2020b. *Public Health Outcomes Framework*. Available at: https://fingertips.phe.org.uk/profile/public-health-outcomes-framework [Accessed 01.12.2020].

Public Health England. 2020c. *Wider Determinants of Health*. Available at: https://fingertips.phe.org.uk/profile/wider-determinants [Accessed 01.12.2020].

Public Health Scotland. 2020a. *What Are Health Inequalities?* Available at: www.healthscotland.scot/health-inequalities/what-are-health-inequalities [Accessed 30.11.2020].

Public Health Scotland. 2020b. *Tools for Monitoring and Evaluation*. Available at: www.healthscotland.scot/tools-and-resources/tools-for-monitoring-and-evaluation [Accessed 01.12.2020].

Public Health Wales. 2013. *Transforming Health Improvement in Wales*. Available at: www.wales.nhs.uk/sitesplus/documents/986/PHW%20Health%20Improvement%20Review%20Final%20Report%20-%20260913.pdf [Accessed 11.03.2022].

Public Health Wales Observatory. 2020. *Life Expectancy and Mortality in Wales*.

Royal College of Paediatrics and Child Health. 2020. *State of Child Health in the UK*. Available at: https://stateofchildhealth.rcpch.ac.uk/evidence/family-and-social-environment/child-poverty/ [Accessed 01.12.2020].

Ruckert, A., Huynh, C., Labonté, R. 2017. Perspectives. Reducing health inequities: is universal basic income the way forward? *Journal of Public Health*; 40(1), 3–7.

Sacks, E., Schleiff, M., Were, M., Chowdhury, A.M., Perry, H. 2020. Communities, universal health coverage and primary health care. Policy and practice. *Bulletin of the World Health Organization*; 98, 773–780.

Salway, S., Mir, G., Turner, D., Ellison, G. T. H., Carter, L., Gerrish, K. 2016. Obstacles to 'race equality' in the English National Health Service: insights from the healthcare commissioning arena. *Social Science and Medicine*; 152, 102–110.

Scottish Community Development Centre. 2020. *Community Capacity Building*. Available at: www.scdc.org.uk/hub/community-capacity-building/ [Accessed 01.12.2020].

Scottish Government. 2020. *Introducing the Scottish Index of Multiple Deprivation 2020*. Available at: www.gov.scot/publications/scottish-index-multiple-deprivation-2020/ [Accessed 01.12.2020].

Scottish Index of Multiple Deprivation. 2020. Available at: https://simd.scot/#/simd2020/BTTTFTT/9/-4.0000/55.9000/ [Accessed 01.12.2020].

Smith, K. E., Anderson, R. 2018. Understanding lay perspectives on socioeconomic health inequalities in Britain: a meta-ethnography. *Sociology of Health & Illness*, 40(1), 146–170.

Social Value Portal. 2020. *Indices of Multiple Deprivation in the UK.* Available at: https://socialvalueportal.com/indices-of-multiple-deprivation-in-the-uk/#:~:text=The%20Indices%20of%20Multiple%20Deprivation%20%28IMD%29%20are%20a,need%2C%20relative%20to%20the%20rest%20of%20the%20country [Accessed 01.12.2020].

Steiner, A. 2016. Assessing the effectiveness of a capacity building intervention in empowering hard-to-reach communities. *Journal of Community Practice*; 24(3), 235–263.

Tawney, R. H. 1931. *Equality.* Allen & Unwin: London.

The Health Foundation. 2017. *How Do Our Education and Skills Influence Our Health?* The Health Foundation: London.

Tudor, H. J. 1971. The inverse care law. *Lance*; 297, 405–412.

Turner, B. S. 1986. *Equality.* Ellis Horwood/Tavistock: London.

United Nations. 1948. *Universal Declaration of Human Rights.* United Nations: New York.

United Nations. 2020. *Sustainable Development Goals.* Available at: www.un.org/sustainabledevelopment/ [Accessed 01.12.2020].

United Nations, Department of Economic Affairs. 2020. *Transforming our world: the 2030 agenda for sustainable development.* Available at: https://sdgs.un.org/ [Accessed 11/03/2022].

van Bergen, A., Hoff, S. J. M., Schreurs, H., van Loon, A., van Hemert, A. M. 2017. Social exclusion index for health surveys (SEI-HS): a prospective nationwide study to extend and validate a multidimensional social exclusion questionnaire. *BMC Public Health*; 17, 253.

Wanless, D. 2004. *Securing Good Health for the Whole Population: Final Report.* HMSO: London.

Welsh Government. 2020a. *Welsh Index of Multiple Deprivation.* Available at: https://gov.wales/welsh-index-multiple-deprivation?lang=en [Accessed 01.12.2020].

Welsh Government. 2020b. *Welsh Index of Multiple Deprivation 2019.* Available at: https://wimd.gov.wales [Accessed 01.12.2020].

Whitehead, M. 2007. A typology of actions to tackle social inequalities in health. *Journal of Epidemiology and Community Health*; 61, 473–478.

Wilkinson, R., Pickett, K. 2009. *The Spirit Level. Why More Equal Societies Almost Always Do Better.* Allen Lane: London.

World Bank. 2019. *High-Performance Health Financing for Universal Health Coverage. Driving Sustainable Inclusive Growth in the 21st Century.* International Bank for Reconstruction and Development/The World Bank: Geneva.

World Bank Group. 2020. *Public Private Partnership Legal Resource Centre: PPPs for the Poor.* Available at: https://ppp.worldbank.org/public-private-partnership/ppps-poor [Accessed 01.12.2020].

World Health Organization. 2019. *World Health Statistics 2019: Monitoring Health for the SDGs, Sustainable Development Goals.* Available at: https://apps.who.int/iris/bitstream/handle/10665/324835/9789241565707-eng.pdf?ua=1 [Accessed 01.12.2020].

World Health Organization. 2020a. *World Health Data Platform.* Available at: www.who.int/data/ [Accessed 01.12.2020].

World Health Organization. 2020b. *Universal Health Coverage*. Available at: www.who.int/news-room/fact-sheets/detail/universal-health-coverage-(uhc) [Accessed 01.12.2020].

World Health Organization. 2020c. *Healthy Cities*. Available at: www.who.int/health promotion/healthy-cities/en/ [Accessed 01.12.2020].

World Health Organization, World Bank, and USAID. 2015. *The Roadmap for Health Measurement and Accountability*. Available at: www.who.int/hrh/documents/roadmap4health-measurement_accountability.pdf [Accessed 11.03.2022].

World Health Statistics. 2020. *Monitoring Health for DDGs. Life Expectancy and Causes of Death*. Available at: www.who.int/publications/i/item/9789240005105 [Accessed 01.12.2020].

9

THE OBESITY EPIDEMIC

LINDA MAGES AND NADINE LITTLER

LEARNING OUTCOMES

By the end of this chapter you will be able to:

- Recognise the current definition and classification of obesity. Understand that they enable standardised objectives on national and international diagnosis, monitoring and research that can inform evidence-based decision making in practice and the development of interventions, services, guidelines and policies.
- Be aware of the global and UK public health policy context on obesity including the implications of epidemiological, demographic and statistical information for health care services. Appreciate that policy is crucial as it sets out plans of action in relation to an issue that has been identified as important, in this case how obesity can be reduced in society.
- Understand the complex multifaceted determinants of obesity across the lifespan as this knowledge informs the development of effective public health interventions that prevent and treat obesity.
- Discuss risk factors and implications that obesity has for the health and wellbeing of individuals and families including in relation to new communicable diseases. Understand that this is important because excess adiposity is recognised as a key risk factor for acute and chronic morbidity and premature mortality.
- Recognise a range of interventions that address obesity and enable lifestyle behaviour change including physical activity and knowledge of the benefits weight loss has for individuals. Appreciate the need for interventions to demonstrate beneficial health outcomes and effective use of resources.

Introduction

Obesity is a significant contemporary health concern affecting all age groups across the lifespan and generating increased healthcare costs. It has been referred to as one of the leading preventable causes of reduced quality of life, illness and death across the population. Tackling the obesity epidemic is key to improving healthy life expectancy and reducing negative impacts on individuals, families and healthcare resources. Discussion of relevant public health policy is integrated throughout this chapter with key terms and case vignettes presented at the end.

Definition and classification of obesity

Obesity is not just cosmetic; it is a chronic non-communicable condition that increases risk of disease, ill health and death. It is a form of malnutrition classified as an over-nutrition problem occurring over time when excess calories and fat (adipose) are consumed in relation to the body's needs for their age, gender, weight and height (Jarvis and Eckhardt, 2020; World Health Organization (WHO) 2018). It is important to have standardised international/national criteria that enable professionals across the world to identify individuals at risk of obesity or who are obese. This supports consistent comparable diagnosis between professionals that can be utilised in research across countries to inform evidence-based clinical decision making and development of interventions, services, guidelines and policies, which over time may change to reflect new knowledge.

Because the classification system used to identify obesity is international, it needs to use measurements that are practicable for professionals working across a range of health and social care settings. The methods of measurement need to provide accurate assessment of adipose amount and distribution that can be used to predict health risk and decide possible interventions. Weight status is classified as 'underweight', 'normal/healthy', 'overweight', 'obesity' and 'extreme obesity' (NHS 2020a). Routine measurements of adiposity used to classify weight status include Body Mass Index (BMI) and waist circumference. Other measurements may include waist-to-height ratio and arm span (Ladwig et al. 2017). An adult with a BMI of $\geq 25\text{kg/m}^2$ is considered overweight, and an adult is considered obese if their BMI is $\geq 30\text{kg/m}^2$. Extreme obesity is classified as $\geq 40\text{kg/m}^2$ (NICE 2014). Using age- and gender-specific growth charts, children are considered overweight if their BMI is $\geq$ the 85th percentile and obese if their BMI is $\geq$ the 95th percentile. 'Tailored' intervention that considers the family situation is recommended for children who have a BMI $\geq$ 91st percentile (NICE 2014).

However, findings from published research on the use of BMI are inconsistent as it does not distinguish between muscle and fat and therefore does not provide an 'accurate measure of body fat content which reflects the proportion of muscle and fat' (Rexford and Lazar 2013, p. 857). Furthermore, it does not account for increases in fat and decreases in muscle with age, differences in fat content according to sex and race, or the distribution of intra-abdominal (visceral) and subcutaneous fat. The latter can predict the risk of obesity-related disease and can be measured using the waist-to-height ratio

(Myung et al. 2019). It is crucial that accurate methods are used to identify people who are at risk of obesity-related health issues and to this end there is evidence that the waist-to-height ratio is the most sensitive measurement and that the BMI is the least sensitive (Myung et al. 2019). Individual demographic and genetic factors, particularly sex, also need to be considered to determine a person's susceptibility to obesity.

There is limited evidence on the use of BMI as a reliable indicator of obesity for children, especially those aged ≤ 5 years (UK National Screening Committee (UK NSC) 2018a). It should be noted that BMI is an indirect measurement of adiposity and in children who are short or tall for their age it may give misleading results (Fayter et al. 2007). Hughes et al. (2011) suggest that gains in weight and BMI occur around 7 to 9 years of age and are not set before the age of 5 compared to Stuart and Panico (2016) who suggest that by 5 years of age growth trajectories indicate children who will become overweight or obese. There is consistent evidence that obese children aged 7 to 11 years have a 4 to 5 times increased risk of obesity in early adulthood (UK NSC 2018b).

UK and global prevalence

The prevalence of obesity is continuing to increase both in the UK and globally. The UK is comprised of four countries: England, Scotland, Wales and Northern Ireland. In England, the data retrieved from the National Child Measurement Programme (NCMP) in 2018/19 (Public Health England (PHE) 2019a) identified an increase in obesity levels in reception children from 9.5% in 2017/18 to 9.7% in 2018/19. Similarly, the number of children who are seriously overweight has increased for ages 10–11 years (Year 6) from 3.2% in 2006/7 to 4.4% in 2019; this suggests there are more than 26,000 children who are obese in England (PHE 2019a).

Parallel to this, NHS Digital (2019) data on 'Obesity, Physical Activity and Diet in England' reports 29% of adults are classified as obese, in comparison to 26% of adults in 2016. Overall there are comparable levels of obesity seen in men (67%) and women (62%), however, morbid obesity is most common in women (NHS Digital 2019). This has resulted in a significant increase in adult obesity from 6.9 million in 1997 to 13 million in 2017 in England (NHS Digital, 2018).

In Scotland, 'two thirds of adults (65%) are overweight and 29% are obese, and the proportion of children at risk of obesity increases with age from 11% between the ages of 2–6 years to 21% between the ages of 12–15 years' (Cheong et al. 2020, p. 4). Whilst in Wales, 60% of the adult population (1.5 million) are overweight or obese, and each year this figure rises by 10,000 (Gething 2019). Similarly, the Health Survey for Northern Ireland 2018/19 (Department of Health 2020) identified 62% of adults are overweight and 25% are obese, and 18% of children aged 2–15 years are overweight and 9% are obese.

From a global perspective, obesity levels have doubled since 1980 with nearly one-third recorded as 'overweight or obese within all ages irrespective of geographical locality, sex, ethnicity and socioeconomic status' (Chooi et al. 2019, p. 6). At this current trajectory, it is estimated that by the year 2030, there will be 1.35 million adults and 254 million children classed as obese worldwide (World Obesity Federation 2019).

Determinants of obesity

To tackle this epidemic, it is necessary to understand the complex aetiology of obesity, which is multi-faceted comprising socio-economic, environmental, biological, psychological and behavioural determinants. Determinants are factors and circumstances that positively or negatively influence health outcomes for individuals and communities, including obesity (Whitehead and Dahlgren 1991). They include employment (Hughes and Kumari 2017), educational attainment (PHE 2019c), health literacy (PHE 2015), and the presence of supermarkets and takeaways (Maguire et al. 2015, PHE 2014a).

Positive determinants protect or promote health and prevent ill health, including obesity, while negative determinants harm or present a barrier to health and can contribute to obesity (Marmot 2010). Diet and exercise are behavioural determinants that can prevent or contribute to obesity and associated chronic disease (García-Dorado et al. 2019). Because behaviour remains a critical determinant of obesity, interventions focus on changing personal choices and responsibilities as they have the potential to reduce associated disease and promote health. However, it is important to appreciate that the environment in which people live influences the choices made (Department of Health and Social Care (DHSC) 2019). It is interesting to note that evidence describes the perceptual difficulty people, including healthcare professionals, experience in detecting obesity and weight gain. Furthermore, as a person's weight increases it has been found that they will underestimate their body size.

Risk and morbidity

There is strong evidence that obesity or being overweight carries increasing risk of developing a range of chronic diseases as an individual's BMI increases (DHSC 2019). It is suggested that being obese can take up to 8 years off a person's life and cause years of disability life years (Grover et al. 2014). Abdominal adiposity causes changes in hormones and other substances released that can result in systemic or local actions associated with insulin resistance and diabetes type 2, pancreatitis, development of metabolic syndrome, cardiovascular disease, liver disease and sleep problems including sleep apnoea. For each $1kg/m^2$ increase in BMI the risk of heart failure may increase to 7% in women and to 5% in men (Haslam, 2014). Raised BMI is a key risk factor for disabling conditions that include osteoarthritis, atherosclerosis, diabetes and stroke (Kritchevsky 2017) and for some cancers (Hooper et al. 2018). Experience of stigma or bullying may impact on a person's self-esteem (Reece et al. 2015) and mental health issues including depression and anxiety are linked to obesity (PHE 2017a).

Obesity can be associated with subfertility and less successful fertility treatment. It raises significant risks during pregnancy for both mother (Denison et al. 2018) and foetal development (Farpour-Lambert et al. 2018, Widen et al. 2019). Risks to the baby include congenital anomalies, stillbirth, premature birth and neonatal death. In the UK, between 10 to 16 women out of every 100 develop gestational diabetes mellitus (GDM) (Diabetes UK 2021).

If high blood sugar levels are not managed they can lead to labour complications, a larger than average baby, low newborn blood sugar levels, and a high risk of the baby being overweight or obese in later life. Compared to women who have a healthy BMI, women with obesity are also at increased risk of miscarriage, pre-eclampsia, venous thromboembolism, anaesthetic complications, postpartum haemorrhage and wound infections (Denison et al. 2018). They are also over-represented among maternal deaths (MBRRACE-UK 2019).

Poverty causes both hunger and obesity, sometimes described as the 'obesity paradox'. This concept is also used to capture the contentious idea that adiposity may have a protective influence on the health and longevity of individuals with established chronic disease (Gupta 2016). For example, studies on the obesity paradox have reported that the lowest mortality among patients with type 2 diabetes and cardiovascular disease was in patients with BMIs of 30 to 35 kg/m² (Haslam 2014). A range of reasons have been suggested to explain the paradox, including that BMI is used inappropriately or that screening for obesity leads to earlier diagnosis and treatment.

Obesity and communicable disease

The impact of the COVID-19 pandemic on the healthcare systems and economies of Europe and the USA has directed attention to the risk posed by obesity for development of severe infection leading to longer duration of illness, secondary infections, complications and hospitalisation (Honce and Schultz-Cherry 2019). During the 2009–2010 H1N1 (Swine Flu) pandemic it was reported across several countries, including Mexico, the USA, New Zealand, Australia, Spain, France and Greece, that evidence identified that obesity has a risk factor for viral infections and of severe disease outcomes from them (von Kerkhove et al. 2011). For SARS-CoV-2 (Coronavirus) an increased prevalence of obesity in patients admitted to intensive care for invasive mechanical ventilation (IMV) has been reported (Simonnet et al. 2020). The UK Intensive Care National Audit and Research Centre (ICNARC 2020) reported that 72% of COVID-19 cases admitted to intensive care units were overweight or had obesity.

Studies of lung function have attributed association of abdominal obesity to impaired ventilation of the lungs and a reduction in lung volume due to the distribution of fat on the chest wall, abdomen and upper airway (Mafort et al. 2016). Increasing abdominal fat also undermines the mechanical effectiveness of the respiratory muscles which can lead to shallow rapid respiration (Park et al. 2012). Furthermore, obesity is shown to manifest a chronic state of low-grade inflammation due to substances released by adipose tissue that can lead to insulin resistance, atherogenesis, high blood pressure and changes in respiratory physiology.

The complex interactions that occur between adipose tissue and the immune system in obesity have been shown to disrupt the immune system's ability to fight infection, for example through dysfunction of white blood cells and decreased antigen response (Abbas et al. 2020). It is known that these substances also result in a diminished immune response to infection (Paich et al. 2013). Although identified as contributing to poor outcomes in H1N1 and COVID-19, it should be noted that knowledge of the impact obesity has on the disease course of respiratory infections is limited. It is interesting to note that evidence has shown an inverse relationship between obesity and mortality from community acquired pneumonia (Földi et al. 2020). These findings have implications for public health emphasis and policy in countries that have a high prevalence of obesity. Because obesity is a predictor of poor prognosis in COVID-19, it is important to remember that it remains a modifiable risk factor.

Behavioural factors

There is overwhelming evidence that health-related behaviours which are embedded in the socio-economic circumstances of children and adults play an important role in obesity. While changing biological and social factors may not be possible, interventions that support behaviour change at an individual level, such as promoting healthy eating and increased physical exercise, can succeed (NICE 2007). We live in an obesogenic society where children and adults eat energy-dense diets, processed and fast foods, large portion sizes, have erratic eating patterns, do not have breakfast and drink high-sugar beverages (Davies 2019, Endalifer and Diress 2020).

The National Diet and Nutrition Survey (PHE 2014b) identified 30% of 4–10-year olds' daily sugar intake was related to sugary drinks, and the Health Survey for England (NHS Digital 2018) data reported only 18% of children aged 5–15 years ate five portions of fruit and vegetables a day. Therefore, it is of no surprise that evidence shows overweight or obese boys consume between 140–500 extra calories and girls have an extra 160–290 calories, in comparison to adults who have an excess intake of between 200–300 calories (Tedstone, 2018).

Aligned to this, there are higher levels of sedentary behaviour and lower levels of physical activity. This is due to people having busy lives where there is more driving, less walking to and from work and school, sedentary roles in the workplace such as driving and office-based roles where people are sitting at a desk or in a car for more than eight hours a day, with 22% of adults being considered as inactive (NHS Digital 2019). Also, there has been an increase in inactive behaviours such as watching television and video gaming, and children and young people are sitting more using their mobile phones to communicate with friends and family. Data from Sport England (2018) found that only 18% of children and young people aged between 5–16 years were taking part in physical activity for 60 minutes a day. This clearly signifies the need to encourage children and young people to get active in their earlier years, otherwise this behaviour of inactivity will continue into their adult years.

Emotional eating, weight bias and stigma

Cultural and psychological factors have been found to impact on wellbeing in relation to body weight and adiposity. Studies not only report social and media pressure to be thin

(Dondzilo et al. 2019) but also raise the issues of emotional eating (MacDougall and Steffen 2017), weight bias (Towell-Barnard 2019) and weight stigma (Vartanian and Porter 2016). Emotional eating can be defined as eating to deal with stress and negative affect; Towell-Barnard (2019) identified its relevance to women who are caregivers of physically or cognitively impaired family members. She found that recognition of emotional eating behaviours in female caregivers could be used to identify those at risk of obesity.

'Weight bias' is described as a negative belief towards individuals because of their weight (Towell-Barnard 2019, p. 8). It is important that health and social care professionals develop awareness and insight of attitudes they may bring to bear in relation to patients, both adults and children, who are overweight or obese (Puhl et al. 2015). A recent study reported how some practitioners expressed insight into their own biases: 'If people have medical complications from their weight, I know that I tend to be less sympathetic' (Halvorson et al. 2019, p. 782). Weight bias can lead to stigma which is associated with a range of negative health and wellbeing outcomes including body dissatisfaction, low self-esteem and depression (Hargens et al. 2013).

According to Goffman (1986), stigmatisation is a social process that occurs when individuals deviate from society's norms. In consequence, they may be designated lower social worth and become a victim of prejudice, bullying and exclusion. It is reported that adolescents who are overweight or obese are more likely to be bullied and experience stigma due to their appearance and because their peers identify them as lazy or incompetent (Koyanagi et al. 2020). Conversely, it has been shown that victimisation of individuals can lead to obesogenic behaviours like impulse eating of calorie-dense foods and drinks (Albaladejo-Blàzquez et al. 2018). Stigma can also be a barrier to prevention and treatment of obesity (Puhl et al. 2018). Individuals may stay at home to avoid bullying, resulting in lower levels of exercise, or may experience sleep problems which have been shown to contribute to obesity (Hargens et al. 2013). Evidence also indicates that individuals who endure weight stigmatisation may develop 'self-stigma' due to 'weight bias internalisation'. This means that they blame themselves for their weight status and apply negative weight-based stereotypes to themselves (Puhl et al. 2018).

Addressing obesity

Introduced as part of the UK government's Childhood Obesity Plan (HM Government 2016), the Soft Drinks Industry Levy requires manufacturers to pay a charge for drinks containing more than 8g of sugar. This has encouraged proactive reductions in sugar by soft drinks manufacturers and recognises the industry's responsibility to enable healthier choices (GOV.UK 2018, 2019). An attempt to curb childhood obesity resulted in Ofcom (the communications regulator) banning adverts for food high in fat, salt and sugar during television time for children under 16 years of age (Ofcom 2006). Health and care professionals have a responsibility to provide evidence-based information to patients and clients on lifestyle risk factors such as obesity. Therefore, they should have knowledge on the most contemporary national guidelines *Obesity: Identification, Assessment and*

Management (NICE 2014) and of policies on healthy eating and physical activity such as *All Our Health: Personalised Care and Population Health* (PHE 2019a).

Public Health England (2019b) recommendations on healthy eating for children (from aged 2 onwards) and adults are encapsulated in *The Eatwell Guide* (NHS 2020b). This provides advice on eating at least five portions of a variety of fruit and vegetables a day, and to include meals with higher fibre starch foods such as potatoes, bread and rice, some dairy and alternatives such as soya drinks, beans, pulses, fish and eggs into their daily dietary intake. The latest physical activity guidelines set out by the UK Chief Medical Officer (DHSC 2019) advises that under-5s should engage in moderate to vigorous physical activity for at least three hours per day, with children and young people aged between 5–18 years undertaking at least one hour of physical activity a day. For adults the recommendation is to participate in 150 minutes' moderate physical activity or 75 minutes' vigorous activity every week.

In conjunction with addressing obesity within England, the other three countries in the UK have also introduced policies and frameworks to tackle this public health crisis, all of which have similar themes. In 2018 the Scottish Government introduced *A Healthier Future – Scotland's Diet and Healthy Weight Delivery Plan* in order to encourage eating well, to maintain a healthy weight and to deliver its ambition to halve childhood obesity by 2030. This vision is focused on five key outcomes (Scottish Government 2018, p. 8):

1   Children have the best start in life, they eat well and have a healthy weight.
2   The food environment supports healthier choices.
3   People have access to effective weight management services.
4   Leaders across all sectors promote healthy weight and diet.
5   Diet-related health inequalities are reduced.

In Wales, the *Healthy Weight: Healthy Wales. Delivery Plan 2020–2022* was introduced by the Welsh Government (2020) as a prevention strategy set out across four themes: Healthy Environments, Healthy Settings, Healthy People and Leadership and Enabling Change which focuses on eight priority areas (Welsh Government, 2020, p. 4):

1   Food and drink environment – healthier options.
2   Creating active environments and spaces.
3   Unlocking potential of the natural environment.
4   Developing healthy, active learning environments which promote emotional wellbeing.
5   Children get the best start in life and a healthy weight starting school.
6   Tackling barriers and reducing health inequalities.
7   Equitable support services to maintain a healthy weight.
8   Building a system of prevention enables leadership at every level.

The framework *A Fitter Future for All. Framework for Preventing and Addressing Overweight and Obesity in Northern Ireland 2012–2022* (DHSSPS 2012) was introduced to 'empower the population of Northern Ireland to make healthy choices to reduce the risk of being overweight and obesity related diseases, by creating an environment which promotes a physically active lifestyle and healthy diet' (DHSSPS 2012, p. 7).

Whilst policies and strategies provide an overarching framework identifying the course of action in tackling obesity, it is important to recognise how health and care professionals can address this public health issue in their role in practice. Health and care professionals have many interactions with patients and clients on a daily basis, which provide an opportunity to introduce Health Education England's (2020) *Making Every Contact Count* approach to behaviour change by starting short 30-second conversations. Public Health England (2017b) has developed the guide *Let's Talk about Weight* to support health and care professionals in having conversations with adults on achieving and maintaining a healthy weight and the benefits to weight loss, as well as referring to weight management services, using a three-step approach to consultations using the following prompts 'ASK', 'ADVISE' and 'ASSIST' (PHE 2017b, p.4).

Aligned to this, health coaching and motivational interviewing skills can be used when working with patients and clients to ensure they have the right knowledge and skills to support them to make behaviour changes through their involvement in their own care (Better Conversation 2020). Both Public Health England and the *British Medical Journal* have developed a range of professional e-learning resources on obesity and motivational interviewing (e-Learning for Healthcare 2020; HENRY 2017, NHS 2020c).

There are also a range of websites and resources to which health and care professionals can signpost patients and clients for evidence-based information on healthy eating and advice on how to increase their physical activity. This begins with the *Start4Life* (PHE 2020a) website which provides advice on healthy eating and exercise during pregnancy, weaning information looking at introducing babies to solid food and tips for healthy meals for toddlers. Once children start school, the *Change4Life* (PHE 2020b) website continues to provide support for parents and carers on making healthy choices, recipes and ways to increase physical activity.

For adults, the NHS Choices (2020) website has produced a weight loss plan, tips for healthy eating and a healthy weight calculator. In 2016 Public Health England launched the 'One You' campaign which provides recipes and tips on creating healthy meals (PHE 2016). There are also trusted health apps such as *ACTIVE10* (PHE 2020c) and *Couch to 5K* (NHS 2017) which encourage adults to increase their physical activity through brisk walking and running. Finally, take some time to review what local services are available in the community you work in, so that you can socially prescribe (signpost and refer) individuals for further support with their behaviour change.

Evaluation

The need for evidence of beneficial impact and cost-effectiveness is emphasised by Local Government and The National Institute for Health Excellence (NICE). Evaluation may be described as a method of 'systematic and objective assessment, analysis, and reporting of information on an on-going programme' (van Koperen et al. 2016, p. 2). Conventionally, experimental research designs such as random controlled trials (RCT) were used to assess the impact of an intervention. However, given the multitude of possible influences it would be difficult to attribute observed outcomes to an intervention.

Interventions and treatment of obesity are complex, multifaceted and sensitive to the political context. They may include intangible benefits that are difficult to quantify such as increased wellbeing and quality of life, or attempt to attribute economic value to efficacy or life-years saved, thereby eliciting ethical debate (Brousselle et al. 2016). There is agreement that RCTs are not always practical or appropriate so Public Health England (2018) advise use of the qualitative and quantitative methods that are most suited to answering requisite evaluation questions. Qualitative methods tend to be 'bottom up' and explore perspectives held by participants using interviews and focus groups to collect information. Quantitative methods include experimental RCTs but are more likely to use surveys and questionnaires. Evaluation is important as it can help to improve interventions, increase accountability and enable dissemination of good practice and successful elements.

Conclusion

Obesity is clearly a key UK and global public health issue that urgently needs addressing (NHS Digital 2018, 2019, WHO 2018) because it increases risk of developing associated chronic diseases and premature death (DHSC 2019). It is important to understand that the social and economic situation of individuals, families and communities is directly linked to their health, with the most disadvantaged experiencing the worst health and most likely to be overweight or obese (Davies 2019, DHSC 2019). Prevention and treatment of obesity focuses on modifiable lifestyle behaviours that require professionals who are trained and resourced to provide advice that supports weight loss (e-Learning for Healthcare (e-LH) 2020, HENRY 2017, NHS 2020c).

Consider the following questions

To consolidate and extend your learning from this chapter consider the questions below.

1. Consider why self-reported height and weight measurements are not reliable.
2. Which determinants do you think have most impact on health and why? Are these the ones that we focus on?
3. What psycho-social issues are associated with being overweight or obese?
4. Within your professional role, list information that might inform an assessment of a person's nutrition.
5. What challenges may arise from running an obesity screening programme in schools?

Key terms

Adiposity: Fat or lipid deposited in the body and is a condition of being overweight or obese.

Android obesity: Increased body fat is located particularly in the abdomen. In women it indicates increased risk of developing type 2 diabetes.

Anthropometric measurements: Values that describe the size, weight and proportions of body fat and skeletal muscle in the human body.

Arm span: Measured from the sternal notch to the tip of the middle finger, multiplied by 2. It is approximately equal to height, useful when it is not possible to measure a person's height.

Body Mass Index (BMI): A marker of ideal weight for height used as an indicator of obesity or undernutrition. NICE (2014) recommend it be used cautiously as it is not a direct measure of adiposity.

Bullying: Defined as repeated aggressive behaviours that can be physical, verbal, cyber based. Bullying acts victimise and exclude individuals and involve a power imbalance that favours the perpetrator.

Gestational diabetes mellitus (GDM): Glucose intolerance during pregnancy which usually resolves shortly after delivery but increases risk of type 2 diabetes and of GDM in future pregnancies.

Gynoid obesity: Fat near the hips, gluteus and quadriceps believed to have less risk than android obesity.

Health coaching: Provides knowledge, skills and confidence for people to become more active in their care, in order to maximise their health and wellbeing.

Health literacy: People have insufficient knowledge, understanding and confidence to access, understand, evaluate, use and navigate health and social care information and services. Poor health literacy is linked to reduced use of preventive services, less success in self-management of long-term conditions, and unhealthy lifestyle.

Invasive mechanical ventilation (IMV): Requires access to the trachea usually via an endotracheal tube that allows a mechanical ventilator to push air/oxygen flow into the patient's lungs to help them breathe. It is a common reason for admission to an Intensive Care Unit.

Life course: This approach looks at long-term effects of health and disease across the whole lifespan during gestation, childhood, adolescence, young adulthood and later adult life.

Metabolic syndrome: A combination of diabetes, high blood pressure and obesity, which carries greater risk of coronary heart disease and stroke.

Motivational interviewing: A person-centred goal-directed method, which enables a person to work through their health issues and develop a plan that works for them.

Obesogenic: An environment or lifestyle that promotes excessive weight gain.

Optimal nutrition: Nutrition consumed can support daily body requirements including any increased metabolic demand due to growth, pregnancy or illness.

Oral glucose tolerance test (OGTT): Glucose is given orally and blood samples taken afterwards to evaluate the efficiency of the body in metabolising glucose.

Over-nutrition: Consumption of nutrients, especially calories, sodium and fat, in excess of daily body needs which can lead to obesity and is a risk factor for long-term conditions.

Pandemic: Refers to infectious diseases affecting a high proportion of people across a wide geographic scale involving entire countries and crossing international boundaries to involve continents and become global. Pandemic is also used to describe non-infectious diseases, such as obesity, or risk behaviours, such as cigarette smoking, that are geographically extensive and may be rising in global incidence but are not transmissible.

Percentile: Children's height and weight is recorded on age and gender specific charts to monitor the rate of growth along 'growth curves' called 'percentile lines'. It is recognised that children come in all shapes and sizes mostly located between the extreme 5th and 95th growth percentiles. The percentile number indicates the percentage of children of that age that a child's measurements exceeds; if a child is on the 50th percentile for height they are taller than 50% of children who are the same age and gender. A steady consistent growth curve is healthy. Sudden drops or increases in a child's growth curve requires an appropriate professional to identify the reasons why.

Population health: This approach aims to improve both physical and mental health outcomes, promote wellbeing and reduce health inequalities across an entire population.

Prevalence: Provides statistics on the number of individuals in a population who are obese.

Sacropenic obesity: Low muscle mass with excess fat due to poor diet and limited exercise resulting in decreased quality of life, physical frailty and increased mortality.

Social prescribing: Often referred to as a 'community referral', this involves health and social care professionals referring people to local non-clinical services.

Undernutrition: Nutrition is inadequate to meet daily needs or added metabolic demands.

Waist circumference: Provides information on the risk of developing long-term health problems. Measurements of $\geq$ 102 cm ($\geq$ 40 inches) in men and $\geq$ 35cm ($\geq$ 88 inches) in women indicate risk. It is measured just above the iliac crests.

Waist-to-hip ratio: Assesses body fat distribution and is an indicator of risk. The waist is measured just above the iliac crests and the hips are measured at the largest circumference of the buttocks.

Further reading

BMJ Learning. 2020. *Management of Obesity.* Available at: https://learning.bmj.com/learning/module-intro/.html?locale=en_GB&moduleId=10056121& [Accessed 07.01.2020].

BMJ Learning. 2020. *Motivational Interviewing in Brief Consultations.* Available at: https://learning.bmj.com/learning/module-intro/motivational-interviewing.html?moduleId=10051582 [Accessed 07.01.2020].

Brown, T., Moore, T. H. M., Hooper, L., Gao, Y., Zayegh, A., Ijaz, S., Elwenspoek, M., Foxen, S. C., Magee, L., O'Malley, C., Waters, E., Summerbell, C. D. 2019. Interventions for preventing obesity in children. *Cochrane Database of Systematic Reviews*, Issue 7. Art. No.: CD001871.

e-Learning for Healthcare (e-LH). 2020. *Obesity: Online Learning for Healthcare and Other Practitioners Working to Tackle Obesity.* Developed in partnership with Public Health England. Available at: www.e-lfh.org.uk/programmes/obesity/ [Accessed 07.01.2020].

ICD-11. 2019. *Coding Tool for Obesity and Obesity Related Conditions in Children and Adults. Obesity. Obesity Related.* Available at: https://icd.who.int/ct11/icd11_mms/en/release [Accessed 07.01.2020].

NHS Digital. 2019. *National Child Measurement Programme 2018/19 School Year*. Available at: https://digital.nhs.uk/data-and-information/publications/statistical/national-child-measurement-programme/2018-19-school-year/final-page [Accessed 09.01.2020].

References

Abbas, A. A., Fathy, S. K., Fawzy, A. T., Salem, A. S., Shawky, M. S. 2020. The mutual effects of COVID-19 and obesity. *Obesity Medicine*; 19.

Albaladejo-Blàzquez, N., Ferrer-Cascales, R., Ruiz-Robledillo, N., Sànchez-Sansegundo, M., Clement-Carbonell, V., Zaragoza-Martí, A. 2018. Poor dietary habits in bullied adolescents: the moderating effects of diet on depression. *International Journal of Environmental Research and Public Health*; 15(8), 1569.

Better Conversation. 2020. *Better Conversation, Better Health, Health Coaching*. Available at: www.betterconversation.co.uk/ [Accessed 10.01.2020].

Brousselle, A., Benmarhnia, T., Benhadj, L. 2016. What are the benefits and risks of using return on investment to defend public health programs? *Preventive Medicine Report*; 3, 135–138.

Cheong, C., Dean, L., Dougall, I., Hinchliffe, S., Mirami, K., Vosnaki, K., Wilson, V., 2020. *The Scottish Health Survey. 2018 Edition Amended in February 2020*. Available at: www.health-ni.gov.uk/sites/default/files/publications/health/hsni-first-results-18-19_1.pdf [Accessed 15.07.2020].

Chooi, Y., Ding, C., Magkos, F. 2019. The epidemiology of obesity. *Metabolism Clinical and Experimental*; 92, 6–10. Available at: https://doi.org/10.1016/j.metabol.2018.09.005 [Accessed 12.01.2020].

Davies, S. C. 2019. *Time to Solve Childhood Obesity*. Department of Health Social Care: London. Available at: https://assets.publishing.service.gov.uk/government/uploads/system/uploads/attachment_data/file/837907/cmo-special-report-childhood-obesity-october-2019.pdf [Accessed 11.03.2022].

Denison, F. C., Aedla, N. R., Keag, O., Hor, K., Reynolds, R. M., Milne, A., Diamond., A. 2018. *Care of Women with Obesity in Pregnancy. Green-top Guideline No. 72*. Royal College of Obstetricians and Gynaecologists: London. Available at: https://obgyn.onlinelibrary.wiley.com/doi/epdf/10.1111/1471-0528.15386 [Accessed 11.03.2022].

Department of Health. 2020. *Health Survey (Northern Ireland) First Results (2018/19)*. Available at: www.health-ni.gov.uk/sites/default/files/publications/health/hsni-first-results-18-19_1.pdf [Accessed 15.07.2020].

Department of Health and Social Care. 2019. *UK Chief Medical Officers' Physical Activity Guidelines*. Available at: https://assets.publishing.service.gov.uk/government/uploads/system/uploads/attachment_data/file/832868/uk-chief-medical-officers-physical-activity-guidelines.pdf [Accessed 11.03.2022].

Department of Health, Social Services and Public Safety (DHSSPS). 2012. *A Fitter Future for All. Framework for Preventing and Addressing Overweight and Obesity in Northern Ireland 2012–2022*. Available at: www.health-ni.gov.uk/sites/default/files/publications/dhssps/obesity-fitter-future-framework-ni-2012-22.pdf [Accessed 15.07.2020].

Diabetes UK. 2021. *Diabetes Statistics*. Available at: www.diabetes.org.uk/professionals/position-statements-reports/statistics [Accessed 15.10.2021].

Dondzilo, L., Rieger, E., Jayawardena, N., Bell, J. 2019. Drive for thinness versus fear of fat: approach and avoidance motivation regarding thin and non-thin images in women. *Cognitive Therapy and Research*; 43(3), 585–593.

e-Learning for Healthcare (e-LH). 2020. *Obesity: Online Learning for Healthcare and Other Practitioners Working to Tackle Obesity*. Developed in partnership with Public Health England. Available at: www.e-lfh.org.uk/programmes/obesity/ [Accessed 07.01.2020].

Endalifer, M. L., Diress, G. 2020. Epidemiology, predisposing factors, biomarkers, and prevention mechanism of obesity: a systematic review. *Journal of Obesity*; 31 May.

Farpour-Lambert, N. J., Ells, L. J., Martinez de Tejada, B., Scott, C. 2018. Obesity and weight gain in pregnancy and postpartum: an evidence review of lifestyle interventions to inform maternal and child health policies. *Frontiers in Endocrinology*; 9, 546.

Fayter, D., Nixon, J., Hartley, S., Rithalia, A., Butler, G., Rudolf, M., Glasziou, P., Bland, M., Stirk, L., Westwood, M. 2007. A systematic review of the routine monitoring of growth in children of primary school age to identify growth-related conditions. *Health Technology Assessment*; 11(22), 1–163.

Földi, M., Farkas, N., Kiss, S., Zàdori, N., Vàncsa, S., Szakó, L., Dembrovszky, F., Solymàr, M., Bartalis, E., Szakács, Z., Hartmann, P., Pàr, G., Eröss, B., Molnár., Z., Hegyi, P., Szentesi, A. 2020. Obesity is a risk factor for developing critical condition in COVID-19 patients: a systematic review and meta-analysis. *Obesity Reviews*; 1–9.

García-Dorado, S. C., Cornselsen, L., Smith, R., Walls, H. 2019. Economic globalization, nutrition and health: a review of quantitative evidence. *Globalization and Health*; 15, 15.

Gething, V. 2019. *Health minister launches ambitious new plan to halt obesity rise in Wales*. Available at: https://gov.wales/health-minister-launches-ambitious-new-plan-halt-obesity-rise-wales [Accessed 15.07.2020].

Goffman, E. 1986. *Stigma. Notes on the Management of A Spoiled Identity*. Simon & Schuster: New York.

GOV.UK. 2018. *Soft Drinks Industry Levy Comes into Effect*. Available at: www.gov.uk/government/news/soft-drinks-industry-levy-comes-into-effect [Accessed 12.01.2020].

GOV.UK. 2019. *Statistics on Obesity, Physical Activity and Diet, England 2019*. Available at: https://digital.nhs.uk/data-and-information/publications/statistical/statistics-on-obesity-physical-activity-and-diet/statistics-on-obesity-physical-activity-and-diet-england-2019 [Accessed 07.01.2020].

Grover, S. A., Kaouache, M., Rempel, P., Joseph, L., Dawes, M., Lau, D. C. W., Lowensteyn, I. 2014. Years of life lost and healthy life-years lost from diabetes and cardiovascular disease in overweight and obese people: a modelling study. *The Lancet Diabetes and Endocrinology*; 3, 114–122.

Gupta, S. 2016. Obesity: the fat advantage. *Nature*; 537(7620), S100–S102.

Halvorson, E. E., Curley, T., Wright, M., Skelton, J. A. 2019. Weight bias in paediatric inpatient care. *Academic Paediatrics*; 19(7).

Hargens, T. A., Kaleth, A. S., Edwards, E. S., Butner, K. L. 2013. Association between sleep disorders, obesity, and exercise: a review. *Nature and Science of Sleep*; 5, 27–35.

Haslam, D. 2014. Obesity in primary care: prevention, management and the paradox. *BMC Medicine*; 12, 149.

Health Education England. 2020. *Making Every Contact Count.* Available at: www.makingeverycontactcount.co.uk [Accessed 10.01.2020].

HENRY. 2017. *Royal Society for Public Health – Accredited Training for Practitioners Working with Young Families.* Available at: https://henry.org.uk/ www.henry.org.uk/sites/www.henry.org.uk/files/2017-12/HENRY-A_Better_Start_case_study.pdf [Accessed 11.03.2022].

HM Government. 2016. *Childhood Obesity: A Plan for Action.* Available at: https://assets.publishing.service.gov.uk/government/uploads/system/uploads/attachment_data/file/546588/Childhood_obesity_2016__2__acc.pdf [Accessed 11.03.2022].

Honce, R., Schultz-Cherry, S. 2019. Impact of obesity on influenza a virus pathogenesis, immune response, and evolution. *Frontiers in Immunology*; 10, 1071.

Hooper, L., Anderson, A. S., Birch, J., Forster, A. S., Rosenberg, G., Bauld, L., Vohra, J. 2018. Public awareness and healthcare professional advice for obesity as a risk factor for cancer in the UK: a cross-sectional survey. *Journal of Public Health*; 40(4), 797–805.

Hughes, A., Kumari, M. 2017. Unemployment, underweight, and obesity: findings from understanding society (UKHLS). *Preventive Medicine*; 97, 19–25.

Hughes, A. R., Sherriff, A., Lawlor, D. A., Ness, A. R., Reilly, J. J. 2011. Timing of excess weight gain in the Avon Longitudinal Study of Parents and Children (ALSPAC). *Paediatrics*; 127(3), e730-6.

Intensive Care National Audit and Research Centre (ICNARC). 2020. *Report on 196 Patients Critically Ill with COVID-19.* Available at: www.icnarc.org/About/Latest-News [Accessed August 2020].

Jarvis, C., Eckhardt, A. (2020) *Physical Examination and Health Assessment.* (8th edn). Elsevier: St Louis, MO.

Koyanagi, A., Veronese, N., Vancampfort, D., Stickley, A., Jackson, S. A., Oh, H., Shin, J. L., Haro, J. M., Stubbs, B., Smith, L. 2020. Association of bullying victimization with overweight and obesity among adolescents from 41 low- and middle-income countries. *Paediatric Obesity*; 15(1), e12571.

Kritchevsky, S. B. 2017. Taking obesity in older adults seriously. *Journal of Gerontology: Series A, Biological Sciences and Medical Sciences*; 73(1), 57–58.

Ladwig, G. B., Ackley, B. J., Makic, M. B. F., Martinez-Kratz, M. R., Zanotti, M. 2017. *Mosby's Guide to Nursing Diagnosis.* (6th edn). Elsevier: St Louis, MO.

MacDougall, M., Steffen, A. 2017. Self-efficacy for controlling upsetting thoughts and emotional eating in family caregivers; *Aging & Mental Health*, 21(10).

Mafort, T. T., Rufino, R., Costa, C. H., Lopes, A. J. 2016. Obesity: systemic and pulmonary complications, biochemical abnormalities, and impairment of lung function. *Multidisciplinary Respiratory Medicine*; 11, 28.

Maguire, E. R, Burgoine, T., Monsivais, P. 2015. Area deprivation and the food environment over time: a repeated cross-sectional study on takeaway outlet density and supermarket presence in Norfolk, UK, 1990–2008. *Health Place*; 33, 142–147.

Marmot, M. 2010. *Fair Society, Healthy Lives.* Marmot Review: London.

MBRRACE-UK. 2019. *Saving Lives, Improving Mothers' Care. Lessons learned to inform maternity care from the UK and Ireland Confidential Enquiries into Maternal Deaths and Morbidity 2015–17.* https://www.npeu.ox.ac.uk/assets/downloads/mbrrace-uk/reports/ MBRRACE-UK Maternal Report 2019- WEB VERSION pdf

Myung, J., Jung, K. Y., Kim, T. H., Han, U. 2019. Assessment of the validity of multiple obesity indices compared with obesity-related co-morbidities. *Public Health Nutrition;* 22(7), 1241–1249.

NHS. 2017. *Couch to 5K.* Available at: www.nhs.uk/live-well/exercise/couch-to-5k-week-by-week/ [Accessed 10.01.2020].

NHS. 2020a. *What is the Body Mass Index (BMI)?* Available at: www.nhs.uk/common-health-questions/lifestyle/what-is-the-body-mass-index-bmi/ [Accessed 07.01.2020].

NHS. 2020b. *The Eatwell Guide.* Available at: www.nhs.uk/live-well/eat-well/the-eatwell-guide/ [Accessed 10.01.2020].

NHS. 2020c. *Start the NHS Weight Loss Plan.* Available at: www.nhs.uk/live-well/healthy-weight/start-the-nhs-weight-loss-plan/ [Accessed 07.01. 2020].

NHS Choices. 2020. *Tips for Healthy Eating.* Available at: www.nhs.uk/live-well/eat-well/ eight-tips-for-healthy-eating/ [Accessed 10.01.2020].

NHS Digital. 2018. *Health Survey for England 2017.* Available at: https://digital.nhs.uk/ data-and-information/publications/statistical/health-survey-for-england/2017 [Accessed 09.01.2020].

NHS Digital. 2019. *Statistics on Obesity, Physical Activity and Diet, England.* Available at: https://digital.nhs.uk/data-and-information/publications/statistical/statistics-on-obesity-physical-activity-and-diet/statistics-on-obesity-physical-activity-and-diet-england-2019 [Accessed 09.01.2020].

NICE. 2007. *Behaviour Change: General Approaches. Public Health Guideline [PH6].* Available at: www.nice.org.uk/guidance/ph6/chapter/1-public-health-need-and-practice [Accessed 07.01 2020].

NICE. 2014. *Obesity: Identification, Assessment and Management. Clinical Guideline [CG189].* Available at: www.nice.org.uk/guidance/cg189 [Accessed 07.01.2020].

Ofcom. 2006. *Television Advertising of Food and Drink Products to Children.* Available at: www.ofcom.org.uk/consultations-and-statements/category-2/foodads_new [Accessed 09.01.2020].

Paich, H. A., Sheridan, P. A. P., Handy, J., Karlsson, E. A., Schultz-Cherry, S., Hudgens, M. G., Noah, T. L., Weir, S. S., Beck, M. A. 2013. Overweight and obese adult humans have a defective cellular immune response to pandemic H1N1 influenza A virus. *Obesity;* 21(11), 2377–2386.

Park, J. E., Chung, J. H., Lee, K. H., Shin, K. C. 2012. The effect of body composition on pulmonary function. *Tuberculosis and Respiratory Diseases;* 72(5), 433–440.

Public Health England. 2014a. *Healthy People, Healthy Places Briefing. Obesity and the Environment: Regulating the Growth of Fast Food Outlets.* Available at: https://assets. publishing.service.gov.uk/government/uploads/system/uploads/attachment_data /file/296248/Obesity_and_environment_March2014.pdf [Accessed 11.03.2022].

Public Health England. 2014b. *National Diet and Nutrition Survey: Results from Years 1,2,3 and 4 (combined) of the Rolling Programme (2008/2009–2011/2012) Executive Summary.* Available at: https://assets.publishing.service.gov.uk/government/uploads/system/uploads/attachment_data/file/594360/NDNS_Y1_to_4_UK_report_executive_summary_revised_February_2017.pdf [Accessed 11.03.2022].

Public Health England. 2015. *Local Action on Health Inequalities. Improving Health Literacy to Reduce Health Inequalities.* Available at: https://assets.publishing.service.gov.uk/government/uploads/system/uploads/attachment_data/file/460709/4a_Health_Literacy-Full.pdf [Accessed 11.03.2022].

Public Health England. 2016. *The Eatwell Guide: How Does it Differ to the Eatwell Plate and Why?* Available at: https://assets.publishing.service.gov.uk/government/uploads/system/uploads/attachment_data/file/528201/Eatwell_guide_whats_changed_and_why.pdf [Accessed 11.03.2022].

Public Health England. 2017a. *Working Together to Address Obesity in Adult Mental Health Secure Units. A Systematic Review of the Evidence and a Summary of the Implications for Practice.* Available at: https://assets.publishing.service.gov.uk/government/uploads/system/uploads/attachment_data/file/591875/obesity_in_mental_health_secure_units.pdf [Accessed 11.03.2022].

Public Health England. 2017b. *Let's Talk about Weight: A Step-by-step Guide to Brief Interventions with Adults for Health and Care Professionals.* Available at: https://assets.publishing.service.gov.uk/government/uploads/system/uploads/attachment_data/file/737904/LTAW_Final_Infographic_Oct_2017_adults.pdf [Accessed 17.03.2022].

Public Health England. 2018. *Guidance. Evaluation Methods.* Available at: www.gov.uk/government/publications/evaluation-in-health-and-well-being-overview/evaluation-methods [Accessed August 2020].

Public Health England. 2019a. *All Our Health: Personalised Care and Population Health.* Available at: www.gov.uk/government/collections/all-our-health-personalised-care-and-population-health [Accessed 09.01.2020].

Public Health England. 2019b. *Childhood Obesity: Applying All Our Health.* Available at: www.gov.uk/government/publications/childhood-obesity-applying-all-our-health/childhood-obesity-applying-all-our-health [Accessed 07.01.2020].

Public Health England. 2019c. *Adult Obesity: Applying All Our Health.* Available at: www.gov.uk/government/publications/adult-obesity-applying-all-our-health/adult-obesity-applying-all-our-health [Accessed 07.01.2020].

Public Health England. 2020a. *Start4Life.* Available at: www.nhs.uk/start4life/weaning/what-to-feed-your-baby/around-6-months/ [Accessed 10.01.2020].

Public Health England. 2020b. *Change4Life.* Available at: www.nhs.uk/change4life/about-change4life [Accessed 10.01.2020].

Public Health England. 2020c. *ACTIVE10.* Available at: www.nhs.uk/oneyou/active10/home [Accessed 10.01. 2020].

Puhl, R. M, Himmelstein, M. S., Quinn, D. M. 2018. Internalizing weight stigma: prevalence and sociodemographic considerations in US adults. *Obesity*; 26, 167–175.

Puhl, R. M., Latner, J. L., O'Brien, K., Luedicke, J. L., Danielstottir, S., Forhan, M. 2015. A multi-national examination of weight bias: predictors of anti-fat attitudes across four countries. *International Journal of Obesity*; 39, 1166–1173.

Reece, L. J., Bissell, P., Copeland, R. J. 2015. 'I just don't want to get bullied anymore, then I can lead a normal life'; insights into life as an obese adolescent and their views on obesity treatment. *Health Expectations*; 19, 897–907.

Rexford, A., Lazar, M. 2013. The health risk of obesity – better metrics imperative. *Science*; 341(6148), 856–858.

Scottish Government. 2018. *A Healthier Future – Scotland's Diet and Healthy Weight Delivery Plan*. Available at: www.gov.scot/publications/healthier-future-scotlands-diet-healthy-weight-delivery-plan/ [Accessed 15.07.2020].

Simonnet, A., Chetboun, M., Poissy, J., Raverdy, V., Noulette, J., Duhamel, A., Labreuche, J., Mathieu, D., Pattou, F., Jourdain, M. 2020. High prevalence of obesity in SARS-CoV-2 requiring invasive mechanical ventilation. *Obesity (Silver Spring)*; 28, 1195–1199.

Sport England. 2018. *Active Lives Children and Young People Survey. Academic Year 2017/18*. Available at: www.sportengland.org/media/13698/active-lives-children-survey-academic-year-17-18.pdf [Accessed 11.03.2022].

Stuart, B., Panico, L. 2016. Early-childhood BMI trajectories: evidence from a prospective, nationally representative British cohort study. *Nutrition and Diabetes*; 26, e198.

Tedstone, A. (2018) *Why we are working to reduce calorie intake*. Available at: https://publichealthmatters.blog.gov.uk/2018/03/06/why-we-are-working-to-reduce-calorie-intake/ [Accessed 10.01.2020].

Towell-Barnard, A. 2019. Weight bias and stigma: how do we really feel about the obese patient? *Journal of Stomal Therapy Australia*; 39(3), 8–10.

UK National Screening Committee (UK NSC). 2018a. *Screening for Obesity in Children ≤5 Years. External Review Against Programme Appraisal Criteria for the UK National Screening Committee (UK NSC)* Version: Draft 2018 update (public consultation document).

UK National Screening Committee (UK NSC). 2018b. *Screening for Obesity in Children of 7-11 Years. External Review Against Programme Appraisal Criteria for the UK National Screening Committee (UK NSC)* Version: Draft 2018 update (public consultation document).

van Koperen, T. M., Renders, C. M., Spierings, E. J. M., Hendriks, A., Westerman, M. J., Seidell, J. C., Schuit, A. J. 2016. Recommendations and improvements for the evaluation of integrated community-wide interventions approaches. *Journal of Obesity*. https://doi.org/10.1155/2016/2385698

Vartanian, L. R., Porter, A. M. 2016. Weight stigma and eating behavior: a review of the literature. *Appetite*; 102, 3–14.

von Kerkhove, M. D., Vandemaele, K. A., Shinde, V., Jaramillo-Gutierrez, G., Koukounari, A., Donnelly, C. A., Carlino, L. O., Owen, R., Paterson, B., Pelletier, L., Vachon, J., Gonzalez, C., Hongjie, Y., Zijian, F., Chuang, S. K., Au, A., Buda, S., Krause, G., Haas,

W., Bonmarin, I., Taniguichi, K., Nakajima, K., Shobayashi, T., Takayama, Y., Sunagawa, T., Heraud, J.M., Orelle, A., Palacios, E., van der Sande, M. A. B., Wielders, C. C. H. L., Hunt, D., Cutter, J., Lee, V. J., Thomas, J., Santa-Olalla, P., Sierra-Moros, M. J., Hanshaoworakul, W., Ungchusak, K., Pebody, R., Jain, S., Mounts, S. W. 2011. Risk factors for severe outcomes following 2009 influenza A (H1N1) infection: a global pooled analysis. *PLoS Medicine*; 8, e1001053.

Welsh Government. 2020. *Healthy Weight: Healthy Wales. Delivery Plan 2020–2022.* Available at: https://gov.wales/sites/default/files/publications/2020-02/healthy-weight-delivery-plan-2020-22.pdf [Accessed 15.01.2020].

Whitehead, M., Dahlgren, C. 1991. What can we do about inequalities in health. *The Lancet*; 338, 1059–1063.

Widen, E. M., Nichols, A. M., Kahn, L. G., Factor-Litvak, P., Insel, B. J., Hoepner, L., Dube, S. M., Rauh, V., Perera, F., Rundle, A. 2019. Pre-pregnancy obesity is associated with cognitive outcomes in boys in a low-income, multi-ethnic birth cohort. *BMC Paediatrics*; 19, 507.

World Health Organization. 2018. *Obesity and Overweight. Key Facts.* Available at: www.who.int/en/news-room/fact-sheets/detail/obesity-and-overweight [Accessed 07.01.2020].

World Obesity Federation. 2019. *Atlas of Childhood Obesity Summary Brief.* Available at: www.worldobesity.org/ [Accessed 12.01.2020].

10

PUBLIC HEALTH AND THE OLDER PERSON

SHIRLEY WILLIS AND CATHRYN SMITH

LEARNING OUTCOMES

By the end of this chapter you will be able to:

* Explore the national and international picture of the older population.
* Understand the theories of ageing.
* Discuss the concept of healthy ageing.
* Explore the impact of loneliness for the older person.

Introduction

The aim of this chapter is to explore the promotion of health in the context of the older adult. It is a popularly held view among the general population that 'old age does not come alone' and indeed it is widely accepted that chronic diseases are largely age related (Carrier 2016), with almost all older adults reporting living with one (or more) long-term conditions (Swerisson and Taylor 2014). Even though some older people will experience old age with support and friendship, for many poor health or disability can mean that this all changes, with the result that people become more dependent on those around them.

The health of the older person is largely a manifestation of the cumulative effects of health behaviours and social influences across the lifespan. With clear evidence of an ageing population globally, the challenge now is to determine how we might best support healthy ageing in the 21st century (McMurry and Clendon 2015) so that older adults can live a fulfilling and rewarding older age.

Defining old age

Defining 'old age' is fraught with difficulty and depends on the perspective from which the definition arises. In Westernised countries the chronological age of 60 or 65 is generally accepted as when a person enters old age. This is largely a political construct and is associated with retirement and receipt of pension benefits in many countries around the world. However, as the World Health Organization (WHO 2002) points out this is an arbitrary measure and does not account for social, environmental or cultural factors and so cannot be applied globally. As Groman (1999) points out, whilst ageing does have a biological element, it is also an experience that is unique to that individual and is influenced by the way that society views and makes sense of old age.

From a sociological perspective, we may need to alter our view of old age to make sense of the demographic changes within the population if we are to support healthy ageing across societies. If 60 is the new 40, then does this mean that 80 is the new 60? This being the case, then the traditional view of old age and the roles of the older person in society will of necessity have to change (Van Teijlingen 2019).

The demographics of ageing

The concept of an ageing population, both nationally and globally, is well documented with the WHO estimating that by 2050 one in five people will be aged 60 or over, equating to 2 billion people worldwide (WHO 2017). From a European perspective the picture is similar, with the number of over 65s projected to double by 2050 in a population that already has the highest median age in the world (WHO 2012). In the UK, the demographic changes within the population reflect this global picture. According to the Office for National Statistics (ONS 2019) in 1997, around one in every six people (15.9%) were aged 65 years and over, increasing to one in every five people (18.2%) in 2017 and is projected to reach around one in every four people (24%) by 2037. More importantly, the over-65 age group is growing faster than any other age group across the UK, primarily due to falls in both birth and death rates which leads to increasing longevity within the population and consequently an ageing population (ONS 2019). See Figure 10.1 for comparison of the elderly population in the UK, Australia, Japan and the USA.

Across all four home nations, it is evident that there is an increasingly older population, and this presents some real opportunities for older people to contribute to society and participate in a meaningful way to benefit the wider community. However, the key factor that determines how older people can interact within society is governed not by their age but by their health (WHO 2017). There is an imperative, then, that the public health agenda needs to recognise and address some of the health challenges faced by older people as there is a real benefit both to the individual and to society as a whole in supporting healthy ageing across the population (Liotta et al. 2018, O'Rourke et al. 2018).

In high-income countries, health systems are often aimed at caring for patients with acute conditions rather than managing the consequences of chronic conditions that are prevalent in older age (Goodwin et al. 2013). If systems are in place these are usually in silos and therefore address each of the issues separately resulting in poly pharmacy and unnecessary interventions (Low et al. 2011, Peron et al. 2011). In low-income countries health systems are limited. Little training is experienced by health workers who may not know how to deal with conditions that are common in older age, such as dementia. Therefore, early diagnosis, treatment and management is often missed (WHO 2015).

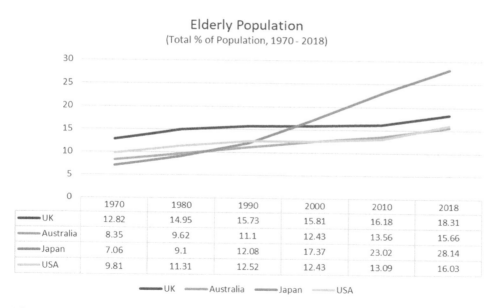

Figure 10.1 Elderly population for selected OECD countries 1970–2018 (OECD 2020)

Contemporary society has been seen to be committed to provide effective services in both health and social care; these services are guided by national and regional policies and frameworks that are diverse and always evolving: the Social Services and Well-being (Wales) Act 2014 (National Assembly for Wales 2014), Public Health England Strategy 2020–2025 (Public Health England 2019a) and the Public Health Wales Strategic Plan 2019–2022 (Public Health Wales 2019) to name a few. The message that is common within all contemporary health and social care policy is that of protecting and improving the health of the population, with particular reference to supporting healthy ageing.

However, with the increasing older population and the increasing life expectancy, important questions arise. Will an ageing population experience good health, with high-quality wellbeing and prolonged periods of social engagement? Or will it be accompanied by illness, loss of independence, disability with added cost to health and social care services? The role of public health is to promote, protect and repair the health of a population (Watkins and Cousins 2010). Given the rise in non-communicable diseases with increasing age, the role that public health must play is as significant to today's ageing society as in the past. In the future we know that the population is living longer, and it is important that it is lived in good health.

The theory of ageing

The theory of ageing is one that is still much debated (Blais 2014) and questions have been raised around the physiological, social and psychological reason as to why people die. Many biological theories (Table 10.1) have been expounded, including the effect of metabolism, stress, free radicals and molecular degradation, genetics and genetic degradation, diet, the role of the immune system and environmental factors in association with cellular breakdown as a consequence of ageing (Trevisan et al. 2019). Perhaps more interestingly from a public health perspective are the psychosocial theories (Table 10.2). Concepts identified within these theories acknowledge the uniqueness of the ageing process to the individual, and consider the adjustments that people make as they age. Insight into this aspect of ageing provides the underpinning basis for many public health interventions to support individuals to achieve healthy ageing and to continue to make a positive and meaningful contribution to society (Trail Ross and Summerlin 2015).

Table 10.1 Biological theories of ageing (Van Teijlingen and Humphries 2019, Edelman et al. 2014)

Biological Theories of Ageing	
Stochastic Theories: events that occur randomly and accumulate over time	**Nonstochastic Theories**: ageing is predetermined
Error Theory	Programmed Theory
Somatic Mutation Theory	Immunological Theory
Free Radical Theory	Neurogenic Control or Pacemaker Theory
Cross-linkage Theory	
Wear and Tear Theory	

Table 10.2 Psychosocial and developmental theories of ageing (Van Teijlingen and Humphries 2019, Edelman et al. 2014)

Disengagement Theory (Cumming and Henry 1961)	Ageing is inevitable and the individual withdraws or disengages from society. There is decreased interaction between the ageing person and society as a whole and the individual slowly withdraws from former roles and activities.
Activity Theory (Havighurst et al. 1963)	Remaining active and involved with society is necessary to achieve life satisfaction in ageing.
Continuity Theory (Havighurst et al. 1968)	The individual continues throughout life in a similar fashion as they have always done in the past. Personality remains constant and this influences role activity and life satisfaction.
Erickson's Development Theory (Erickson 1982)	Predetermined order of development and specific tasks are associated with specific periods across the lifespan. For older adults, the developmental stage is integrity versus despair.
Tornstam's Theory of Gerotranscendance (Tornstam 1989)	Ageing is viewed as the movement from birth to death and maturation towards wisdom.

The view that ageing will inevitably lead to physical and psychological decline is one that is widely held. From a bio-medical perspective, ageing may be seen as the physical manifestation of an increasing life expectancy. Old age is often perceived as a 'problem' with any potential solutions placed firmly within the medical agenda (Van Teijlingen 2009). However, in reality ageing is an ongoing process across the lifespan and is multi-factorial in nature with psychological and social factors that interact with the inevitable underlying biological changes (see Figure 10.2). Ageing is often viewed by Western societies in a negative way, although this cannot be applied universally as in many cultures

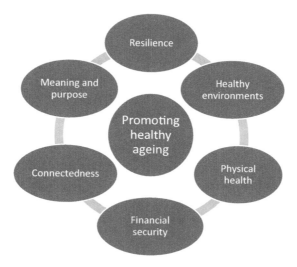

Figure 10.2 The complexity of healthy ageing (adapted from Public Health England 2019b)

the elderly are revered for their life experiences. Conversely, WHO (2017) takes the view that ageing is a valuable if often challenging process, but that society as a whole benefits from having an older population.

Healthy ageing

Public health has seen a marked improvement in life expectancy over the last 100 years, yet health inequalities persist across populations. While there is a shift in distribution of population towards older age, there is insufficient evidence to suggest that the older population are in fact living with better health than their predecessors. It is suggested that in the UK, men aged 65 can expect to live only about half of their remaining life expectancy without disability (10 out of 19 years), whilst for women only 10 out of their expected 21 years is likely to be lived free of any disability (Office for National Statistics 2018a). This then must be the public health challenge to be addressed and leads us to ponder the question whether the increasingly ageing population is a symbol of successful health service provision or a burden requiring costly health interventions to maintain.

It is evident that society can benefit greatly from a healthy, active and participative older population (WHO 2015, 2017), but the impact of the wider social determinants of health (Dahlgren and Whitehead 1993) across the lifespan do affect the functional ability and capacity of the individual in older age. Whilst the biopsychosocial model of health is well recognised and provides the basis for much of the public health agenda, it could be argued that for the older person the psychological element becomes increasingly important in terms of promoting overall health. This approach focuses on the promotion of social activity and engagement and remaining physically active in order to make a meaningful contribution to society.

Loneliness

Social isolation itself is well recognised as a prevalent and urgent public health issue (Lasgaard et al. 2016). Loneliness is a problem across the population, but older people may be seen as particularly at risk. The ONS (2018b) suggests that whilst loneliness may strike at any point across the lifespan, older homeowners living alone with long term health conditions are particularly at risk. Social life for the older person changes dramatically as the individual's peer group becomes diminished, and widowhood compounds this further (Christiansen et al. 2016). The late Jo Cox MP (2017) identified the impact that loneliness can have on individuals and on society as a whole and suggested that tackling loneliness is a 'generational challenge' if we are to achieve a 'less lonely, more connected' world recognising the multifactorial nature of loneliness across the lifespan and in older age more specifically.

Loneliness may be defined as 'a negative, distressing emotional response to a discrepancy between one's desired and actual social relationships' (Peplau and Perlman 1982). Lasgaard et al. (2016) make the distinction between loneliness and social isolation suggesting that whilst these are not synonymous, there is a relationship in terms of the quality and quantity of social contact. Loneliness is a very subjective experience that is unique to the individual and Jopling (2015) makes the distinction that social isolation is a more objective state that can be measured in the context of the number and quality of social interactions.

For some, older age can appear as a 'golden opportunity' to do all the activities that have previously been constrained by the need to work and care for children or elderly relatives. However, for many, older age can appear as a perfect storm of life events associated with loss and negativity. Retirement can signify the loss of social identity, social support networks and of purpose and meaning to some individuals. The loss of a spouse or loved one through death and the gradual decline of the individual's peer group can lead to social isolation and loneliness accompanied by the loss of independence and purpose in life (Figure 10.3). The consequences for the mental and physical health of the individual of this combined assault is significant (see Figure10.4).

The impact of loneliness on health

The impact on health in older age of the experience of loneliness at any point across the lifespan, including childhood and adolescence, should not be underestimated (Caspi et al. 2006). There is a significant body of evidence to support the concept of loneliness as a risk factor for poor physical and mental health in the older adult (Caspi et al. 2006, Hawkley et al. 2010, Luanaigh and Lawlor 2008, Pressman et al. 2005). Furthermore, Holt-Lunstead and Smith (2015) argue that loneliness as a risk factor should be considered alongside inactivity and obesity as a predictor of mortality.

It is clear that people deal with loneliness differently and this is determined by a multitude of factors including gender, personality and capacity for resilience (McMurry and Clendon 2015). Women tend to rely on wider friendship networks and value their homes and independence. Men, on the other hand, often find it difficult to stay at home

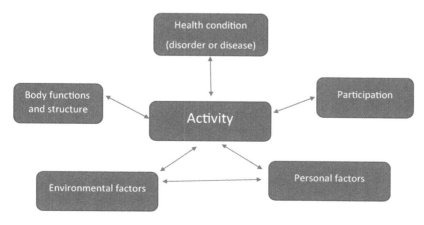

Figure 10.3 Model for disability and ageing (adapted from WHO 2002)

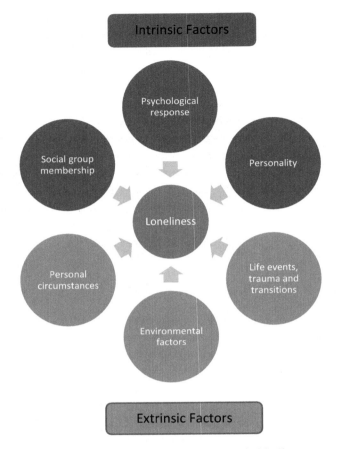

Figure 10.4 Pathways into loneliness (Goodman et al. 2015)

but find it challenging to join new social groups. Men have a tendency to rely on fewer long-standing friendships and this in turn limits their opportunities to socialise within a wider social circle. This then needs to be considered from a public health perspective when considering services that aim to address loneliness in older age and to encourage the older person to engage in social activities.

Challenges for the older LGBTQ population

In 2017 the UK saw an increase in the percentage of lesbian, gay and bisexual individuals to 2% of the overall population (ONS 2019). Even though this percentage represents a small minority of the population some individuals are reluctant to identify their sexuality and therefore that percentage could be much higher. Furthermore, men are more likely to identify their sexuality than women, and similarly younger people are more likely to identify this than the older generation (ONS 2019), so there is a real concern that the older LGBTQ population is at risk of going unnoticed and therefore unsupported by public health services. For the population of adults aged 50 years and over it was reported that nearly 2% of females reported as LGB compared to nearly 3% for males (ONS 2019). This then poses a challenge for public health services as the LGBTQ community remains a sector of the population that is likely to be 'hidden' and potentially reluctant to access services.

Globally, there is in general some reluctance around disclosing sexuality, with a strong leaning towards seeing sexuality as a private affair. Whilst health and social care services in Western democracies, privacy and confidentiality is valued and protected, in countries where social protection and legal acknowledgement for the LGBTQ community is limited or absent, the health of this population has been adversely affected by the impact of discrimination. In addition, for the LGBTQ in older age, there has been a failure of health and social care services to meet the needs of this group with the absence of any recognition of LGBTQ issues in old age (AGE Platform Europe and ILGA-Europe 2012). Even in countries that offer legal rights, the experiences reported show that older LGBTQ people experience a variety of health inequalities. Yet it is odd to think that these health inequalities occur in a health and social care service where privacy is valued and protected; nevertheless, some LGBTQ people have misgivings about sharing information with medical providers about sexual practices due to concerns over confidentiality and stigma.

Research in relation to the needs of older LGBTQ people is a growing area (Fredriksen-Goldsen et al. 2010, Ward et al. 2010), yet healthcare policies and procedures seem to overlook the distinctive needs of older LGBTQ people (Ward et al. 2010). Within the National Health Interview Survey (NHIS 2013–2014) it was found that lesbian, gay and bisexual individuals over the age of 50 had a higher prevalence of chronic conditions, mental distress and disability compared to heterosexual individuals of a similar age. Similarly, transgender older adults had a higher risk of disability, poor health outcomes and elevated risk of victimisation (Fredriksen-Goldsen et al. 2014). This therefore poses the question of the demand on the delivery of the public health agenda, and how health professionals care for these individuals now and in the future.

The older LGBTQ community and health care

Within the LGBTQ community is a wide range of people from different socioeconomic backgrounds, ethnicities and age and therefore should be seen as a heterogeneous group rather than a homogenous one. There has been a long history of discrimination linked to health care, and a lack of awareness by health care professionals has resulted in this community facing many challenges, one being attaining a high level of good health due to the challenges in accessing culturally competent health care services (Ard and Makadon 2012). The older generation within health care are nearly all assumed to be heterosexual and therefore when it comes to accessing services the older LGBTQ population is recurrently invisible. This can add to the social isolation that some older people experience due to the fear of prejudice and lack of visibility (Power et al. 2010).

So why is it that growing older affects the LGBTQ community in a disproportionate way? To answer part of this question we will look at the fact that this community does not always have access to the same circle of family and friends support that many take for granted. Stonewall (2011) found that LGBTQ people were more likely to live alone and have little support from family and friends compared to heterosexual people. The problem of loneliness and social isolation in older age for this group is compounded and poses an additional challenge for public health services. This therefore leans itself to the importance of the availability of external services for older LGBTQ people, as they are twice as likely to rely on these services compared to their heterosexual peers. Fundamentally it is also important to realise the continued gap in the provision of these community services for the LGBTQ community, which tend to focus primarily on younger people. Traditional services for the older person tend to be quite generic to meet the needs of the majority, with the result that LGBTQ people can feel unwelcome.

Moving into a care home is an emotional process for any person; the process to get to that stage can be a gradual one or one of quick transition. There is a misguided assumption that everyone who resides in a care home is heterosexual. It is estimated that in a 120-bed care home 8 of those residents would be from an LGBTQ community (Heath 2012, Age Concern 2006). To add to this, almost half of LGBTQ people do not feel comfortable in 'coming out' to their carers, with nearly 70% claiming they would not be able to be themselves in a care home setting (Stonewall 2011). Equally the fear of rejection causes profound anxieties when considering residential care (Stein et al. 2010). Within the literature the fears around the need for residential care is seen as a social reality; attitudinal research suggests that residential care home staff attitudes towards older people's sexual activity is varied. There were also many issues around the possibility of care home staff being discriminatory towards older LGBTQ people, with many providers demonstrating limited awareness and understanding of sexual orientation (Commission for Social Care Inspection 2008). Within the UK mostly all care home managers were found to be more permissive in their attitudes than the care home staff who carry out the direct care (Bouman et al. 2007), this could result in isolation and loneliness in a place that should be full of warmth and safety (Ward et al. 2010).

We should be reluctant to advocate a 'how to work with LGBTQ older adults' approach to the development of public health services, as this can imply that this population group have different health care needs. There is a risk that this approach would further add to the divide that already exists and sustain the social divisions between different groups whilst overlooking diversity within the wider community. Instead we should not assume a person's identity or sexual preference and instead encourage and support individuals through the path they take.

Tackling the issue

So the imperative to address loneliness in older age is well established, but the challenge for public health services now is in identifying the lonely and socially isolated within the general population. Put simply: how do you engage with a group that is already socially isolated? In contemporary society it is easy to assume that everyone is connected through the medium of social media platforms, but from an ethical perspective of social justice this is a dangerous assumption to make.

Whilst it would be erroneous to assume that all elderly people are lonely and socially isolated, it is clear that loneliness is a significant risk for older people and does have an impact on the physical and mental health of the individual. The development of strategies to increase the social activity and participation within society has been a key driver in developing public health policy (see Figure 10.5), and in turn to address the social inequalities that still exist in our 21st century society (Marmot 2011, 2018).

According to Dickens et al. (2011) the evidence for the effectiveness of public health interventions aimed at addressing loneliness and social isolation is ambiguous at best. Generally, interventions can be categorised into those which are delivered one-to-one or in a group, and may either focus on engagement with specific activities or those that offer support and signposting information. O'Rourke et al. (2018) go further and propose that in reality it is very difficult to determine whether interventions aimed at reducing loneliness and social isolation actually achieve their stated aims. However, it is interesting to note that Calder et al. (2018) consider that there is evidence to support the view that changes to lifestyle in older age can be effective in improving a wide range of issues including cognitive health, immune function and vascular health. Improving the health of the individual in this way could as a consequence allow the individual to become more socially active and therefore less lonely and isolated. But the challenge remains to identify a range of interventions to meet the needs of this complex group who may see themselves as 'too old' to make a difference.

WHO (2015) consider that the aim of healthy ageing is to address two issues for the individual as they age: their intrinsic capability and their functional ability. As with the generally accepted definition of health, healthy ageing needs to be seen in a much broader context than just the absence of disease. Intrinsic capability refers to the physical

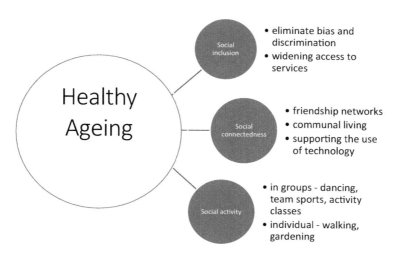

Figure 10.5   Model for health ageing

and mental capabilities. For some this may be retained into their 80s and 90s, whilst for others this might be compromised at a much earlier age. However, from the perspective of public health, it is the functional ability of the individual that might be the key to ageing well. The interaction of the individual with their environment determines their functional ability, and it is the development and maintenance of their functional ability that enable wellbeing in older age.

Conclusion

Public health has a responsibility to ensure that the particular health needs of the older population are considered if we are going to support an older population who are active and engaged with society. It is evident that the older population is growing globally, and this could pose a challenge for the provision of health and social care services. The psychosocial theories of ageing are particularly relevant to the provision of public health, and it is clear that this might be particularly important for addressing loneliness and meeting the needs of the vulnerable older population.

Consider the following questions

1. Thinking of your local area what services and activities are available for the older person in the community. What might be the barriers and facilitators impacting on the uptake of these services and activities?
2. Reflecting on your current practice, what changes might you consider in order to meet the needs of the older LGBTQ community?

Key terms

Primary care; public health; loneliness; LGBTQ; Ageing; older age; healthy ageing

Further reading

Centre for Ageing Better. 2020. *An Old Age Problem? How Society Shapes and Reinforces Negative Attitudes to Ageing*. Available at: https://ageing-better.org.uk/publications/old-age-problem-how-society-shapes-and-reinforces-negative-attitudes-ageing?gclid=EAIaIQobChMIsueDxdHB9gIVqe_tCh3yEg9MEAAYASAAEgJfN_D_BwE [Accessed 12.03.2022].

Centre for Ageing Better. 2020. *Summary: State of Ageing in 2020*. Available at: https://ageing-better.org.uk/summary-state-ageing-2020 [Accessed 12.03.2022].

Chew-Graham, C., Ray, M. 2016. *Mental Health and Older People: A Guide for Primary Care Practitioners*. Springer International Publishing: Cham.

Eckstrand, K., Ehrenfeld, J. (Eds). 2016. *Lesbian, Gay, Bisexual and Transgender Healthcare: A Clinical Guide to Preventive, Primary and Specialist Care*. Springer International Publishing: Cham.

Nay, R., Garrett, S., Fetherstonhaugh, D. 2014. *Older People: Issues and Innovations in Care*. (4th edn). Churchill-Livingstone Elsevier: Chatswood, Australia.

References

Age Concern. 2006. *The Whole of Me..: Meeting the Needs of Older Lesbians, Gay Men and Bisexuals Living in Care Homes and Extra Care Housing*. Age Concern: London.

AGE Platform Europe and The European Region of the International Lesbian, Gay, Bisexual, Trans and Intersex Association. 2012. *Equality for older lesbian, gay, bisexual, trans and intersex people in Europe*. [online] Available at: https://www.ilga-europe.org/resources/policy-papers/joint-policy-paper-equality-older-lesbian-gay-bisexual-trans-and-intersex [Accessed 13.04.2022].

Ard, K. L., Makadon, H. J. 2012. *Improving the Healthcare of LGBT People*. Fenway Institute: Boston, MA.

Blais, K. 2014. Older adult. In C. Edelman, E. Kudzma, C. Mandle (Eds), *Health Promotion Throughout the Lifespan*. (8th edn). Elsevier: St Louis, MO.

Bouman, W. P., Arcelus, J., Benbow, S. M. 2007. Nottingham Study of Sexuality and Ageing (NoSSA II). Attitudes of care staff regarding sexuality and residents: a study in residential and nursing homes. *Sexual and Relationship Therapy*; 22(1), 45–61.

Calder, P., Cardif, S., Christopher, G., Kuh, D., Langley-Evans, S., McNulty, H. 2018. A holistic approach to health ageing; how can people live longer healthier lives? *Journal of Human Nutrition and Dietetics*; 31, 439–450.

Carrier, J. 2016. *Managing Long-Term Conditions and Chronic Illness in Primary Care – A Guide to Good Practice*. (2nd edn). Routledge: Abingdon.

Caspi, A., Harrington, H., Moffitt, T. E. et al. 2006. Socially isolated children 20 years later: risk of cardiovascular disease. *Journal of Developmental and Behavioural Paediatrics*; 27(6), 514.

Christiansen, J., Breinholt, Larsen F., Lasgaard, M. 2016. Do stress, health behaviours and sleep mediate between loneliness and adverse health conditions among older people? *Social Science and Medicine*; 152, 80–86. http://dx.doi.org/10.1016.j.cocscimed.2016.01.020

Commission for Social Care Inspection. 2008. *Putting People First. Equality and Diversity Matters 1: Providing appropriate services for lesbian, gay and bisexual and transgender people*. Commission for Social Care Inspection: Norwich.

Cox, J. 2017. Combatting loneliness one conversation at a time. *The Jo Cox Foundation*. Available at: www.jocoxfoundation.org/loneliness_commission [Accessed 06.06.2020].

Cumming, E., Henry. W., 1961. *Growing Old*. Basic Books: New York.

Dahlgren, G., Whitehead, M. 1993. *Tackling Inequalities in Health: What Can We Learn and What Has Been Tried?* The King's Fund: London.

Dickens, A., Richards, S., Graves, C., Campbell, J. 2011. Interventions targeting social isolation in older people: a systematic review. *BMC Public Health*; 11, 647. https://biomedcentral.com/1471-2458/11/647

Edelman, C., Kudzma, E., Mandle, C. 2021. *Health Promotion Through the Lifespan.* (8th Edn). Elsevier: St Louis, MO.

Erikson, E.H. 1982. *The Life Cycle Completed: A Review.* New York: W.W Norton.

Freidricksen-Goldsen, K., Kim, H.J., Barjen, S., Balsam, K.F., Mincer, S.L. 2010. Disparities in health-related quality of life: a comparison of lesbians and bisexual women. *American Journal of Public Health*; 100, 2255–2261. doi: https://doi.org/10.2105/AJPH.2009.177329

Freidricksen-Goldsen, K., Simoni, J., Kim, H.J., Lehavot, K., Walters, K., Yang, J., Hay-Ellis, C. 2014. Teh Health Equity Promotion Model: Reconceptualization of Lesbian, Gay, Bisexual and Transgender (LGBT) Health Disparities. *American Journal of Orthopsychiatry*; 84(6), 653–663. doi: 10.1037/ort0000030

Goodman, A., Adams, A., Swift, H. 2015. *Hidden Citizens: How Can We Identify the Most Lonely Adults?* The Campaign to End Loneliness: London. Available at: www.campaigntoendloneliness.org/wp-content/uploads/CEL-Hidden-People-Exec-Summary-final-1.pdf [Accessed 23.06.2020].

Goodwin, N., Sonola, I., Thiel, V., Kodner, D. L. 2013. *Coordinated Care for People with Complex Chronic Conditions: Key Lessons and Markers for Success.* The King's Fund: London. Available at: www.hqsc.govt.nz/assets/General-NEMR-files-images-/nick-goodwin-co-ordinated-care-kingsfund-Nov-2013.pdf. [Accessed 20.10.2019].

Groman, M. 1999. Development and rights of older people. In J. Randal et al. (Eds), *The Ageing and Development Report: Poverty and Independence in the World's Older People.* Earthscan: London.

Havighurst, R. L., Neugarten, B. L., Tobin, S. S. 1963. Disengagement, personality, and life satisfaction in the later years. In P. Hansen (Ed.), *Age with a Future.* Munksgard: Copenhagen.

Havighurst, R. L., Neugarten, B. L., Tobin, S. S. 1968. In B. L. Neugarten (Ed.), *Middle Age and Ageing.* University of Chicago Press: Chicago, IL.

Hawkley, L., Thisted, R., Masi, C., et al. 2010. Loneliness predicts increased blood pressure: 5 yr crossed-lagged analysis in middle aged and older adults. *Psychology of Aging*; 25(1), 132–141.

Heath, H. 2012. Supporting sexuality and intimate relationships. *Nurse Residential Care*; 14(9), 475–477.

Holt-Lunstad, J., Smith, T. 2015. Loneliness and social isolation as risk factors for mortality; a meta analytic review. *Perspectives of Psychological Science*; 10, 227–237.

Jopling, K. 2015. *Promising Approaches to Reducing Loneliness and Isolation in Later Life.* Age UK/Campaign to End Loneliness: London. Available at: www.campaigntoendloneliness.org/wp-content/uploads/Promising-approaches-to-reducing-loneliness-and-isolation-in-later-life.pdf [Accessed 23.06.2020].

Lasgaard, M., Friis, K., Shelvin, M. 2016. 'Where are all the lonely people?' A population-based study of high-risk groups across the life span. *Society of Psychiatry and Psychiatric Epidemiology*; 51, 1371–1384. doi: 10/1007/s00127-016-1279-3

Liotta, G., Ussai, S., Illario, M. et al. 2018. Frailty as the future core business of public health: report on the activities of the A3 Action Group of the European Innovation Partnership on Active Health Ageing (EIP on AHA). *International Journal of Environmental Research and Public Health*; 15(12), 2843– 2869.

Low, L. F., Yap, M., Brodaty, H. A. 2011. Systematic review of different models of home and community care services for older persons. *BMC Health Serv. Res.*; 9(11), 93.

Luanaigh, C., Lawlor, B. 2008. Loneliness and health of older people. *International Journal of Geriatric Psychiatry*; 23, 1213–1221.

Marmot, M. 2011 *Fair Society Healthy Lives*. Institute of Health Equity: London.

Marmot, M. 2018. *Health Inequity in England: The Marmot Review 10 Years On*. Institute of Health Equity: London. Available at: www.health.org.uk/sites/default/files/upload/publications/2020/Health%20Equity%20in%20England_The%20Marmot%20Review%2010%20Years%20On_full%20report.pdf [Accessed 29.06.2020].

McMurry, A., Clendon, J. 2015. *Community Health and Wellness*. (5th edn). Elsevier Australia: Chatwood.

National Assembly for Wales. 2014. *Social Services and Well-being Act*. National Assembly for Wales: Cardiff.

National Health Interview Survey (NHIS). 2013. [online] Available at: https://www.cdc.gov/nchs/nhis/nhis_2013_data_release.htm [Accessed 13.04.2022].

O'Rourke, H., Collins, L., Sidan, S. 2018. Interventions to address social connectedness and loneliness in older people. *BMC Geriatrics*; 18, 214. https://doi.org/10.1186/s12877-018-0879

Office for National Statistics. 2018a. *Health State Life Expectancies, UK: 2015 to 2017*. Office for National Statistics: London. Available at: www.ons.gov.uk/peoplepopulationandcommunity/healthandsocialcare/healthandlifeexpectancies/bulletins/healthstatelifeexpectanciesuk/2015to2017 [Accessed 19.06.2020].

Office for National Statistics. 2018b. *Loneliness – What Characteristics and Circumstances Are Associated With Feeling Lonely*? Office for National Statistics: London. Available at: www.ons.gov.uk/peoplepopulationandcommunity/wellbeing/articles/lonelinesswhatcharacteristicsandcircumstancesareassociatedwithfeelinglonely/2018-04-10 [Accessed 06.06.2020].

Office for National Statistics. 2019. *Overview of the UK Population 2019*. Office for National Statistics: London. Available at: www.ons.gov.uk/peoplepopulationandcommunity/populationandmigration/populationestimates/articles/overviewoftheukpopulation/august2019 [Accessed 30.08.2019].

Peplau, L., Perlman, D. 1982. Perspectives in loneliness. In L. Peplau, D. Perlman (Eds), *Loneliness: A Sourcebook of Current Theory Research and Therapy*. Wiley: New York.

Peron, E. P., Gray, S. L., Hanlon, J. T. 2011. Medication use and functional status decline in older adults a narrative review. *American Journal of Geriatric Pharmacotherapy*; 9(6), 378–391.

Power, L., Bell, M., Freemantle, L. 2010. *A National Study of Ageing and IV (50 plus)*. Terrance Higgins Trust: London.

Pressman, S., Cohen, S., Miller, G., et al. 2005. Loneliness, social network size, and immune response to influenza vaccination in college freshman. *Health Psychology*; 24, 297–306.

Public Health England. 2019a. *Public Health England Strategy 2020–2025*. Public Health England: London.

Public Health England. 2019b. *A Menu of Interventions for Productive Healthy Aging*. Public Health England: London.

Public Health Wales. 2019. *Public Health Wales Medium Term Strategic Plan 2019–2022*. Public Health Wales: Cardiff.

Stein, G. L., Beckerman, N. L., Sherman, P. A. 2010. Lesbian and gay elders and long-term care: identifying the unique psychosocial perspectives and challenges. *Journal of Gerontological Social Work*; 53(5), 421–435.

Stonewall. 2011. *Lesbian, Gay and Bisexual People in Later Life*. Stonewall: London. Available at: http://tinyurl.com/oj6y7pu [Accessed 11/03/2022].

Swerisson, H. Taylor, M. 2014. Public health for an ageing society. In R. Nay, S. Garrett, D. Fetherstonhaugh (Eds), *Older People: Issues and Innovations in Care*. (4th edn). Elsevier Australia: Sydney.

Tornstam, L. 1989. Gero-transcendance: A Reformulation of the Disengagement. *Theory Ageing*; 1, 55–63.

Trail Ross, M. E., Summerlin, E. B. 2015. Senior health. In M. Nies, M. McEwan (Eds), *Community/Public Health Nursing*. (6th edn). Elsevier: St Louis, MO.

Trevisan, K., Christina-Perira, R., Silva-Amaral, D., Aversi-Ferreira, T. A. 2019. Theories of aging and the prevalence of Alzheimer's disease. *Biomed International*. Available at: https://doi.org/10.1155/2019/9171424 [Accessed 11.03.2022].

Van Teijlingen, E. 2019. Social aspects of ageing. In E. Van Teijlingen, G. Humphries (Eds), *Psychology and Sociology Applied to Medicine*. (4th edn). Elsevier: Edingburgh.

Ward, R., Pugh, S., Price, E. 2010. *Don't Look Back? Improving Health and Social Care Service Delivery for Older LGB Users*. Ewulit and Human Rights Commission: Manchester.

Watkins, D., Cousins, J. 2010. *Public Health and Community Nursing – Frameworks for Practice*. (3rd edn). Balliere Tindall Elsevier: Oxford.

World Health Organization. 2002. *Proposed working definition of an older person in Africa for the MDS Project*. Available at: www.who.int/healthinfo/survey/ageingdefnolder/en/ [Accessed 18.10.2019].

World Health Organization. 2012. *Strategy and Action Plan for Healthy Ageing in Europe*. World Health Organization: Geneva.

World Health Organization. 2015. *World Report on Ageing and Health*. World Health Organization: Geneva.

World Health Organization. 2017. *Global Strategy and Action Plan on Ageing and Health*. World Health Organization: Geneva.

11

SUBSTANCE USE AND PUBLIC HEALTH

IAIN MCPHEE

─────────── LEARNING OUTCOMES ───────────

By the end of this chapter, you will be able to:

- Understand key terms such as the difference between substance use, and substance abuse.
- Identify the core elements of a disease concept of addiction (dependence).
- Understand how healthcare professionals can support clients with an addiction from a public health perspective.

Introduction

This chapter begins with a broad overview of what is meant by problem use of substances and explores distinctions between use, misuse and abuse. By discussing the distinction between use and abuse, the moral judgements underpinning the term 'abuse' are revealed. The elements that underpin the addiction concept are identified and introduced to understand how and in what way substance use problems and related harm can be understood. The utility of the addiction concept in defining or diagnosing addiction as a disease (dependence syndrome) uses a case study of Mr. B, a user of tobacco who prior to cutting down and eventually stopping, describes all of the hallmarks of 'addiction' related to his use of tobacco. Finally, evidence based interventions that are useful in reducing harms associated with problematic substance use are discussed.

Defining substance use

While there are many tens of thousands of substances that can be classified in terms of their legal status or therapeutic value, it is useful to identify functional reasons why people use a substance. Analgesics reduce pain, depressants reduce anxiety and aid sleep, stimulants lift mood and energy levels, and psychedelics alter how the mind processes information.

As there is no standard definition of a drug or substance that is uncontested, or makes some form of normative judgement, such as good or bad, moral or immoral, legal or illegal, a general description of a drug refers to a substance that can be used to modify a chemical process or processes in the body, or treat an illness, and relieve a symptom, or be used to enhance a performance or ability, or to alter states of mind. The term 'substances' in an attempt to reduce the prejudice associated with the word 'drug' includes legal and illegal, medical, and non-medical drugs and while not exhaustive will include: alcohol, opioids, cannabinoids, sedatives or hypnotics, cocaine, other stimulants including caffeine, hallucinogens, tobacco, and volatile solvents, and other hallucinogens.

In understanding substance use as a problem, it is necessary to define what the problems associated with the use of substances are. These problems can be summarised as legal, physical, psychological and social.

Legal

The primary UK legislation controlling the manufacture, possession and distribution of drugs is the Misuse of Drugs Act 1971. The Act classifies drugs into categories from A to C, making possession, sale or supply a criminal offence. Excluded from this classification are the legally available drugs alcohol and tobacco, prescription drugs and the sale of over-the-counter medications.

There are legal restrictions placed on the availability of many substances; for example one must be over 18 in the UK to purchase alcohol, and over 16 to purchase cigarettes and tobacco products. The availability of alcohol and tobacco are controlled by a system of licensing, overseen by local authorities throughout the UK. Some over-the-counter medicines are regulated by the vendor. The purchase of codeine for pain management requires that the vendor asks pertinent questions about who will use the drug while making the purchaser aware of any addictive potential.

Physical

There are physical consequences of using some drugs, particularly those classed as 'psychoactive' that can in certain amounts produce a state of intoxication. Alcohol, for example, can lead to intoxication, and resultant 'drunk' behaviour that could lead to an accident, or be linked to a criminal act such as a public disorder offence. In addition, drugs such as alcohol, opiates and nicotine can produce 'withdrawal' symptoms which can be mild or severe, and in the case of long-term hazardous drinking of alcohol can be life threatening, requiring medical intervention.

Psychological

The consequences of using psychoactive substances that intoxicate or produce euphoria can be reinforcing; that is, the pleasure associated with their use can be the salient factor that leads to repeated use and even habitual use of a substance. In addition, decision making can be negatively affected, where the use of the drug becomes a primary factor in avoiding the distress of craving or withdrawal. This can result in difficulty in reducing use or achieving or maintaining abstinence.

Social

Social consequences can be both positive and negative. For example, in the UK alcohol is widely available, and it has many uses in social gatherings. While some cultures and religions do observe abstinence as a requirement of faith, in general terms alcohol is often considered a 'social' drug. However, the use of some drugs, because of their legal status, can result in social consequences that are negative, and a criminal record can be the result of possession of a drug controlled within the Misuse of Drugs Act 1971. The social consequences of using controlled drugs can lead to stigma and this stigma, particularly if linked to a criminal offence, can result in discrimination.

In addition to the physical, psychological and social consequences of using a substance, there are definitions that refer to 'medical' and 'legal' harms associated with use. The WHO international classification of disease (ICD-10) section that describes mental and behavioural disorders, alcohol dependence is described as:

> ...a disorder of regulation of alcohol use arising from repeated or continuous use of alcohol. The characteristic feature is a strong internal drive to use alcohol, which is manifested by impaired ability to control use, increasing priority given to use over other activities and persistence of use despite harm or negative consequences. These experiences are often accompanied by a subjective sensation of

urge or craving to use alcohol. Physiological features of dependence may also be present, including tolerance to the effects of alcohol, withdrawal symptoms following cessation or reduction in use of alcohol, or repeated use of alcohol or pharmacologically similar substances to prevent or alleviate withdrawal symptoms (ICD-10, chapter 5: https://icd.who.int/browse10/2019/en#

This definition of the habitual use of alcohol includes the core elements of a disease concept of addiction referred to as a 'dependence syndrome'. Craving is characterised by 'a strong urge', linked to a 'loss of control' over consumption and an inability to modify patterns of use despite adverse consequences. Also included in this definition are the terms 'tolerance' and 'withdrawal', which we will refer to later in this chapter. For a contemporary overview of how and in what way substance use problems are understood, defined, and diagnosed you can refer to the ICD-10 or the upcoming ICD-11. (International Classification of Diseases (ICD) (who.int)

The use of drugs

Having noted the difficulty in defining what a drug or substance is in an attempt to avoid stigma and discrimination, there are also some challenges in estimating the use of substances in the United Kingdom (UK) population.

The patterns and prevalence on the use of drugs is documented in most nation states. In the four nations of the UK, the use of alcohol, tobacco and drugs that are controlled by legal means are regularly collected and collated. In Europe, the European Monitoring Centre for Drugs and Drug Addiction (EMCDDA) publishes the patterns and prevalence of the use of drugs throughout Europe and publish annually on the drug situation in the UK (EMCDDA 2020). The use of drugs can have consequences in several areas of life, noted as social, legal, physical and psychological. As the use of drugs can result in harm, in particular psychoactive substances that have powerful effects on the mind and body, they can become a cause for concern. While there is no distinction made in countries within the UK between use and abuse, the prevalence of use and problematic use of substances are regularly published.

Prevalence

The term 'prevalence' refers to the proportion of a population who have used a drug over a particular time period. In general population surveys, prevalence is measured by asking respondents in a representative sample drawn from the population to recall their use of drugs.

The three most widely used recall periods are: lifetime (ever used a drug); last year (used a drug in the last twelve months); last month (used a drug in the last 30 days). Prevalence information obtained from a representative sample can be used to estimate prevalence in the population.

In addition to survey data, some data is collected from A&E, from specialist statutory (NHS) and non-statutory treatment centres, and criminal justice agencies. The percentage of the population who do not take part in these surveys and data gathering activities of various agencies is estimated.

Drug use estimates in England and Wales

The UK government national survey known as the Crime Survey for England and Wales (CSEW) examines the extent and trends in illicit drug use among a sample of 16- to 59-year-olds. The CSEW measures non-problematic drug use for the drug types and population it covers. However, it does not provide estimates of problematic drug use (PDU), as many such users may not be a part of the household resident population which is covered by the survey, or they may lead such chaotic lifestyles that they are unlikely to take part in the survey.

Around 1 in 11 (9.4%) adults aged 16 to 59 report the use of a drug in the last year. This equates to around 3.2 million people. Around 1 in 5 (20.3%) adults aged 16 to 24 report use of a drug in the last year, which equates to around 1.3 million people. However, the regular or problematic use of an illegal drug is uncommon in the general population (Office for National Statistics (ONS) 2019).

Scotland

The Scottish Crime and Justice Survey (SCJS) results since the 1980s indicates that problem drug use (PDU) is uncommon among the general population, with cannabis being the most commonly reported drug used (NHS Digital 2018).

Scotland experiences a high prevalence of problem drug use and drug deaths compared to the rest of the UK (ONS, 2020). The number of individuals with problem drug use in Scotland is estimated to be in the range 55,800 to 58,900. The rate of problem drug use amongst males and females was highest in the 25 to 34 years age group (Information Services Division 2019).

The Information Services Division (ISD), the data-gathering agency for NHS Scotland, estimates problem use of opioids and benzodiazepines, which are the drugs most commonly reported as misused by service providers. Research also reveals that drug harms are unevenly distributed in Scotland, with the majority of PDU and incidence of drug related death (DRD) over-represented among users who reside in areas of deprivation (McPhee and Sheridan 2020; ISD 2020).

Northern Ireland

In Northern Ireland, the Department of Health provides data on alcohol, tobacco and use of controlled drugs, and the prevalence of gambling separately. The drug prevalence survey in Northern Ireland indicates wide regional and age variations in reported lifetime use and inferred regular (used last month) prevalence.

What government data from each of the four nations in the UK indicates is that while there are regional and age variations, regular use of drugs controlled within the Misuse of Drugs Act 1971 are uncommon in the four countries that comprise the UK population.

The EMCDDA annual reports produces data that indicates that among people who use drugs, the patterns of use range from experimental to habitual and dependent consumption. Cannabis is the most commonly used drug with a prevalence of use about five times that of other substances. The use of heroin and other opioids remains relatively uncommon in the general population, although it may be concentrated in some geographical locations. However, opiates and opioids are the drugs most commonly associated with harmful forms of use, including injecting. The extent of stimulant use and the types that are most common vary across the UK, and evidence reveals an increase in injecting stimulant type substances (cocaine, amphetamine and some new psychoactive substances (NPS)) occurring throughout the UK (EMCDDA, 2020, p. 14).

The use of tobacco

The reported sales and use of tobacco in the UK is declining (NHS Digital 2020), though it remains a cause for concern among pregnant women, young people and older people who have used tobacco for a long period. Data from the ONS indicates that in 2019, 14.1% of people aged 18 years and above smoked cigarettes, which equates to around 6.9 million people in the population, based on estimates from the Annual Population Survey (APS).

Of the four nations, 13.9% of adults in England smoked, 15.5% of adults in Wales, 15.4% of adults in Scotland and 15.6% of adults in Northern Ireland, 16% of men smoked compared with 13% of women. Those aged 25 to 34 years had the highest proportion of current smokers (19.0%). In the UK, around 1 in 4 (23.4%) people in routine and manual occupations smoked (this is around 2.5 times higher than people in managerial and professional occupations), and 5.7% of respondents said they currently used an e-cigarette, which equates to nearly 3 million adults in the UK population (ONS, 2019, ONS 2020).

The use of alcohol

Alcohol is a legally available substance and can be purchased by anyone over 18 in the UK. Survey data collated by Alcohol Change UK (https://alcoholchange.org.uk/alcohol-facts/fact-sheets/alcohol-statistics) indicates that the amount of alcohol consumed per person in the UK changes over time. After reaching a peak in the mid-2000s, consumption has been falling steadily, particularly among young people. Most recently the average consumption per adult based on sales of alcohol is about 9.7 litres of pure alcohol per year, which equates to 18 units a week: this is approximately two and a half units of alcohol per person per day. Average consumption figures are useful but limited. They show roughly what is happening across the UK population; however, specific individuals or social groups may consume more or less than the average.

It is the case that most people use alcohol in a risk-free manner, without many problems, while others find it difficult to stop drinking when they feel they want to. The language used to define alcohol harms can be confusing. Terms such as 'problem drinking', 'addiction' or 'alcoholic' are often used interchangeably, without much agreement on what these terms mean.

The terminology and language we use to describe social, criminal issues and health conditions influences and reflects our attitudes and approaches to addressing them (McPhee, 2013). Indeed it is apparent that the terms we commonly use can result in stigma, which can become discrimination. Kelly et al. (2016) provide a superb overview of the impact of the stigmatizing terms we use to describe problems with the use of substances (see Kelly, Saitz & Wakeman, 2016).

Units consumed can be useful in defining harm and risk associated with drinking. One unit of alcohol is defined as a half pint of beer, a small glass of wine or a pub measure of spirit alcohol. It is commonplace to describe different patterns of drinking in terms of increasing risk associated with number of units consumed. There are a range of risks that tend to increase with consumption. It is possible to assess levels of risk associated with amount of alcohol consumed, as well as taking stock of behaviours that occur while intoxicated. The problems associated with the use of alcohol can be identified using screening tools that document use in units, such as the Alcohol Use Disorders Identification Test (AUDIT), which assesses the amount and pattern of units consumed and harms associated with drinking. Information on the AUDIT approved by the WHO can be accessed at this web address: www.who.int/publications/i/item/audit-the-alcohol-use-disorders-identification-test-guidelines-for-use-in-primary-health-care.

For example, normal drinking can be defined as someone with an AUDIT score of between 8 and 15. A woman drinking up to 14 units a week, or a man drinking up to 21 units a week, generally speaking suggests low risk of harm. The National Institute for Health and Care Excellence (NICE) have useful definitions of harmful and hazardous drinking that refer to the units of alcohol consumed (see https://www.nice.org.uk/guidance/ph24/chapter/7-Glossary#harmful-drinking-high-risk-drinking).

The harms associated with the use of alcohol do not fall neatly into categories associated with amounts consumed. For example, someone who reduces their consumption from 50 units a week to 20 will achieve a significant reduction in potential harm, even though potentially categorised as 'at risk'. No system of harm or risk recognition or diagnostic criterion is perfect, as most human activity is extremely complex; however, the use of diagnostic criterion linked to patterns of use and calculations of units consumed help identify those individuals who might benefit from reducing their use and those who might benefit from complete abstinence.

Trying to work out if someone has a problem with their use of alcohol or not can reinforce the idea that alcohol problems are a simple issue of diagnosis. However, diagnosis is complex, with varying degrees of use patterns, and levels or categories of harm to consider. Recognising the harm associated with habitual use of alcohol is important, for example if one subscribes to the idea that the habitual use of alcohol is a disease; however, this concept reinforces the notion that there are just two types of alcohol user: those with a disease and those without.

The term 'alcoholism' implies that alcohol addiction is a disease that one is either suffering from or not. This idea remains widely accepted and is the underpinning philosophy of Alcoholics Anonymous (AA) that began in 1930s in North America after a period of alcohol prohibition. In North America, for various reasons, the belief that addiction is a 'chronic relapsing disorder' has become widely accepted, however, outside of the USA this remains controversial (see the Stanton Peele website for a useful historical overview of how addiction and dependence are conceptualised: https://peele.net/lib/index04.html).

Understanding the disease concept/addiction

A person who displays an inability to control their use to a degree that is harmful to themselves and others is commonly described as being 'addicted'. It is apparent that the definition of substance abuse, or measures of harm, and the diagnostic criterion for addiction or dependence share a number of common factors. Addiction is recognised or diagnosed by a person's reported heightened and habituated need for a substance; by the intense suffering that results from discontinuation of its use; and by the person's willingness to sacrifice all (to the point of self-destructiveness) for substance use (Peele 1995; NICE 2018). There are 'core' elements that underpin most common definitions and classifications of addiction or dependence and are present in the ICD-10 definition of alcohol dependence (https://icd.who.int/browse10/2019/en#).

Tolerance

Over time, users describe experiencing drug tolerance, which is interpreted as requiring more of a substance to achieve the pleasure or outcome desired. In general terms tolerance will depend on several factors, such as the type of drug used, the health and wellbeing of the individual who uses it, and the cultural setting in which the use takes place. Tolerance can be understood as a continual process rather than a single state, which can change over time after periods of reduced use or abstinence.

Craving

Craving refers to the physical and psychological discomfort users experience when they are unable to access a substance that they use regularly. For some this is overwhelming, although can reduce over time, while for others, craving is non-existent.

Withdrawal

Withdrawal is often linked to craving, and users report that with some drugs, the experience of withdrawal is so unpleasant that the user avoids it at all costs, leading to an inability to cut down or stop. Withdrawal can be extremely unpleasant for some and almost nonexistent for others. This means that there is a subjective element to this concept. Some users report no physical withdrawal symptoms from drugs such as cocaine or amphetamine, while habitual users of opiates report unpleasant physical symptoms. Problems experienced by users of alcohol who stop drinking abruptly include being at risk of seizures that require medical intervention, such as the short-term use of benzodiazepines, to minimise these risks.

The elements of the disease concept of addiction

The disease concept of addiction has influenced definitions of harmful use and abuse. While it is possible to define alcohol dependence or addiction by, for example, the regularity of units consumed and the negative health consequences associated with habitual use, to make a distinction between risky, hazardous and dependent use, dependence or addiction can be classified as a disease when linked to the following core elements in Table 11.1.

Diagnosing addiction/dependence

While not exhaustive, these basic or core elements of a disease concept form the basis of all diagnostic measures of addiction or dependence.

Users of tobacco routinely report how 'addictive' or habit forming the use of nicotine is, and how difficult it is to cut down or stop. The case study that follows introduces Mr. B, a smoker of tobacco. Throughout the case study are numbered comments relating to Table 11.2 that explain his journey from initiation to dependence. Mr. B explains the ease with which he started smoking, and the difficulty in cutting down. When reading through the case study, try to understand the behaviour of Mr. B, what he thinks about his use of tobacco, and using the elements of the disease concept of addiction try to evaluate if Mr. B's use of tobacco meets all of the elements of a disease concept.

Table 11.1   The elements of the disease concept of addiction

Discrete Entity: It being 'discrete' suggests that one is either addicted or not addicted, that is recognised or diagnosed relatively easily. Those who experience difficulty in stopping or cutting down believe themselves to be different from other people who may be able to use alcohol for example without problems.

Abnormal Craving: Describes an overwhelming desire or urge to use a substance. When craving is experienced, obtaining and consuming the substance supersedes all other activities and responsibilities – it is in this sense 'abnormal'. Craving is often linked to tolerance, and refers to the belief that more of a drug is required to achieve a desired state, such as intoxication or a reduction in negative withdrawal symptoms.

Loss of Control: The ability to choose when and how to consume the substance is lost. Once loss of control is experienced, uncontrolled or habitual use despite negative consequences can become a norm.

Irreversibility: This view is fundamental in explanations of addiction or dependence that have a biological cause. Irreversibility implies that changes at a cellular level prevent a return to non-problematic patterns of use. What is inferred from this element is that once control has been lost, it can only be regained by abstinence.

Progressiveness: Negative health consequences inevitably become worse resulting in deteriorating mental and physical health.

Case study: Mr. B, a born smoker

I was born under a hospital bed during an air raid in London. Even the midwife smoked. My father smoked when he visited, and mum had 'fags' beside the bed. It was war time, so no one cared too much. I went home to a smoker's house and lived my early years in what would now be regarded as 'second-hand' smoke abuse. In those days everyone smoked, you were odd if you didn't – 'Really, you don't smoke? Give it a try, go on ...'

I remember rerolling my father's used tobacco. Truly disgusting, but I knew I had to persevere. That's how I started, and of course I was told I couldn't smoke until I was 16, but I wasn't going to wait. This was a rite of passage, growing up stuff, and I progressed to buying packs of fives having scraped up enough pennies with a few mates. I smoked through my secondary school days quite openly. I was 'cool'. It was 'cool'. There were your 'working class' fags: Players, Weights; posh brands like American Camels, State Express; and exotics like Sobranie and Gauloise. Your choice of cigarette spoke volumes about you.

In my late teens while working I could smoke properly. Cigarettes and a lighter beside my bed, one before sleep and then to clear my lungs first thing in the morning. It was important to have a full pack as soon as possible because the thought of running out was not a pleasant idea, and even getting down to a near-empty packet, the last two or three brought on anxiety: 'Would I have enough to get through the rest of the day before I could get to a shop? Could I borrow one from another worker if I ran out?' (1)

Being prevented from having a 'puff' was such an acute sense of loss as to be avoided at all costs, even if it meant scrounging butts from ash trays and going back to childhood and rerolling what could be salvaged. To say it was the norm understates the hold it had on society and individual – and me. Smoking was a routine; it was a pause between tasks; it was like punctuation during the day.

Everything about tobacco use was crafted by experts to enhance the look, the feel, the choices, the elegance, the ruggedness. Accessories like the coveted gold lighter, silver cigarette cases, even the packs were a work of specialists, just cardboard but how well constructed, how well designed, how it fit into the hand and how it gave you guilt when near empty. The whole smoking experience was addictive, and the thought of risk didn't come into the equation for many years. (2)

Smoking was as ingrained a part of life and society as the pint of milk on the doorstep, the bus to work, pictures at the cinema once a week and putting on your trousers in the morning. The nation, indeed, the world smoked – advertised too, encouraged, manipulated, socially engineered and we just didn't understand we were junkies, and the pushers were creating more habit-forming tobaccos, easier to inhale, lying and deceiving in print and Parliament and we didn't feel a thing, except a cough.

The cough: can't be an issue. Look at all those glamourous movie stars smoking with true elegance and panache. Sports personalities, TV adverts extolling 'easy on the throat' (no one told us that three 'Marlboro Men' died of throat cancer advertising that brand). When I did get a cough, the recommendation was to change brands.

I had no idea I was hooked, addicted. It was years before I woke up. I couldn't go a few hours without a 'drag' and I was coughing more. (3)

I tried to give up. So many times, that I can't count. Cutting down; changing to supposedly lighter brands. The excuses: just one won't hurt; 'Can I cadge a smoke mate, I'm giving up'.

All followed by failure and self-loathing because I was weak. It was then that I saw smoking as some kind of demon inside that smoked, not me, and that demon punished me every time I tried and failed by making me smoke more. That was how I pictured the enemy of addiction. (4)

This went on for ten years or so until I came to the sudden realisation that my failure was related to the word 'trying'. Failure was a built-in option because 'trying' makes allowances. (5)

It all came to a head when, following a coughing bout after running up some steps and of course lighting a cigarette, I asked myself if this was the one that would kill me. (6)

I stopped trying to give up smoking and instead I simply stopped. That's it: no drama in the event to relate, I just became a non-smoker. Instantly. I gave up when I was 60 because I didn't want to be a dead smoker. I'm in my late 70s now and from time to time I feel something is missing when I have a coffee, finish a meal, or just stand contemplating a view. It (craving) only lasts seconds. Nearly 20 years has passed since I held a cigarette, that's how powerful the cigarette experience was. (7)

I don't remember a serious craving, but I missed the punctuation in the day, the feel of a cigarette in my fingers, the presence of the pack, having a coffee on its own and that was difficult for a week or so, but it did not compare to the trauma of trying to give up. (8)

There is a confession to add here though. That sense of loss while having a coffee has been made up by chocolate; I make sure I have a few bars in stock. It would be silly to run out, wouldn't it? Have you noticed the packaging on chocolate? Opening a bar and peeling back the silver paper ... (9)

Table 11.2   Interpreting the case study of Mr. B

1. Mr. B describes being aware of *craving*, and in avoiding *withdrawal* he makes sure he always has a supply of cigarettes.

2. It is apparent that Mr. B has not (at this time) *contemplated* changing his behaviour.

3. Mr. B is contemplating change and reports negative consequences of his smoking. He describes himself as being addicted to nicotine but makes a distinction between tobacco users and heroin users. He has the urge to use (experiences craving).

4. He describes numerous attempts at giving up and describes feeling bad after each *relapse*. He reports that he cannot go a few hours without a repeated dose (tolerance). His use continues despite adverse health consequences (coughing).

5. Mr. B describes repeated attempts at giving up, and as relapse is considered a failure, it negatively affects his self-esteem. Here he clearly expresses frustration at his inability to exert *control* over his use.

6. Mr. B has reached a point where he contemplates *action* by making a decision to stop. He indicates that he is able to *maintain* his new behaviour.

7. After almost fifty years of tobacco use Mr. B indicates that 20 years after stopping (despite several relapses), the temporary subjective experience of tobacco *craving* remains.

8. It is interesting that Mr. B has learned from previous attempts at cutting down and stopping. Experiencing relapse led eventually to him acquiring knowledge about high risk situations. This new information on risk changes his attitude to smoking that led to his preferred behavioural outcome – abstinence.

9. One question you might ask at this point. Is Mr. B reporting being addicted to chocolate? Does a craving for this substance infer that he is a chocolate addict?

Note from the case study that Mr. B uses language that is recognisable from certain key terms and phrases in the definition of dependence used by the WHO International classification of diseases (ICD-10). By reading over the case study again, this time work out from Table 11.3 if the language and terms used by Mr. B enable smoking to be identified or diagnosed as a disease.

Mr. B describes craving, repeated relapse, withdrawal, and a cycle of using and stopping that clearly impacts on his self-esteem. What is most striking, however, is that the subjective negative experiences of withdrawal and craving do lead to numerous relapses and difficulty stopping. What is clear is that eventually Mr. B stopped, after numerous relapses. While his preferred outcome was abstinence, could Mr. B be described or diagnosed as an addict using the elements of the disease model?

Beyond the elements of the disease concept of addiction that are used in making a diagnosis, there are other ways of understanding 'dependence' that focus on reducing harm, without necessarily linking this to abstinence. The following section introduces the reader to the 'stage of change' model known as the trans theoretical model (TTM) and the principles of 'motivational interviewing' that can be helpful and work well with screening tools such as the AUDIT to help identify harms and risk and aid in helping clients recognise and work towards reducing the harm associated with the use of substances.

Table 11.3 Is the disease concept useful in diagnosing smoking as a disease?

Discrete Entity: The population can be divided neatly into smokers and non-smokers. However, the only thing that differentiates smokers from non-smokers is the behaviour itself. This element is limited to describing users from non-users.

Abnormal Craving: Smokers do report that craving is uncomfortable. However Mr. B does not describe this experience of craving as overwhelming.

Loss of Control: Mr. B does indicate that for around ten years he never contemplated change, however he does not report feeling that he lost control due to craving or withdrawal.

Irreversibility: Many smokers do experience relapse, and state that they returned to smoking as if they had never stopped. There does seem to be some subjective value in this element. However, this element similar to 'discrete entity' merely categorises those who have regained control, from those who describe having lost control over the ability to make behavioural changes. In this sense it has limited use.

Progressiveness: Examining the consequences of smoking, it is possible to conclude that some diseases such as cancer are progressive. However, it is doubtful whether the use of tobacco (behaviour) itself is progressive, as most smokers do reach a level of use that suits their needs. Most people do not smoke until they lose consciousness but find a level of the drugs that suits their level of tolerance. So as a reference to tolerance, this has some subjective value. However it has limited use in identifying smoking as a behaviour becoming progressively 'worse'.

The health professional's role in supporting a client with substance use problems

There is clearly utility in the addiction concept in determining the severity of dependence an individual experiences in using substances. While adherents of the disease concept would suggest that abstinence is the best way to prevent further harms from occurring, from a harm reduction perspective, reducing harms associated with the use of substances is as important, if not more so, than stopping use. It is in this area that the addiction concept creates division between adherents of the disease concept who support and promote abstinence as a definition of successful outcome, and anyone not achieving or agreeing with this, is considered to be in 'denial'.

A method of communication that avoids this type of confrontation scenario is motivational interviewing (MI), developed by Miller and Rollnick in 1991. As a technique, MI aids the change process by expressing acceptance of a client's stage of change, or when they might be expressing ambivalence with regards to making behaviour changes. MI builds on humanistic theories, regards capability for exercising free choice and changing through a process of self-actualisation. The therapeutic relationship is equal though directive, with the goal of eliciting self-motivational statements and behavioural change from the client to enhance motivation for positive change (Miller and Rollnick 1991).

Motivational interviewing is a counselling style based on the following assumptions:

- Ambivalence about change is normal.
- The alliance between you and your client is a collaborative partnership to which you each bring important expertise.
- An empathic, supportive, yet directive style of communication provides conditions for behaviour change.

In their book *Motivational Interviewing: Preparing People to Change Addictive Behavior* Miller and Rollnick state:

> The strategies of motivational interviewing are more persuasive than coercive, more supportive than argumentative. The motivational interviewer must proceed with a strong sense of purpose, clear strategies, and skills for pursuing that purpose, and a sense of timing to intervene in particular ways at incisive moments. (1991, pp. 51–52)

Miller and Rollnick (1991) set out five general principles for MI:

1 Express empathy through reflective listening.
2 Develop discrepancy between clients' goals or values and their current behaviour.
3 Avoid argument and direct confrontation.
4 Adjust to client resistance rather than opposing it directly.
5 Support self-efficacy and optimism.

Having respect for and acceptance of an individual struggling with substance use encourages a nonjudgmental, collaborative and supportive relationship. Note how different this is from demanding that someone stops, and that if they do not agree that they must stop, that they are in denial.

Client motivation is a strong predictor of change, and this approach puts primary emphasis on providing support for client motivation for change. Therefore, even if clients do not stay for a long course of treatment (as is often the case with problematic substance use), using MI can be helpful in the process of behaviour change, as it has research evidence that links its use to client motivation.

Prochaska and DiClemente's (1983) work on smoking led to the development of their stage of change model, which at its inception was important in helping both users and therapists in understanding why relapse occurred (see Table 11.4).

You can use the stage of change model as a guide, allowing a visual understanding of where an individual might be in relation to their experience of being dependent on a substance or behaviour. This allows you as a practitioner to understand behaviour change as a process rather than an event (which is the underpinning philosophy of the addiction concept) and allows one to offer support and aid movement between stages. What makes the cycle of change so useful is that in discussing relapse as a process in behaviour change, one can help a client recognise the risk factors that led to relapse and make efforts in decision making and behaviour to reduce harm. Relapse is often considered a failure, particularly if dependence is considered a disease, however using the cycle of change, and linking discussion about and relapse to the principles of MI, the public health professional can positively impact on client motivation to make changes to their behaviour.

The core principles of MI, being non-confrontational and non-judgmental, are also extremely useful in helping someone experiencing difficulty with the use of a substance to contemplate change, or if having decided, helping them stay motivated to maintain that decision to change.

Table 11.4 Transtheoretical model (TTM)

There are six stages in the trans-theoretical model of behaviour change (Prochaska and DiClemente, 1983).

The stages of change describe addiction as a process rather than a discrete category of behaviour.

Pre contemplation: client is not aware or concerned that their substance use is an issue.

Contemplation: client becomes aware that substance use results in negative consequences.

Decision/determination: the client decides to change behaviour and begins to make appropriate plans.

Action: the client has decided to make changes to behaviour (cutting down, or stopping).

Maintenance: refers to making considerable effort to maintain the decision to change behaviour.

Relapse: clients find maintenance of behaviour change difficult and revert to previous patterns of use. In this model, this is considered a temporary part of the behaviour change process. Relapse is considered part of the stages of change, rather than an end point, or failure.

The stages of change model developed by Prochaska and DiClemente is conceptualised as a circle or spiral beginning with pre-contemplation (no change); contemplation (considering change); preparation (planning change); action (engaging with an intervention or decision to change); maintenance (maintaining change). 'Relapse' is part of the cycle or process of behaviour change.

Relapse from this perspective is considered useful in gathering information about how relapse occurs, without considering it a failure to maintain abstinence. The stage of change model can be used with a client-centred style of communicating such as MI, and goes beyond naming disagreement as denial and allows a professional to gather information in a non-challenging manner. In understanding and discussing what causes relapse and using this information to avoid or cope with risk factors can help avoid relapse and reduce harm. More importantly, discussing relapse allows the client to consider if they are truly contemplating behaviour change and working towards cutting down or stopping. The model is useful, and by asking a series of questions using the principles of MI and listening actively, with purpose, it is possible to work out if a client should engage in therapy, or treatment, or if information is required (if they are at the pre-contemplating stage) and wait for them to move beyond pre-contemplation to contemplating change, and taking action (Prochaska and DiClemente 1983).

The stages of change and MI are examples of what are known as 'brief interventions'. Brief interventions are relatively easy to administer by non-specialists, in non-clinical settings.

Specialist treatment in relation to long-term use of substances such as alcohol, heroin, and tobacco may require a detox, particularly in relation to substances that have associated unpleasant and even life-threatening withdrawal symptoms such as prolonged hazardous alcohol use.

These brief interventions are also collectively known as 'harm reduction' interventions, which address the harms associated with drinking alcohol, smoking or injecting substances and have strong evidence of efficacy. Harm reduction interventions can include giving advice on the safe use of a substance, including illegal drugs, advice on safe injecting, and offering advice on cutting down smoking and alcohol use. Abstinence is not the objective from a harm reduction perspective, and while desirable, the focus is on reducing harms. An additional resource that you may find helpful can be found on the WHO website relating to brief interventions that can be useful for public health professionals: The ASSIST-linked brief intervention for hazardous and harmful substance use Manual for use in primary care: http://apps.who.int/iris/bitstream/handle/10665/44321/9789241599399_eng.pdf;jsessionid=ACD1EED263DB22A9D92F6FED62C3A229?sequence=1.

Conclusion

Making distinctions between substance use and abuse reveals that some judgements are being made whenever any use is defined as abuse. Attempting to be non-judgmental can be very useful in building trust and rapport between you and an individual who is seeking help from you in relation to their use of substances. As the use of some substances can be stigmatising, and link to discrimination, there can be considerable shame and guilt associated with their use. Adopting a non judgmental approach to this use can be very helpful in building trust.

In describing the various harms that result from the use of alcohol, and the ways in which risk and harm is understood, we reveal the array of terms used to identify or diagnose problems associated with its use. The difficulty that clients report in cutting down or stopping in relation to the use of substances is captured by the elements of the addiction concept in an attempt to categorize harm and understand and define risk. However, as the exercise using the case study of Mr. B has highlighted, defining the behaviour (smoking tobacco) as a disease is a challenge, even if the habitual use of tobacco does result in potentially life-threatening diseases.

The case study of Mr. B was used to test the utility of the concept in relation to smoking and was useful in understanding the harms that result from use. The case study revealed some of the processes of behaviour change that occur over time. In the brief overview of the stages or process of change, the stage of change or trans theoretical model (TTM) is useful in revealing the various stages that clients experience with the use of a substance. There is utility in the TTM to target specific interventions to an individual's stage of change and helping them decide the best outcome, either providing information if they are not yet ready to change (pre contemplator), or in helping them to achieve abstinence or cutting down use to reduce harm.

When the TTM is used in combination with a basic non-judgmental and directed supportive language approach to assessment that underpins Motivational Interviewing (MI), this demonstrates the important role for public health specialists in helping people cut down or stop the use of substances. Read over Mr. B's case study one more time. You will discover that it is possible to understand the stages of change that he experienced, particularly when he was describing relapse, and how the principles of MI can be used to help clients who describe and experience similar difficulty with their use of substances, to recognise that changing behaviour is possible.

CONSIDER THE FOLLOWING QUESTIONS

1. What are the negative consequences of describing use of substance as substance abuse?
2. What are the main elements of the disease concept of addiction that serve to identify or diagnose substance use problems?
3. How well do the components of a dependence syndrome explain the long-term use of tobacco?
4. What interventions and assessment tools can public health professionals use to facilitate behaviour change and reduce harmful substance use and consequences?

Key terms

A&E: Accident and Emergency.

AA: Alcoholics Anonymous.

Addiction: A state where loss of control over ability to stop or cut down on something that is problematic results in negative consequences. Addiction may be diagnosed if certain elements are identified during an assessment.

APS: Annual Population Survey.

AUDIT: Alcohol Use Disorder Inventory Tool.

BI: Brief interventions.

Craving: A state of physical or psychological discomfort.

CSEW: Crime Survey for England and Wales.

Dependence: A state of addiction or dependence. The term is often used interchangeably with **addiction**.

EMCDDA: European Monitoring Centre for Drugs and Drug Abuse.

ISD: Information Services Division of NHS Scotland.

MI: Motivational interviewing.

NHS: National Health Service.

NICE: National Institute for Health and Care Excellence.

NPS: New psychoactive substances.

ONS: Office for National Statistics.

PDU: Problem drug user(s).

SCJS: Scottish Crime and Justice Survey.

TTM: Trans-theoretical model (stage of change model).

UK: United Kingdom.

WHO: World Health Organization.

Further reading

Department of Health and Social Care. 2016. *Guidance: Alcohol Consumption: Advice on Low Risk Drinking*. Available at: https://www.gov.uk/government/publicatio ns/alcohol-consumption-advice-on-low-risk-drinking [Accessed 12.03.2022].

National Institute for Health and Care Excellence (NICE). 2010. *Alcohol-use Disorders: Prevention*. Available at: www.nice.org.uk/guidance/ph24/chapter/7-Glossary [Accessed 12.03.2022].

World Health Organization. n.d. *Alcohol, Drugs and Addictive Behaviours Unit: Terminology and Classifications*. Available at: www.who.int/teams/mental-health-and-substance-use/alcohol-drugs-and-addictive-behaviours/terminology [Accessed 12.03.2022].

References

European Monitoring Centre for Drugs and Drug Addiction (EMCDDA). 2020. *European Drug Report 2020: Key Issues*. Publications Office of the European Union: Luxembourg.

Information Services Division. 2019. *Drug Use and Misuse Statistics in Scotland*. ISD, Scottish Government: Edinburgh.

Kelly, J. F., Saitz, R., Wakeman, S. 2016. Language, substance use disorders, and policy: the need to reach consensus on an 'addiction-ary'. *Alcoholism Treatment Quarterly*; 34(1), 116–123.

McPhee, I., 2013. *The Intentionally Unseen: Illicit and Illegal Drugs Use in Scotland: Exploring Drug Talk in the 21st Century*. Lambert Academic Publishing.

McPhee, I., Sheridan, B. 2020. AUDIT Scotland 10 years on: explaining how funding decisions link to increased risk for drug related deaths among the poor. *Drugs and Alcohol Today*; 20(4), 313–322. https://doi.org/10.1108/DAT-05-2020-0024

Miller, W. S., Rollnick, S. 1991. *Motivational Interviewing: Preparing People to Change Addictive Behavior*. Guilford Press: New York.

Mold, A. 2018. Framing drug and alcohol use as a public health problem in Britain: past and present. *Nordisk Alkohol Nark*; 35(2), 93–99. Available at: www.ncbi.nlm.nih.gov/pmc/articles/PMC6130767/ [Accessed 01.03.2021].

National Institute of Clinical Excellence (NICE). 2018. *Alcohol Use Disorders, Diagnosis, Assessment and Management of Harmful Drinking and Alcohol Dependence*. Available at: www.nice.org.uk/guidance/cg115/documents/alcohol-dependence-and-harmful-alcohol-use-full-guideline2 [Accessed 01.03.2021].

NHS Digital. 2018. *Statistics on Drug Misuse: England*. Available at: https://digital.nhs.uk/data-and-information/publications/statistical/statistics-on-drug-misuse/2020 [Accessed 01.03.2021].

NHS Digital. 2020. *Statistics on Smoking – England*. Available at: https://digital.nhs.uk/data-and-information/publications/statistical/statistics-on-smoking/statistics-on-smoking-england-2020 [Accessed 21.03.2022].

Office for National Statistics. 2019. *Drug Misuse: Findings from the 2018 to 2019 CSEW*. HMSO: London.

Office of National Statistics. 2020. *Deaths Related to Drug Poisoning in England and Wales: 2019 Registrations, Deaths Related to Drug Poisoning in England and Wales – Office for National Statistics (ons.gov.uk)*, London [Accessed 01.11.2021].

Peele, S. 1995. *Diseasing of America: How We Allowed Recovery Zealots and the Treatment Industry to Convince Us We Are Out of Control*. Lexington Press: Lanham, MD.

Prochaska, J. O., DiClemente, C. C. 1983. Stage and process of self-change of smoking: towards an integrative model of change. *Journal of Consulting and Clinical Psychology*; 51(3), 390–395. Available at: https://doi.org/10.1037/0022-06x.51.3.390 [Accessed 27.10.2020].

World Health Organization. 1994. *Lexicon of Alcohol and Drug Terms: A Technical Document Publication*. WHO: Geneva. Available at: https://www.who.int/publications/i/item/9241544686 [Accessed 01.03.2022].

12
MENTAL HEALTH

ALEX NUTE

━━━━━━━━━━━━ LEARNING OUTCOMES ━━━━━━━━━━━━

By the end of this chapter you will be able to:

- Consider the differences between mental health and mental disorder according to the dual continuum model and make links to inequality and social deprivation as determinants of mental health.
- Compare the aims and objectives of universal, selective and indicated prevention public mental health interventions.
- Understand the centrality of mental health promotion and prevention within a public health framework.
- Gain awareness of global and national policies and clinical pathways to identify appropriate public mental health interventions across the lifespan.
- Recognise early symptoms of psychosis, anxiety and depression.

Introduction

This chapter will provide an overview of public mental health practice as a primer for deeper understanding of this broad field. It begins by situating mental wellbeing at the heart of public health approaches and introduces models and practice frameworks to help understand how health promotion and prevention work is undertaken in practice.

A lifespan approach will be presented with real life examples of policies and initiatives that address inequalities in health and their impact on the mental health of individuals and communities. New ideas and challenges such as those posed by the COVID-19 pandemic will be introduced to stimulate further reading and action on mental health promotion.

Setting the scene

The impact of poor mental health presents a global challenge for people of all ages, societies and to public health. Depression and anxiety disorders are among the leading contributors to health burden worldwide (Global Burden of Disease (GBD) 2019), and in the UK 74% of respondents to a survey reported feeling overwhelmed by stress in the previous year (Mental Health Foundation 2021). The cost of mental ill health to the UK economy is around £35 billion each year in terms of sickness absence, staff turnover and lost productivity (Centre for Mental Health 2017).

Achieving good mental health must then be recognised as a core component of societal and individual wellbeing, though a commonly agreed definition of what that actually is remains elusive and shrouded in cultural and political discourse. It can, however, be agreed that mental health represents more than just the absence of disorder. The World Health Organization Comprehensive Mental Health Action Plan describes a broad conceptualisation of mental health as 'a state of well-being in which the individual realises his or her own abilities, can cope with the normal stresses of life, can work productively and fruitfully, and is able to make a contribution to his or her community' (WHO 2021, p.1), providing a platform for the global objectives it identifies for achievement by 2030.

This kind of formalisation of mental health as an holistic, positive construct helps to define it as more than just another piece of a public health jigsaw as it is integral to the effective functioning of individuals and communities (WHO 2004). 'Mental wellbeing' can be brought within the public health framework despite the difficulties in assessing or quantifying it or establishing it as an end-goal of person-centred interventions; mental health is a resource for living and a community asset from fulfilment of potential to community flexibility and resilience, and public mental health strategy should therefore act to promote it.

Public mental health

Public mental health arises from the same principles as wider public health practice, helping to situate it within the overall understanding of health as an issue for societal mobilisation (Acheson 1988). Public mental health practice involves the promotion of wellbeing and the prevention of disorder (in practice there can be considerable overlap here) as well as effective treatment and care and recovery should they arise.

While access to secondary mental health services may still be largely bound up with formal psychiatric assessment and diagnosis of mental disorder, the hegemony of the biological model which medicalised understanding and the response to mental distress through the 20th century is giving ground to a less positivist 'recovery-oriented' approach that emphasises building on strengths and generating 'resilience'. Recent developments in primary care provision mark a shift of focus away from only decreasing symptoms to include a more individualised consideration of human experience and self-management, with importance placed on understanding and acceptance, growth and personal empowerment.

The considerable benefits that the bio-medical model has provided through advances in medication and health technologies now fit within a 'bio-psychosocial' model that extends appreciation of the determinants of mental health around systemic, social and environmental influences along with genetic and biological risk factors. This has helped to generate an expansion in the available treatment options for mental disorders which can be seen, for instance, in the growth of evidence-based psychological interventions and their adoption into clinical guidance and pathways published by the National Institute for Health and Care Excellence (NICE).

Tudor (1996) proposes a 'dual continuum' that helps differentiate mental health promotion and prevention from interventions for mental disorders, and so establishes a conceptual framework for public mental health practice that can be inclusive of both working to mitigate losses and to move toward growth (see Figure 12.1).

The two dimensions illustrate that presence of a diagnosable mental disorder is not necessarily indicative of psychological and emotional function, that although there is a

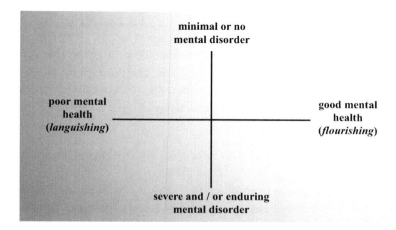

Figure 12.1 The dual continuum model (adapted from Tudor 1996, and Keyes 2005)

correlation between mental disorder and poor mental health, people with an established diagnosis will nevertheless encounter a range from good to poor mental health or wellbeing. Outcomes on the wellbeing continuum are of relevance to public health as they are reliant on two fluctuating and distinct aspects: 'hedonic' and 'eudaimonic' contents and functions. Put simply hedonic happiness is founded in experiences that inspire joy and pleasure, and allow for actions that meet needs and wants. Eudaimonic happiness is a more general sense of satisfaction and achievement, and actualisation of this through inspiration and action. Both contribute to the personal sense of mental wellbeing (Huta 2015).

The experience of good mental health makes a significant contribution to quality of life and the health of individuals and communities. Where attributes and skills promoting emotional health and positive thinking are aligned with good social relationships and a sense of purpose or 'coherence', a growing body of evidence suggests outcomes for longevity, employment status, criminality, healthy living styles and pro-social behaviours can be predicted (Friedli 2009).

This dialogue between the person and their environment suggests that hedonia and eudaimonia, and therefore position on the axis of wellbeing, are open to the influence of a wide range of determinants.

Common determinants of mental wellbeing

- Family structure and dynamics.
- Equality and oppression.
- Education and employment.
- Community and relationships.
- Lifestyle and biomedical health.
- Housing and environment.
- Trauma and attribution styles.

The propensity for people and communities to be either 'flourishing' or 'languishing' (Keyes 2005) according to the effect of these determinants establishes their priority for sustainable action through health and social care policy. The Ottawa Charter for Health Promotion (WHO 1986) identifies five key areas for action to drive a positive orientation on the wellbeing continuum:

1 **Building healthy public policy** to create an integrated, multi-agency effort to challenge inequality and improve wellbeing across the lifespan.
2 **Create supportive environments** in communities, workplaces, educational settings and at home to create a 'socioecological approach to health' (1986, p. 2).
3 **Strengthen community action** through empowerment, *co-production*, learning and setting locally relevant priorities.

4   **Develop personal skills** and knowledge in areas from psychoeducation, anxiety management and building resilience.
5   **Reorient health services** to the pursuit of wellbeing, meaning recovery-oriented secondary services and a stronger presence in primary care, alongside mental health promoting activities and prevention.

Pickett and Wilkinson (2013) build a convincing case for the impact of inequality on happiness and wellbeing by presenting data from a broad range of research illustrating that more people experience mental illnesses in societies that exhibit greater inequality. Citing the work of James (2007) and Frank (1999), they show how a culture that prioritises acquisition and normative understandings of success creates aspirations that the majority of members will not attain, at the same time as marginalising personal relationships and a sense of connectiveness among other attributes that could actually bring them happiness.

In England the Fair Society, Healthy Lives review (Marmot 2010) notes that the distribution of health across society falls on a gradient that directly correlates with social status, opening up a discussion of relevance to the UK as a whole. Poverty creates barriers to preventative measures whether they be affirming social activities, classes, time for personal development and access to resources supporting of growth or more structural issues arising from poor quality housing, employment and nutrition. The challenges facing public health in the 21st century identified by the WHO (n.d.) reflect the scale of the work that lies ahead.

Main challenges facing public health in the 21st century

- Family structure and dynamics.
- Economic crisis.
- Widening inequalities.
- Ageing population.
- Increasing levels of chronic disease.
- Migration and urbanization.
- Environmental damage and climate change.

(WHO n.d.)

The complex interplay of social determinants, individual risk and protective factors, and environmental influences suggest that public mental health policy will be most effective where national, local and individual approaches are informed by an 'ecological framework' that encompasses these key areas.

A framework for intervention

Mrazek and Haggerty (1994) proposed a spectrum of interventions supporting mental health that spans treatment of disorder and subsequent maintenance of recovery, along with a three-category framework of 'universal', 'selective' and 'indicated' prevention interventions. When delivered in partnership between health and social care agencies and the third sector, these preventative interventions deliver effective public health outcomes of benefit to the individual and the wider community (Marmot 2010).

Barry (2013), however, argues that this framework presents interventions that focus only on avoiding or managing loss associated with disorder and puts forward a modified spectrum to include promotion of wellbeing, adding competence, empowerment, supportive environments and resilience as overlapping concepts inspiring of good mental health.

Mental health evolves throughout the lifespan (WHO 2021). This chapter will move forward as a primer for understanding public mental health using a lifespan approach to review how key public mental health measures can target priority mental health conditions. Barry's (2013) modified framework will be applied to real world exemplars to demonstrate how health promoting and preventing interventions can be applied to the broad field of public mental health and disorder.

Early years

Across the UK maternal mental health policy and pathways have emphasised the importance of early experiences in predicting future mental health outcomes. Effective public mental health programmes start working with the youngest infants and their caregivers through the preventative methods of healthy child programmes and interventions, many of which involve the promotion of competence and secure attachment.

The psychological theory of attachment describes how the relationship between the parent or guardian and infants in the first few years of development is a crucial indicator of future mental health and wellbeing (Bowlby 1969). The establishment of a trusting bond with a primary caregiver provides the infant with a 'safe base' to make positive predictions about future relationships and is predictive of better outcomes in personal resilience, self-esteem, academic performance and social behaviours. Conversely insecure attachment, where an affective bond does not develop, can lead to long-term experience of depression and anxiety, poor coping strategies and emotional dysregulation that affect relationships and quality of life. Please see Chapter 6 for an extensive table of attachment classifications.

Presentation of insecure attachment

- Poor eye contact.
- Aversion to touch.
- Problems with conduct.
- Emotional distancing.
- Separation anxiety.

Good-quality parenting programmes follow principles of 'primary prevention' to reduce the incidence and severity of developmental concerns and build future resources for wellbeing and resilience. For public mental health practice, primary prevention aims to ensure the strongest possible start in life through adoption of broad strategies to challenge health inequalities as well as those that focus on reducing adverse childhood experiences (ACEs) by building healthy relationship and parenting skills.

Programmes that promote secure attachment begin with recognition and appropriate responding to the emotions and behaviours of infants. A toolkit developed by the Parent-Infant Foundation (Bateson et al. 2019) provides an example of how an evidence-based framework for developing better parent–infant relationships can first consider the psychological needs of the caregiver. The framework explores issues resulting from unresolved trauma or anxiety that may be affecting confidence and engagement to build a strengths-based approach to empathic responding, warmth, contact and capacity to change.

Interventions to promote attachment build in intensity from the encouragement of nurturing physical contact between caregiver and infant to more formal interventions such as counselling, cognitive behaviour therapy and other brief psychological interventions where the assessment of needs suggest a more intensive approach is required.

Estimates suggest that up to one in five maternal caregivers experience disruption to their mental health through the perinatal period (Faculty of Public Health and Mental Health Foundation 2016), with specialist multi-disciplinary and multi-agency teams providing enhanced support and supervision in the community and where necessary inpatient settings (see Chapter 7).

Service provision for perinatal mental health can incorporate 'secondary prevention' work to reduce the impact of established mental disorder on the parenting relationship. Perinatal mental health services can play a key role in monitoring parental mental health and providing early access to effective support and interventions to minimise ACEs. This work can begin in the prenatal or pregnancy planning period for parents and caregivers with a previous history of mental disorder.

Prevention work can also focus on the transition from infant settings to primary school to ensure the best chance of engagement with early education. Home-based school readiness programmes that build confidence, concentration and attention to purposeful tasks can be complemented by targeted induction activities helping children and parents become familiar with environments and expectations, and sharing knowledge of their developmental experiences to that point (Roberts 2014).

Children and young people

Following transition into full-time education, the influences on health and wellbeing extend beyond the home. Relative deprivation and parenting styles do continue to have considerable influence over health and wellbeing, but formative opportunities emerge to promote empowerment through a positive sense of identity, resilience, acquisition of knowledge and relationships to enable active participation in society (WHO 2021).

The journey from childhood to adolescence and young adulthood is characterised by change. Physical growth is mirrored by an expansion of social and emotional experiences that can lead to less healthy outcomes, with up to 50% of mental disorders beginning before the age of 14 (WHO 2021).

In 2018 it was estimated that one in four children will present as experiencing poor mental health (National Assembly for Wales 2018) with significant challenges to wellbeing arising from new media and environmental concern adding to the extant determinants encompassing poverty, family separation, racism, neglect and abuse.

NICE (2009a) provides guidance for educators and health and social care professionals on working collaboratively with families along with whole-school and curriculum approaches to promote wellbeing in secondary education. School-based interventions (see Table 12.1) are implemented at a local level in the UK with guidance drawn from national level mental health and education strategies allowing for some flexibility in approach to meet the needs of the population.

The scaffolding that educational performance provides for future prospects, and the development of life skills including those promoting of positive mental health, affirm the goal of wellbeing as a key impact area for schools. Preventative work with this age group can also link to interventions where addressing behaviours such as bullying, school avoidance, self-harm, substance use and criminality, may require joining a multi-agency approach where risk is considered to be high.

Indicated prevention interventions target people with early signs and symptoms of disorder who are at high risk. A first episode of psychosis is a distressing and potentially life-changing event that typically occurs at the crossroads between adolescence and young adulthood (Kirkbride et al. 2017) and carries the risk of developing into an enduring experience of bi-polar disorder, schizophrenia and other related disorders.

Early warning signs of psychosis

- Problems with concentration
- Suspicion or paranoia
- Changes in sleep pattern and appetite
- Unease and social withdrawal
- High expressed emotion or blunted affect
- Poor hygiene and lack of interest
- Increasingly odd ideas / behaviours
- Responding to unseen stimuli

Table 12.1 Examples of school-based interventions

Whole-school approaches	Embedded curriculum areas
Pro-social actions	Emotional literacy
Peer mentoring	Sex and relationships
Building resilience	Alcohol, tobacco and drugs
Pastoral support	Digital literacy and safety
Safeguarding	Respecting diversity

Evidence suggests that long-term outcomes are affected by the initial duration of untreated psychosis (DUP) (McFarlane 2011) characterised by these early warning signs, making early detection and intervention vital.

The initial response to a suspected first episode of psychosis is a multi-disciplinary assessment and intensive symptomatic treatment with anti-psychotic medication led by a specialist child and adolescent mental health service (CAMHS) or early intervention service (EIS) (NICE 2016). Following initial treatment, care planning for first episode psychosis moves forward to offer indicated preventative interventions comprising relapse prevention, psychoeducation, educational and vocational support, social inclusion work and individual/family psychosocial interventions.

These kinds of partnership working between health, social care, education and families can help build strengths and resilience as they approach the transition to the next step on their life course.

Adult mental health

The emphasis placed on developing emotional strength and resilience in early life in fact serves to illustrate the importance of moving to the next stage of life equipped to flourish and build personal assets. Beginning work, starting families and adapting to changing circumstances can be opportunities for growth and fulfilment or times when those strengths are tested. With one in six people in the UK experiencing symptoms at any given time, public mental health policy can reach into all aspects of adult life and make a difference through the practice of prevention and promotion.

One key area of practice is to confront and reduce the stigma associated with poor mental health. Stigma can be broken down into three linked elemental problems of knowledge, attitudes and behaviours that give rise to ignorance, prejudice and discrimination (Thornicroft et al. 2007). Table 12.2 provides examples of the potential social and individual consequences of stigmatisation.

'Social marketing' uses commercial marketing techniques as a methodology to promote social change that can be employed as an effective tool for mental health promotion. Between 2017 and 2019 a national third-sector campaign Time to Change, led by charities Mind and Rethink Mental Illness, used a multimedia social marketing strategy to target men in skilled manual and administrative roles who were detached from

Table 12.2 Elements of stigmatisation (adapted from Thornicroft et al. 2007)

Elements of Stigma	Problems of Knowledge	Problems of Attitudes	Problems of Behaviour
Outcome	Ignorance	Prejudice	Discrimination
Reaction	Shunning	Fear	Rejection
Impact	Social isolation	Self-stigmatisation	Deprivation
	Limitation of Community	Limitation of Help-seeking	Limitation of Equality

an understanding of mental health. The campaign's messaging focused on behaviour change and provision of support, with evaluation of the project showing significant improvements in the knowledge and understanding of the target group and importantly an increased confidence in how to advise a friend to seek help (González-Sanguino et al. 2019).

Stigma can have profound effects on experiences of work as Marmot (2010) points out that people with mental health problems are more likely to be unemployed or in poorly paid low-status roles. Supporting organisations and occupational health professionals to challenge structural discrimination and promote supportive environments can mean accessing opportunities to build social networks, personal capital and resilience alongside stimulating and rewarding employment (Faculty of Public Health and Mental Health Foundation 2016).

The workplace is a potentially stressful environment with workload pressure, relationships with colleagues, feelings of powerlessness or role ambiguity and lack of support potentially driving maladaptive responses and negative mental health outcomes. The Covid-19 pandemic has seen the cost of poor mental health to UK employers rise to £53-56 billion per year (Deloitte 2022) and employers have a statutory responsibility to prevent the demands that can positively motivate performance from developing into anxiety and disorders such as generalised anxiety disorder (GDA), a long-term condition with potentially debilitating psychological and physiological symptoms (see Table 12.3).

Universal prevention interventions aim to reduce disorder and improve wellbeing for whole populations rather than targeting areas of specific risk. Universal interventions in the workplace could involve:

- Identification of risk factors through stress risk assessment (Health and Safety Executive n.d.).
- A focus on causes of stress and consideration of adjustments such as flexible working (NICE 2009b).
- Promoting inclusive and supportive management styles (Chartered Institute of Personnel and Development 2021).

Complementing these prevention strategies with opportunities strengthen personal resources through development, and support will further encourage people to flourish in positive working environments. This mirrors the approaches of tertiary prevention

Table 12.3 Symptoms of generalised anxiety disorder

Psychological symptoms	Physiological symptoms
Apprehension and dread	Fatigue
Difficulty concentrating	Headache
Catastrophising	Nausea
Irritability	Aches and pains
Restlessness	Palpitations
Feeling overwhelmed	Dizziness
Avoidance	Sleep disturbance

interventions which aim to reduce the impact of long-term and complex health problems through building self-management skills and ability. Tertiary interventions can also comprise programmes to support, train and potentially redeploy staff to maximise productivity and job satisfaction.

Later life

Global populations are ageing rapidly, with estimates suggesting that by 2050 one in every five people will be aged over 60 and that approximately 15% of older adults will experience mental disorder (WHO 2017) pointing to increasing challenges in meeting the health and social care needs of this group.

The promotion of resilience through active and healthy ageing has been relatively neglected in policy and strategy and under-resourced in practice. Age Concern and the Mental Health Foundation (2006) identify five key areas of influence that promoting activities need to focus on to help mitigate the risk of languishing in later years and grow an appreciation of older generations as a community asset.

Key factors affecting health and wellbeing of older adults

- Being valued and not discriminated against.
- Participating in meaningful activity.
- Replacing isolation with good relationships.
- Keeping well and avoiding illness.
- Being financially secure.

The WHO (2017) frame this within a wider deterministic and human rights-based perspective, citing the need for strategies to ensure access to resources that will provide programmes of community development for health and social care targeting the most vulnerable and provision of secure and supportive housing. Promoting positive mental wellbeing for older people in care homes has been the focus of a quick guide for managers developed by NICE and the Social Care Institute for Excellence (2020). Four themes are identified to frame activities promoting wellbeing:

- Respecting personal identity.
- Providing physical, social and leisure activities.
- Assessing and supporting health and mental wellbeing.
- Ensuring access to healthcare.

Older adults are more likely to live with disability and chronic illness, and the cumulative effects of problems with mental health over a lifespan can have profound impacts in later years (Friedli 2009). Poverty, social isolation, loneliness and loss become more common determinants of health in older age groups and people become more vulnerable to abuse at home and in institutional care settings.

Together these factors can put older people at increased risk of developing depression. Table 12.4 provides a diagnostic framework for depression (NICE 2009c), though it is important to note that some associated symptoms are commonly experienced by older adults at a sub-threshold level.

Psychiatric morbidity is a key indicator of suicide risk, with psychosis, substance misuse and primarily depression related to suicide ideation and attempt. Reported suicide accounts for 1.4% of all premature deaths worldwide (Brådvik 2018), though the true figure may be much higher. In 2018 the highest risk groups for suicide in the UK were males and females aged 45 to 49 years, though rates are also significant for the oldest age groups for both (Office for National Statistics 2018).

National suicide prevention strategies across the UK are founded in an ecological approach to public health in order to reduce suicide. They focus on selected and indicated high-risk groups that include users of secondary mental health care and specific occupational groups beneath a universal framework of interventions. Selective prevention interventions target people at higher risk of developing depression or other major mental disorders; these could be people from socially deprived areas, families with a history of substance misuse or neglect, prison communities or people with biomedical vulnerability.

The Mental Health First Aid training programme is an example of a preventative framework that has featured in strategies for England, Scotland, Wales and Northern Ireland. Over 12 hours the workshops aim to equip staff working in health and social care as well as the wider public to recognise the warning signs of mental distress and respond with support and advice to seek out ongoing help. Cross-cultural evaluation of the programme has shown it to be effective in boosting confidence in both recognition of and responding to mental disorder even in crisis situations and reduces stigmatising attitudes (Morawska et al. 2012).

Table 12.4 Recognising depression (NICE 2009c)

Diagnosis of Depression (NICE 2009b)	
Key symptoms: • **persistent sadness or low mood** • **marked loss of interests or pleasure**	**Associated symptoms:** • disturbed sleep (decreased or increased compared to usual) • decreased or increased appetite and/or weight • fatigue or loss of energy • agitation or slowing of movements • poor concentration or indecisiveness • feelings of worthlessness or excessive or inappropriate guilt • suicidal thoughts or acts

One or more **key symptoms** have been noted on most days, most of the time for at least two weeks. Add to the number of **associated symptoms** to determine if an episode is:
• mild (less than five total)
• severe (most/all symptoms impacting on day-to-day functioning)
• or somewhere in between (moderate)

Building mental health literacy and help-seeking behaviours are cornerstones of mental health promotion and the prevention of disorder, and the positive outcomes of public mental health work across the lifespan are evidence of the potential benefits they can provide for people and communities.

Mental health for all

These strategies and exemplars provide a flavour of current practice and areas for development that represent a wealth of good practice and complexity that could not be contained in this chapter. Perhaps the most critical area warranting further exploration is the role of collaboration in building potential for flourishing and cohesive communities.

Community regeneration is not limited to investment in physical spaces and economies. Achieving and maintaining good mental health across the lifespan means promoting activities that build protective factors of connectedness, access to good quality support and resilience, and universal, selective and indicated preventative interventions to reduce incidence of mental disorder. The influence of social settings on health and wellbeing behaviours is profound, and local gateway projects that encourage professionals to reach out to under-represented and low engagement areas can help break down barriers of understanding and distrust by providing opportunities for hard-to-reach communities and those providing services to co-create social capital in the community space.

Taking a social justice approach re-establishes the connection between community and wellbeing over the current emphasis on individualised pathology that otherwise undervalues social determinants of mental health (Friedli 2009). Public mental health interventions that take into account the intersectionality of wellbeing with the diversity of community profiles arising from ethnicity, sexuality, refugee status, gender and gender identity, culture, religion, chronic illness, homelessness, veterans' health, substance misuse and criminality can help build prevention strategies that are culturally sensitive, avoid 'conceptual equivalence' and so encourage help-seeking behaviours.

The global COVID-19 pandemic that arrived in the UK in early 2020 placed an unprecedented burden on all sectors of health and social care, applying further pressure on other specific key priorities such as NHS waiting lists and mental health services. The well-documented public health response applied universal, selective and indicated prevention interventions through a tiered framework responding to rates of transmission and hospitalisation. Social distancing and lockdown measures to limit the spread of the coronavirus had predictable adverse effects in terms of social, psychological and opportunity harms through a process of 'collateral damage' (Bavli et al. 2020) illustrated by significant increases in incidence of depression (Office for National Statistics 2021), suicidal thoughts and feelings and inability to cope with the stress of the pandemic (Mental Health Foundation 2021).

Devolved administrations around the UK provided public health guidance tailored to each population's mental wellbeing offering promoting and preventing advice and routes to help and support, while third-sector groups have pointed to the opportunities that recovery from the pandemic provides to ensure 'parity of esteem' for mental health in future public health strategy and with a core focus on tackling the pre-existing inequalities the pandemic further exposed.

Concepts around what constitutes good health have moved on from normative theories to those that focus on the individual and their ability to self-actualise as members of communities using mental health promotion to reduce the social gradient. New ways of thinking are emerging in community based strategies, some of the most evolutionary are the growth of recovery colleges that train students in self-management and peer support, social prescribing and time banking, mindfulness and bodywork classes and book prescription initiatives that provide access to evidence-based manualised self-help advice. Walking and wellness groups, green gyms and ideas clustered around 'ecotherapy' are linking behavioural activation, social inclusion and peer support for people managing anxiety and working through trauma.

Caution is wise, however, as for instance for every example of a validated online self-directed or interactive therapeutic resource that decolonises wellbeing from biomedical hegemony, there are several more that live beyond the borders of the evidence-base in an infodemic of quick-fix but ultimately lame wellbeing literature. In the 10-year review of progress since the Marmot Review (2010) the authors note that the call to prioritise strategy on tackling health inequality has not been answered by the national government (Marmot et al. 2020).

Ultimately, as Hanlon and Carlisle (2013) note, the most profound message that emerges from wellbeing research is to spend more time and energy improving relationships, and less on the desire to increase standards of living.

Conclusion

This chapter has introduced the principles and practice of public mental health to improve the health and wellbeing of universal populations, selective groups and indicated individuals using primary, secondary and tertiary models of prevention. A modified model of public mental health interventions was used to show how interventions can be targeted across the lifespan.

It has included frameworks for targeting and delivering health promotion interventions to develop competence, empowerment, supportive environments and resilience and provided examples of policies and approaches to illustrate real world applications. Future challenges and opportunities were presented to identify areas for further exploration and action.

CONSIDER THE FOLLOWING QUESTIONS

1. Construct your own definitions of universal, selective and indicated preventions. What examples of public mental health interventions can you research or construct for each?

2. Take a moment to consider where you would place yourself on the two dimensions of the dual continuum. What helps you to move your centre toward flourishing?
3. How could wellbeing be promoted to help create a positive environment in your workplace, college or school?
4. What mental health promotion activities are you aware of in your local neighbourhood? What other interventions may be of benefit and how could they be introduced?
5. What are the most significant challenges that public mental health policy needs to address over the next five years?

Key terms

Anxiety: A feeling of stress and dread that can be a feature of everyday life or acutely distressing to the point of panic. Anxiety can lead to negative appraisals of self, others and future prospects and lead to avoidant behaviour or complex conditions such as obsessive-compulsive disorder, post-traumatic stress disorder or generalised anxiety disorder.

Attachment: The emotional bond that develops between infant and parent/caregiver in the first few years of development.

Bio-psychosocial: A model or approach to mental health care which takes into account an holistic range of biological, psychological and social factors when assessing needs and intended outcomes of care.

Co-production: A collaborative model of service design and delivery which involves communities and service users in the identification of need, planning, commissioning and application of health and social care initiatives.

Conceptual equivalence: The assumption that ideas, beliefs and truths have the same meaning in other cultural contexts, potentially leading to a mismatch in what is meant and what is heard, or what is needed and what is delivered.

Depression: A persistent feeling of sadness or low mood, marked loss of interests and pleasure that affects day-to-day functioning and relationships.

Dual continuum: A conceptual model that differentiates mental heath (wellbeing) and mental illness (disorder) as related and scaling phenomena.

Ecological framework: A model of public health that recognises the complexity of environmental determinants of health behaviours and influences on outcomes.

Ecotherapy: A broad approach to therapeutic and prevention interventions that centres on activity, connectivity and green spaces.

Eudaimonic happiness: Happiness that results from an overall sense of satisfaction and achievement.

Flourishing: A positive sense of place and purpose which allows for personal development and satisfaction with life.

Hedonic happiness: Happiness derived from pleasurable and joyful experiences.

Indicated preventive interventions: Prevention interventions that target people with early signs and symptoms of disorder who are at high risk.

Languishing: The subthreshold experience of low mood, low motivation and disinterest indicative of poor mental health.

Mental wellbeing: Positive emotional, cognitive and social functioning that allows for personal resilience and self-actualisation.

Parity of esteem: Giving equal priority to mental health and physical health.

Perinatal mental health services: A specialist multi-disciplinary team providing care and treatment for mothers experiencing mental disorder.

Public mental health: The promotion of wellbeing and the prevention of disorder and effective treatment, care and recovery should they arise.

Primary prevention: Population level actions to reduce the incidence of disorder.

Psychosis: A cluster of symptoms affecting feelings, perceptions and behaviour that include hallucinations, delusions and problems with thinking, and associated with major mental disorder.

Recovery: A process of moving away from poor mental health or disorder that begins with a holistic view of the person and their strengths and emphasises the individual nature of the journey and goalsetting. Recovery depends on three components: commitment to progress; whole-person approach; empowerment and self-management (Hafal 2009).

Resilience: The ability to cope with stress and bounce back from adversity.

Secondary prevention: Intervening in the early stages of disease to prevent disorder from developing.

Selective preventive interventions: Preventive interventions targeted at an at-risk group or individual to prevent further symptoms from developing.

Social marketing: A process that uses commercial marketing techniques to promote positive health and social behaviours.

Suicide: An intentional act to prematurely end a person's own life.

Universal preventive interventions: Population level preventive interventions that are not targeted on the basis of individual risk and focus on equality and understanding.

Further reading

Brown, J. S., Learmonth, A. M., Mackereth, C. J. 2015. *Promoting Public Mental Health and Well-being: Principles into Practice*. Jessica Kingsley: London.

Goldie, I. 2013. *Public Mental Health Today: A Handbook*. Pavilion: Brighton.

Knifton, L., Quinn, N. (Eds). 2013. *Public Mental Health Global Perspectives*. McGraw-Hill Education: Maidenhead.

Newton, J. 2012. *Preventing Mental Ill-Health: Informing Public Health Planning and Mental Health Practice*. Routledge: Abingdon.

References

Acheson, D. 1998. *Independent Inquiry into Inequalities and Health (Acheson Report)*. The Stationery Office: London.

Age Concern and the Mental Health Foundation. 2006. *Promoting Mental Health and Well-being in Later Life: A First Report from the UK Inquiry into Mental Health and Well-being in Later Life*. Age Concern and the Mental Health Foundation: London.

Barry, M. 2013. Adopting a mental health promotion approach to public mental health. In I. Goldie (Ed.), *Public Mental Health Today: A Handbook*. Pavilion Publishing: Brighton.

Bateson, K., Lang, B., Hogg, S., Clear, A. 2019. *Development and Implementation Toolkit*. Parent–Infant Foundation: London.

Bavli, I., Sutton, B., Galea, S. 2020. Harms of public health interventions against COVID-19 must not be ignored. *BMJ*; 371, m4074.

Bowlby, J. 1969. *Attachment and Loss*. Basic Books: New York.

Brådvik, L. 2018. Suicide risk and mental disorders. *International Journal of Environmental Research and Public Health*; 15(9), 2028.

Centre for Mental Health. (2017). *Mental Health at Work: The Business Costs Ten Years On*. Centre for Mental Health: London.

Chartered Institute of Personnel and Development. 2021. *Mental Health in the Workplace*. Available at: www.cipd.co.uk/knowledge/culture/well-being/mental-health-factsheet [Accessed 22.12.2021].

Deloitte. 2022. *Mental health and employers: The case for investment – pandemic and beyond*. Deloitte: London.

Faculty of Public Health and Mental Health Foundation. 2016. *Better Mental Health for All: A Public Health Approach to Mental Health Improvement*. Faculty of Public Health and Mental Health Foundation: London.

Frank, R. 1999. *Luxury Fever*. Free Press: New York.

Friedli, L. 2009. *Mental Health, Resilience and Inequalities*. World Health Organization (Europe): Copenhagen.

Global Burden of Disease. 2019. Disease and Injuries Collaborators. Global burden of 369 diseases and injuries in 204 countries and territories, 1990–2019: a systematic analysis for the Global Burden of Disease Study 2019. *Lancet*; 396, 1204–1222.

González-Sanguino, C., Potts, L. C., Milenova, M., Henderson, C. 2019. Time to change's social marketing campaign for a new target population: results from 2017 to 2019. *BMC Psychiatry*; 19, 417.

Hafal. 2009. *My Recovery: A Step-by-step Plan for People With Serious Mental Illness*. Hafal: Neath. Available at: https://mnpmind.org.uk/wp-content/uploads/2021/09/Hafal-My-recovery.pdf [Accessed 12.03.2022].

Hanlon, P., Carlisle, S. 2013. Positive mental health and wellbeing: connecting individual, social and global levels of wellbeing. In L. Knifton, N. Quinn (Eds), *Public Mental Health Global Perspectives*. McGraw-Hill Education: Maidenhead.

Health and Safety Executive. n.d. *Work-related stress and how to manage it*. Available at: www.hse.gov.uk/stress/risk-assessment.htm [Accessed 22.12.2021].

Huta, V. 2015. An overview of hedonic and eudaimonic well-being concepts. In L. Reinecke, M. Oliver (Eds), *Handbook of Media Use and Well-being*. Routledge: New York.

James, O. 2007. *Affluenza*. Vermilion: London.

Keyes, C. 2005. Mental illness and/or mental health? Investigating axioms of the complete state model of health. *Journal of Consulting and Clinical Psychology*; 73, 539–548.

Kirkbride, J., Hameed, Y., Ankireddypalli, G. et al. 2017. The epidemiology of first-episode psychosis in early intervention in psychosis services: findings from the Social Epidemiology of Psychoses in East Anglia [SEPEA] Study. *American Journal of Psychiatry*; 74, 143–153.

Marmot, M. 2010. *Fair Society, Healthy Lives: The Marmot Review: Strategic Review of Health Inequalities in England Post-2010*. Department for International Development: London.

McFarlane, W. 2011. Prevention of first episode psychosis. *The Psychiatric Clinics of North America*; 34(1), 95–107.

Mental Health Foundation. 2021. *Coronavirus: Mental Health in the Pandemic. Wave 12 – September 9-16-2021*. Available at: www.mentalhealth.org.uk/our-work/research/coronavirus-mental-health-pandemic [Accessed 10.01.2022].

Morawska, A., Fletcher, R., Pope, S., Hethwood, E., Anderson, E., McAuliffe, C. 2012. Evaluation of mental health first aid training in a diverse community setting. *International Journal of Mental Health Nursing*; 22, 85–92.

Mrazek, P., Haggerty, R. (Eds). 1994. *Reducing Risks for Mental Disorders: Frontiers for Preventive Intervention Research*. National Academy Press: Washington, DC.

National Assembly for Wales. 2018. *Mind Over Matter: A Report on the Step Change Needed in Emotional and Mental Health Support for Children and Young People in Wales*. National Assembly for Wales: Cardiff.

National Institute for Health and Care Excellence (NICE). 2009a. *Social and Emotional Wellbeing in Secondary Education*. National Institute for Health and Care Excellence: London.

National Institute for Health and Care Excellence (NICE). 2009b. *Mental Wellbeing at Work (PH22)*. National Institute for Health and Care Excellence: London.

National Institute for Health and Care Excellence (NICE). 2009c. *Depression in Adults: Recognition and Management. Clinical Guideline [CG90]*. National Institute for Health and Care Excellence: London.

National Institute for Health and Care Excellence (NICE). 2016. *Psychosis and Schizophrenia in Children and Young People: Recognition and Management (Clinical Guideline [CG155])*. National Institute for Health and Care Excellence: London.

National Institute for Health and Care Excellence & Social Care Institute for Excellence (NICE). 2020. *Promoting Positive Mental Wellbeing for Older People: A Quick Guide for Registered Managers of Care Homes*. National Institute for Health and Care Excellence: London.

Office for National Statistics. 2018. *Suicides in the UK: 2018 Registrations*. Available at: www.ons.gov.uk/peoplepopulationandcommunity/birthsdeathsandmarriages/deaths/bulletins/suicidesintheunitedkingdom/2018registrations [Accessed 21.12.2021].

Office for National Statistics. 2021. *Coronavirus and Depression in Adults, Great Britain: July to August 2021*. Available at: www.ons.gov.uk/peoplepopulationandcommunity/ wellbeing/articles/coronavirusanddepressioninadultsgreatbritain/julytoaugust2021 [Accessed 21.12.2021].

Pickett, E., Wilkinson, R. 2013. *Inequality: An Underacknowledged Source of Mental Illness and Distress*. In L. Knifton, N. Quinn (Eds), *Public Mental Health Global Perspectives*. McGraw-Hill Education: Maidenhead.

Roberts, J. 2014. *Improving School Transitions for Health Equity*. Institute for Health Equality: London.

Thornicroft, G., Rose, D., Kassam, A., Sartorius, N. 2007. Stigma: ignorance, prejudice or discrimination? *British Journal of Psychiatry*; 190, 192–193.

Tudor, K. 1996. *Mental Health Promotion*. Routledge: London.

World Health Organization. 1986. *Ottawa Charter for Health Promotion*. Available at www. who.int/teams/health-promotion/enhanced-wellbeing/first-global-conference [Accessed 22.03.2022].

World Health Organization. 2004. *Promoting Mental Health: Concepts, Emerging Evidence, Practice (Summary Report)*. World Health Organization: Geneva.

World Health Organization. 2017. *Mental Health of Older Adults*. Available at: www. who.int/news-room/fact-sheets/detail/mental-health-of-older-adults [Accessed 21.12.2021].

World Health Organization. 2021. *Comprehensive Mental Health Action Plan 2013–2030*. World Health Organization: Geneva.

World Health Organization. n.d. *Public Health Services*. Available at: www.euro.who.int/ en/health-topics/Health-systems/public-health-services/public-health-services [Accessed 21.12.2021].

13

ORAL HEALTH

KATE PHILLIPS

LEARNING OUTCOMES

By the end of this chapter you will be able to:

- Understand the role oral health plays in a person's overall health, including their psychosocial wellbeing.
- Understand the prevalence and aetiology of common oral diseases which include dental decay and periodontal disease.
- Have clarity on the role social and economic division play in oral diseases in regards to health inequalities.
- Consider the wider social and environmental conditions that influence oral health behaviour choices and oral health literacy, including the key behavioural risk factors predisposing individuals and the influencing wider determinants of health.
- Critically analyse the public health preventative approach to oral health promotion from a social and political perspective.

Introduction

Oral health is referred to as the 'ability to speak, smile, smell, taste, touch, chew, swallow and convey a range of emotions through facial expressions with confidence and without pain, discomfort and disease of the craniofacial complex' (FDI World Dental Federation 2020, p. 1). This aspect of health, although often not prioritised, remains an integral element of an individual's overall health, wellbeing and physical and social functioning (Shedlin et al. 2018). Whilst improvements in living conditions have contributed to an increasing life expectancy, this alternatively is counter-producing significant challenges in relation to the prevalence of non-communicable diseases (NCD), which includes the prevalence of oral diseases (Fukai et al. 2017). The increasing incidence of oral disease is predominantly associated to key behavioural risk factors involving the increased intake of dietary sugars, excessive tobacco and alcohol exposure and a lack of exposure to fluoride to strengthen teeth (Jacobsen 2019). These behavioural risk factors, which are also attributed to other common NCD such as diabetes, cardiovascular disease and cancers, are posing a significant public health challenge across the lifespan. They are also significantly attributed to the socio-economic circumstances in which individuals live, creating unfair oral health differences between differing population groups which is referred to as health inequality. These unfair differences occur due to the social and environmental conditions in which individuals live, which includes conditions such as their level of income, level of educational attainment and access to health services. These conditions can influence or limit the healthy choices that an individual can make in relation to their oral health. To address these potential influences and reduce this burden of disease, public health action now focuses on a proactive preventative and health promoting approach as opposed to a reactive treatment paradigm (Watt et al. 2019).

The ethos of this approach is underpinned from a global political perspective through the implementation of the World Health Organization's (WHO 2019a) Oral Health Programme and within the Tokyo Declaration on dental care and oral health for health longevity (WHO 2015). This global political direction recognises that oral health is a fundamental right across the lifespan and the risk factors associated with oral disease are common to other NCD. This poses responsibility on policy makers to implement a 'common risk factor approach' (Fukai et al. 2017) to promote oral health and integrate this into the NCD prevention and control development agenda. This agenda will focus on tackling risk factors that occur due to the economic, environmental and social circumstances in which individuals live. However, this preventative approach to oral health must be individualised as the risk factors differ across the lifespan due to age-related oral physiology and differing environmental and behavioural risk factors. Within this chapter the risk of oral disease and the influencing determinants will be critically explored from both a child and adult perspective. This will focus on the development of dental decay and periodontal disease as highly prevalent oral diseases and an exploration of the evidence-based preventative approach to oral health that will reduce this burden of disease.

Oral health in children

A healthy oral cavity is an integral element of health and wellbeing from birth. The FDI World Dental Federation (2020) defines oral health as being free from facial discomfort and pain, oral infection, sores, tooth decay or loss. Including the ability to suck, bite chew and promote the optimum conditions for age appropriate speech development. Yet these conditions are not inevitable and a reality for a growing number of the population with the development of dental decay (also referred to as 'dental caries') becoming the most prevalent non-communicable disease in children. The WHO (2019b) confirm that 60–90% of school-aged children globally have compromised oral health wellbeing due to the presence of dental decay, with 486 million children suffering from this disease within their primary dentition. From a national perspective, within the UK the incidence of oral disease varies across the four geographical regions and within differing socio-economic groups (Godson and Seymour 2019). The Children's Dental Health Survey commissioned by the Health & Social Care Information Centre (2015) operates oral health surveillance decennially of children aged 5, 8, 12 and 15 years residing in England, Wales and Northern Ireland. In Scotland this epidemiological evidence is collected annually via the National Dental Inspection Programme which measures the incidence of oral disease in Primary 1 and Primary 7 children (Information Services Division 2019a). Although these two surveys operate differing sampling methods, both epidemiological surveys use the DMFT Index to identify prevalence, which refers to measuring the number of Decayed, Missing and Filled Teeth across the sample population. Table 13.1 compares the prevalence of 5 and 8 year-olds who have clinical decay experience in England, Wales

Table 13.1 The prevalence of child dental decay across the four nations

Region	% of 5-year-olds affected by clinical decay experience in 2013	Mean number of teeth affected	% of 12-year-olds affected by clinical decay experience in 2013	Mean number of teeth affected
England (Holmes et al. 2015)	31	1.8	32	1.9
Wales (Porter et al. 2015)	41	2.4	52	2.7
Northern Ireland (Ravaghi et al. 2013)	40	2	57	2.8
Region	% of Primary 1 children with obvious decay experience in 2018	Average number of teeth affected	% of Primary 7 children with obvious decay experience in 2019	Average number of teeth affected
Scotland (Information Service Division 2018; Information Service Division 2019b)	29	1.14	20	0.42

and Northern Ireland. In Scotland the prevalence is identified for both Primary 1 and Primary 7 children to offer some comparison. The prevalence of clinical decay is statistically higher across Wales and Northern Ireland in both identified age groups; however, all four nations have identified a significant incidence for a disease which is mostly preventable.

Although improvements in the prevalence of dental decay has been identified across the four nations from previous recorded epidemiological studies from those referenced, these statistics continue to be significantly higher across all the four nations in areas of high social and economic deprivation, clearly highlighting unfair oral health differences across the population. The Children's Dental Health Survey identified that 'in 5 year olds, four tenths (41%) of those eligible for free school meals had obvious decay experience in primary teeth, compared to three tenths (29%) of other children of the same age' (Health & Social Care Information Centre 2015, p. 4). Hence children disadvantaged by socio-economic deprivation are at an increased risk of experiencing oral health difficulties. This can be critically interpreted more clearly by having an understanding of the key behavioural risk factors predisposing individuals to the risk of dental decay and the influencing wider determinants of health.

Behavioural risks factors

The aetiology of dental decay occurs primarily due to the consumption and frequency of food and drinks that are high in sugars. When sugary foods enter the mouth, the natural bacteria and the microbial biofilm, which is the plaque that builds on the tooth surface, metabolises the dietary sugars into lactic acid (Godson et al. 2018). This acidic pH level within the mouth demineralises the enamel of the teeth, causing the tooth structure to break down. Saliva offers a protective barrier by clearing food debris from the oral cavity and neutralising the acid to support the structure of the tooth enamel to remineralise (Felton and Chapman 2014, Godson et al. 2018). However, the frequent consumption of sugary drinks and foods can increase the process of demineralisation, compromising the protective mechanism of the saliva which causes the teeth to cavitate and dental decay to develop (Felton and Chapman 2014, Daly and Smith 2015). To promote the gingival health and inhibit the process of demineralisation, tooth brushing is recommended twice a day with fluoride toothpaste to remove the microbial biofilm from the tooth surface and any food debris in and between the teeth compromising the natural pH level within the mouth. Fluoride is a chemical element which strengthens and hardens the tooth enamel, enriching the process of remineralisation and making the teeth more resistant to cavitation (Dalal et al. 2019). The increasing prevalence of dental decay can therefore be attributed to poor dietary and oral hygiene practices. These include the frequent snacking on sugary foods and the prolonged contact of sweetened drinks on the teeth, accompanied by a lack of access to therapeutic levels of fluoride through an appropriate toothbrushing routine which should start as soon as the first primary tooth emerges at around 6 months of age (Godson and Seymour 2019).

Although the primary dentition are naturally exfoliated and replaced by the permanent dentition during early childhood, the presence of tooth decay is often not viewed as concerning to parents (Warrilow et al. 2019). Nevertheless, the eruption of the primary dentition has an essential role in the healthy development and function of the oral cavity. They support the development of speech and dietary behaviours and provide a space for the natural growth and alignment of the permanent dentition (Infant & Toddler Forum 2010). The presence of dental decay in the primary dentition not only predisposes the permanent dentition to decay but can have a detrimental impact on a child's physical, emotional, cognitive and social development. Children can experience excessive pain, swelling and potential infection. These symptoms can compromise nutritional intake, growth and sleeping behaviours which can have a detrimental impact on concentration levels, speech development and long-term developmental and academic progression (Forward 2014; Godson et al. 2018).

The presence of dental decay can also alter a child's oral aesthetics. As children grow older and enter school this can have a negative effect on their self-esteem and confidence in social situations when expressing emotions such as smiling or laughing (Voogd 2014). They may become the victim of teasing and bullying from their peers, which can affect their emotional and social wellbeing. Time away from school may be necessary to manage the oral symptoms and seek necessary dental treatment. Dental treatments such as extractions are often required to be performed under anaesthetic or sedation, which elevates the treatment risk to a developing child (Warrilow et al. 2019). The early removal of the primary dentition can also lead to malalignment of the permanent dentition and the need for extensive orthodontic provision during adolescence. Alternatively, if left untreated dental decay has the potential to put a child at risk of developing fatal systemic complications, such as respiratory conditions and sepsis (Forward 2014). These are unnecessary risks and consequences of an oral disease which is preventable with the implementation of key oral health-enhancing behaviours established from birth. These key behaviours are documented in Table 13.2.

Influencing determinants of health

The prevalence of dental decay can also be understood from a wider social and economic perspective. Dalghren and Whitehead's (1991) model of the main health determinants (see Figure 13.1) illustrates three interlinking spheres that have a direct influence on an individual's health and create the conditions in which a person lives. These conditions can directly influence an individual's oral health literacy and oral health enhancing behaviours. They are classified as individual lifestyle factors, social and community networks and socio-economic, cultural and environmental conditions. This model when applied to oral health wellbeing can support conclusions to be drawn to translate how social determinants can influence this aspect of health and adherence to recommended preventative key oral health behaviours, as seen in Figure 13.1.

Parents or carers who are experiencing economic disadvantage and struggling to meet their family's financial needs may not prioritise the need to purchase oral hygiene products, such as toothbrushes or toothpaste, or opt to buy cheaper alternatives which potentially do not have the recommended concentration of fluoride. Dietary behaviours are also influenced by financial pressures, with the general preconception that healthy nutritious food sources are more expensive (Warrilow et al. 2019). A review of the British Nutrition

Table 13.2 Key oral health-enhancing behaviours for children and adults (Public Health England 2017a: contains public sector information licensed under the Open Government Licence v3.0)

Key Oral Health Enhancing Behaviours for Children (Public Health England 2017a). (Cited in Godson & Seymour 2019)

Toothbrushing

Expose teeth to fluoride as soon as the first tooth erupts in the mouth by toothbrushing with an appropriate fluoride toothpaste:

0–3 years – Use a smear of fluoride toothpaste containing 1000 ppm

3–6 years – Use a smear or peas sized amount of fluoride toothpaste containing more than 1000 ppm

7+ years – Use a fluoride toothpaste containing 1350–1500 ppm

Toothbrushing should occur at two periods during the day, one being at night when the saliva levels are generally low. Toothbrushing should be supervised until the age of 7 years. Rinsing should be avoided following brushing to maintain fluoride concentration levels within the oral cavity.

NB: Children 0–6 years at high risk of decay can use a fluoride toothpaste containing 1350–1500 ppm.

Dietary principles

Breast-feeding should be encouraged from birth as per Unicef baby friendly guidelines.

Reduce the consumption and frequency of dietary food and drinks containing sugar.

The use of a free-flow cup should be encouraged for drinks from 6 months of age.

Only water and milk should be offered in a bottle.

Bottle use should be discouraged from 1 year of age.

Dental attendance

Register with the dentist and attend regular preventative check-ups as recommended. The first dental visit should occur at 6 months.

Key oral health behaviours for adults to prevent dental caries and periodontal disease (Public Health England 2017a).

Tooth brushing

Brush each tooth and the gum line with a fluoride toothpaste (1350–1500ppm) twice a day.

This should occur at the last thing at night and on another occasion during the day.

To maintain fluoride concentration levels in the oral cavity rinsing should be avoided following brushing.

High risk individuals identified by a dental practitioner may be advised to use a fluoride mouthwash between brushing.

Remove plaque daily with floss, tape or interdental brushes as advised by a dental practitioner.

Dental attendance

Dental registration and attendance is recommended for ongoing preventative advice and treatment.

Dietary intake

Reduce the amount and frequency of sugars within the dietary intake, including drinks containing sugar.

Tobacco and alcohol consumption

Smoking or chewing any form of tobacco should be avoided.

Alcohol consumption should be reduced to recommended safe levels, classified as 14 units per week, consumed evenly over three or more days.

Foundation briefing paper on diet and school children (Weichselbaum and Buttriss 2014) identified that children disadvantaged by economic deprivation were more likely to consume processed foods and non-diet drinks which increased their overall daily intake of sugar. Parents have a detrimental influence on the development of their child's oral health behaviours from birth. However, the parental stress attributed to social and economic deprivation may hinder a parent's ability to perceive their child's susceptibility to oral health

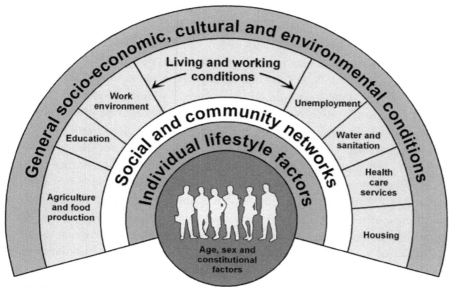

Source: Dahlgren and Whitehead, 1991

| INDIVIDUAL LIFESTYLE FACTORS: |
| Dietary intake high in sugar content and frequency. |
| Lack of exposure to fluoride. |
| Poor toothbrushing and oral hygiene routine. |

| SOCIAL & COMMUNITY NETWORKS: |
| Increased local availability of processed foods and sweetened drinks. |
| Low oral health literacy. |
| No exposure to water fluoridation. |
| Employment contractual restrictions to take paid leave to access dental provision and care. |

| SOCIO-ECONOMIC, CULTURAL & ENVIRONMNETAL CONDITIONS: |
| Unequitable access to local NHS dental services. |
| Limited transport links to efficiently access dental healthcare services and cost- effective nutritious food produce. |

Figure 13.1 The main determinants of health (Dahlgren and Whitehead 1991)

difficulties and prioritise a ritualistic routine of oral health behaviours. Lower education levels may also result in a lack of awareness of the aetiology of dental decay, attributing to general poor oral health literacy. This can include a lack of parental self-confidence and self-efficacy to establish a regular tooth-brushing routine with their child. Within differing communities there may be inequality in the access to preventative NHS dental resources, forcing some families to potentially travel long distances to access dental care which may be outside of their financial means and available transport links.

Oral health improvement programmes

In accordance with the FDI World Dental Federation Vision 2020 (Glick et al. 2012), governments have the responsibility to implement public health policies that advocate oral health preventive programmes which improve oral health literacy and reduce disease levels related to this aspect of health. In the UK, the National Institute for Health and Care Excellence (NICE) (2016) has been instrumental in recommending quality public health provision to reduce the risk of oral health difficulties in children which involves the promotion of key oral health behaviours as seen in Table 13.2. This is reflective of the public health provision outlined within the Health & Social Care Act (2012) and Local Authorities now have a professional responsibility to implement oral health improvement programmes that will target early years settings, including schools in localities where there is an increased risk of oral disease. The improvement plans should outline provision that promotes the establishment of evidence based oral health behaviours such as 'supervised toothbrushing schemes and fluoride varnish programmes' (NICE 2016, p.7). Programmes such as this support children to develop the skills and the routine of toothbrushing, which occurs during supervised sessions within the early years school setting. It also provides children with daily exposure to fluoride. These interventions facilitate the development of a supportive healthy environment which offers the skills and resources required to empower children to develop key evidence based preventative oral health behaviours and enhance their oral health literacy. Eden et al. (2019) has suggested that school-based oral health interventions can be effective as they target children at a time when their attitudes and habits around health behaviours are still developing. Children are also a great influence on their parent's knowledge and attitudes so have the potential to modify their oral health behaviours at home. It is envisaged that healthy oral habits developed in the early years can support these behaviours to be become ritualistic throughout life (see Table 13.3).

In England, with 333 Local Authorities in situ, there are significant variations in relation to the oral health interventions delivered across the English population to respond to the varied prevalence of oral health needs across differing communities. In 2017, Public Health England (PHE 2017b) reported that 77% of Local Authorities have commissioned oral health improvement programmes targeted at the 0–5 year age group. Of these, 51% include supervised toothbrushing programmes in early years school settings as recommended by NICE (2016), and 46% had implemented the provision of toothbrushes and toothpaste. The provision of free toothbrushes and toothpaste ensures that these resources are also available at home irrespective of financial barriers in order to empower toothbrushing behaviours to continue within the home environment. Oral health programmes have also been implemented across the other three UK nations; these are known as 'Happy Smiles' in Northern Ireland (Integrated Care 2018), 'Designed to Smile' in Wales (Welsh Assembly Government 2008) and 'ChildSmile' in Scotland (Scottish Government 2018). All three programmes operate independently but the main underpinning ethos of the initiatives is to empower children identified as high risk to develop good oral health and dietary behaviours through the provision of oral health education and skills development, including the provision of support to navigate dental service provision. Children between the ages of 3–6 years entering into a targeted early years setting situated in localities experiencing high levels of socio-economic deprivation are provided with free oral hygiene

Table 13.3 Key oral health-enhancing behaviours for children and adults (Public Health England 2017a): contains public sector information licensed under the Open Government Licence v3.0)

Key Oral Health Enhancing Behaviours for Children (Public Health England 2017a). (Cited in Godson & Seymour 2019)

Toothbrushing

Expose teeth to fluoride as soon as the first tooth erupts in the mouth by toothbrushing with an appropriate fluoride toothpaste:

0–3 years – Use a smear of fluoride toothpaste containing 1000 ppm

3–6 years – Use a smear or peas sized amount of fluoride toothpaste containing more than 1000 ppm

7+ years – Use a fluoride toothpaste containing 1350–1500 ppm

Toothbrushing should occur at two periods during the day, one being at night when the saliva levels are generally low. Toothbrushing should be supervised until the age of 7 years. Rinsing should be avoided following brushing to maintain fluoride concentration levels within the oral cavity.

NB: Children 0–6 years at high risk of decay can use a fluoride toothpaste containing 1350–1500 ppm.

Dietary principles

Breast-feeding should be encouraged from birth as per Unicef baby friendly guidelines.

Reduce the consumption and frequency of dietary food and drinks containing sugar.

The use of a free-flow cup should be encouraged for drinks from 6 months of age.

Only water and milk should be offered in a bottle.

Bottle use should be discouraged from 1 year of age.

Dental attendance

Register with the dentist and attend regular preventative check-ups as recommended. The first dental visit should occur at 6 months.

Key oral health behaviours for adults to prevent dental caries and periodontal disease (Public Health England 2017a).

Tooth brushing

Brush each tooth and the gum line with a fluoride toothpaste (1350–1500ppm) twice a day. This should occur at the last thing at night and on another occasion during the day.

To maintain fluoride concentration levels in the oral cavity rinsing should be avoided following brushing.

High risk individuals identified by a dental practitioner may be advised to use a fluoride mouthwash between brushing.

Remove plaque daily with floss, tape or interdental brushes as advised by a dental practitioner.

Dental attendance

Dental registration and attendance is recommended for ongoing preventative advice and treatment.

Dietary intake

Reduce the amount and frequency of sugars within the dietary intake, including drinks containing sugar.

Tobacco and alcohol consumption

Smoking or chewing any form of tobacco should be avoided.

Alcohol consumption should be reduced to recommended safe levels, classified as 14 units per week, consumed evenly over three or more days.

products such as toothpaste and toothbrushes and empowered to take part in a supervised toothbrushing activity. This is accompanied by age-appropriate oral health education and the provision of educational materials for parents to support and transfer the development of these oral health behaviours from the school setting into the home environment.

Oral health in the adult population

The protection of the oral cavity as expected throughout childhood also remains an integral aspect of health and wellbeing in adulthood. However, oral diseases continue to debilitate almost half of the global population, with 3.5 billon people affected by oral diseases (WHO 2019b). This could be directly attributed to the high levels of dental decay in the child population which may directly predict the oral health behaviours and the quality of this aspect of health throughout adulthood. Nevertheless, the breakdown of the tooth surface as a result of dental decay remains the most prevalent non-communicable disease worldwide in the adult population, with a similar aetiology reflective of dental decay in children as analysed above. This includes the mirroring of behavioural risk factors such as a high dietary sugar intake and limited exposure to fluoride due to not adhering to evidence-based oral health behaviours (see Table 13.2). As well as dental decay, adults are also at an increased risk of developing peridontal disease, and this remains the 11th most prevalent disease globally (WHO 2019b). Peridontal disease is defined as 'the inflammation of the peridontium (the supporting structure of the tooth)' (Felton and Chapman 2014, p. 41). This condition is attributed to non-adherence to oral hygiene routines such as toothbrushing which increases the presence of the bacterial biofilm on the tooth surface (plaque) resulting in inflammation of the tissues surrounding the teeth (Jacobsen 2019). The continued presence of this bacterial biofilm surrounding the tooth surface can result in an inflammatory response to the gingival tissues which causes redness and bleeding and is classified as 'gingivitis' (Robinson and Marshman 2017). This pattern of disease is often perceived and accepted as an inevitable consequence of ageing but it can be prevented through adherence to appropriate preventative evidence-based lifestyle behaviours reinforced through oral health education (Daly and Smith 2015) as documented in Table 13.2.

Dental registration and access to routine dental examinations can ensure that periodontal disease is diagnosed and preventative treatment is prescribed to reduce the ongoing negative effects of this disease, which can include gum recession, unstable tooth structure and potential tooth loss (Daly and Smith 2015). Prompt diagnosis and preventative treatment is crucial as the early onset of this disease can be asymptomatic, progressing to irreversible damage to the tooth structure and the periodontium. Smoking or chewing tobacco and excessive alcohol consumption is also a significant contributing risk to developing periodontal disease, dental decay and oral cancers. Due to the addictive nature of these substances and the potential challenges and barriers influencing this lifestyle choice, the use of more specialist support may be required, such as the prescription of nicotine replacement therapy to empower individuals to make oral health-enhancing behaviour changes. Nevertheless, healthcare professionals have a professional responsibility to explore these individual behaviours and provide opportunistic advice and signpost to additional smoking cessation or alcohol support services as required (PHE 2017a). This approach to public health has been explored further in Chapter 11.

The most up-to-date national statistics (Steele et al. 2011) that analyses population groups from England, Wales and Northern Ireland decennially has identified that in

2011, 23% of the adult population had evidence of primary decay evident on the surface of a tooth; 31% had obvious decay present in the roots of teeth or dental crowns indicating the need for restorative intervention, with the average number of teeth affected as 2.7. The Scottish Adult Oral Health Survey 2016–2018 presents a differing picture (Information Services Division 2019b); however, these results are not directly comparable due to the differing sampling data collection methods used. In Scotland, 67% of the population were reported to have a functional dentition, which is classified as the presence of 21 undiseased teeth. Furthermore, statistical data across the four nations continues to suggest that adults experiencing social and economic deprivation have an increased vulnerability to dental decay and oral disease (Robinson and Marshman 2017).

Influencing determinants of health

The social and environmental circumstances that create barriers to the protection of the oral cavity can again be interlinked to Dahlgren and Whitehead's (1991) model (see Figure 13.1). Population groups experiencing deprivation may not have the oral health literacy to prioritise this aspect of their health and wellbeing. Financial pressures may make accessing and affording preventative dental treatment unachievable (Shedlin et al. 2018). Dental anxiety is also a recognised barrier to accessing regular dental provision, especially if individuals are experiencing oral disease and the need for invasive restorative treatment (Hakeberg and Wide 2018). Time taken off from work to manage symptoms or seek treatment could contribute to a financial implication or economic inequity and opportunities for promotion, widening the social inequalities that already exist (Robinson and Marshman 2017). Oral disease and decay also has the potential to cause severe pain, facial swelling and social isolation. Altered oral aesthetics due to these symptoms and tooth loss can cause embarrassment and avoidance of social engagements which can negatively impact a person's confidence and self-esteem (Hakeberg and Wide 2018).

A preventative approach to oral health

To address the oral health needs of the UK population there has been a politically driven refocus of primary dental services during the 21st century across all the four nations. Dental practitioners now have a professional responsibility to promote the oral health and wellbeing of their practice population (PHE 2017a) and ensure the provision of dental treatment takes a more 'needs led preventative focused approach' (Welsh Government 2017 p.4). Dental practitioners are now proactive in supporting behaviour change and empowering their practice population to take control of their oral health and increase their perceived susceptibility to oral disease. Dental treatment plans therefore include oral education and preventative advice tailored to the individual needs of the patient following an oral assessment and consideration of the clinical pathways within *Delivering Better Oral Health: An Evidence-based Toolkit for Prevention* (PHE 2017a) (see Table 13.2). The population are encouraged to commence a lifetime routine of visiting the dentist from as early as the age of one, for preventative treatment at least every six months. This health-promoting intervention will only target groups of the population that are proactive in addressing their oral health needs and are registered with a dental practitioner and attend for regular dental examinations. Individuals experiencing social and environmental barriers may only access dental treatment and advice in an emergency due to affordability, dental anxiety or accessibility. For those individuals forced to be reactive in relation to their dental health and wellbeing, the NICE (2016) guidelines recommend dental practitioners empower this vulnerable population group to build a positive relationship with dental services and understand the benefits of regular attendance and support their navigation of local dental provision.

Healthcare professionals also have a professional responsibility to empower individuals to make behaviour changes and be proactive rather than reactive in relation to their oral health (Shedlin et al. 2018). NICE (2016) guidelines recommend that the assessment of the oral health needs of individuals receiving health and social care should be a fundamental aspect of care, and the implementation of care plans should incorporate the provision of oral hygiene and referral to dental expertise as required. For children this will include empowering parents/carers to develop the oral health literacy to implement the key oral health-enhancing behaviours to reduce the risk of their children developing dental decay. Nonetheless, the provision of education alone will be ineffective without exploring the social and environmental factors that are influencing an individual's attitudes and behaviours towards their oral health wellbeing (Robinson and Marshman 2017). Only then can health education be tailored to address the individual circumstances and barriers that influence effective behaviour change related to oral health routines and behaviours (PHE 2017a). Targeted oral health interventions may therefore be required to address the individual challenges that individuals encounter in implementing oral health-enhancing behaviours. This could include supporting dental registration, teaching skills related to toothbrushing, as well as the promotion of meal routines to reduce daily sugar intake and the preparation of healthy meals on a budget. This is a recognised evidence-based approach known as 'Making Every Contact Count' whereby practitioners engage in conversations with individuals regarding their lifestyle risk factors to support positive behaviour change (NICE 2020). It is also the philosophy of health promotion that is illustrated within the Ottawa Charter (WHO 1986) as the process of empowering individuals to take control over the social and environmental conditions that influence their health and have the self-efficacy to make healthy lifestyle choices which will safeguard their overall health and wellbeing.

COVID-19 and oral health

Due to the COVID-19 pandemic access to routine preventative dental treatment has been restricted, with many dental practices closing across the UK to adhere to lockdown restrictions and reduce the potential risk of transmitted infection from oral examinations and procedures. Access to dental care has been restricted to emergency treatment, usually carried out in identified regional locations. This has potentially widened oral health inequalities further, in particular for those population groups who normally may have difficulties navigating the provision of healthcare services. The General Dental Council (2020) have reported that dental practitioners have experienced an increase in the population's demand for dental expertise post-lockdown, resulting in the need for services to be prioritised according to patient need. This has resulted in a continued rise in the demand for dental expertise and as a consequence worsening oral health difficulties may transpire. Alternatively, individuals may actively continue to avoid dental care due to a continued fear of transmitted infection. Therefore, the practitioner's role in promoting oral health and supporting the population to navigate dental services provision and address their oral health needs continues to be a healthcare priority to reduce widening oral health inequalities.

Conclusion

Oral health is a fundamental aspect of a person's overall health and wellbeing. However, epidemiological evidence suggests oral disease continues to affect a significant number of the population from cradle to grave. A preventative proactive approach is required to tackle the common associated risk factors such as poor oral hygiene, poor dietary practices, tobacco use and alcohol consumption. This requires consideration of the complex social and environmental challenges that directly influence these risk factors and create oral health inequalities. Political action is targeted at preventative interventions that support oral health literacy, particularly within the early years, through the socialisation of oral health behaviours when routines are establishing to stabilise these lifestyles choices throughout adulthood. Healthcare professionals are in a unique position to ensure that oral health wellbeing is integrated into every opportunistic contact with clients to promote key evidence-based oral health behaviours and reduce the prevalence of oral disease.

Consider the following questions

Having read the chapter take time to think about the following:

1. What oral health interventions for children and adults are implemented within your area of practice?
2. What social determinants can healthcare practitioners influence in practice to promote oral health?
3. What key oral health messages will you as a healthcare professional deliver in practice?

Key terms

Demineralisation: Calcium and phosphate ions are lost from the tooth enamel when the pH acidic level in the mouth rises due to the metabolism of dietary sugars by the microbial biofilm which is present on the tooth surface (Godson et al. 2018, WHO 2022).

Dental caries: The breakdown of the tooth enamel due to the frequent process of demineralisation, also known as tooth decay.

Determinants of health: A person's physical characteristics that directly influence health outcomes including genetic inheritance, age and gender. This also includes the wider social and environmental conditions in which a person lives that has a direct influence on their health and lifestyle behavioural choices (Dahlgren and Whitehead 1991).

Gingival health: The quality of the tissues (gums) that support and protect the tooth structure.

Gingivitis: An inflammatory response of the gingival tissues which causes redness and bleeding (Robinson and Marshman 2017).

Making Every Contact Count (MECC): A brief health promotion evidence-based intervention that is delivered opportunistically by healthcare professionals during routine contacts with clients or patients. The intervention empowers clients and patients to engage in conversations about their health, which includes lifestyles choices related to diet, exercise, smoking, alcohol and emotional health and wellbeing (NICE 2020).

Non-communicable disease: A disease which is not infectious and contracted from another person. It is attributed and influenced by an individual's environment or lifestyle choices and predominantly preventable.

Oral disease: A condition of the mouth which affects the health of the teeth, the bone and the supporting tissues and may result in symptoms such as pain, inflammation or infection. Common conditions include dental decay (**dental caries**), periodontal disease and oral cancers (Centers for Disease Control and Prevention 2020).

Permanent dentition: The secondary teeth, of which there are 32 in total, replace the primary dentition from approximately 5 years of age (Felton and Chapman 2014).

Primary dentition: Consists of 20 teeth that primarily erupt into the oral cavity at differing time intervals from 6–30 months of age (Felton and Chapman 2014). They are also referred to as 'deciduous' or 'baby' teeth and are naturally replaced by the permanent dentition.

Remineralisation: Calcium and phosphate ions are absorbed back into the tooth surface when the acid in the mouth is neutralised by the protective action of saliva and the regular exposure to fluoride (Felton and Chapman 2014).

Further reading

FDI World Dental Federation. 2019. *Facts, Figures and Stats Oral Disease: 10 Key Facts.* Available at: www.fdiworlddental.org/oral-health/ask-the-dentist/facts-figures-and-stats [Accessed 06.03.2020].

National Institute for Health & Care Excellence (NICE). 2020. *Making Every Contact Count.* Available at: https://stpsupport.nice.org.uk/mecc/index.html [Accessed 02.03.2020].

World Health Organization. 2018. *Oral Health.* Available at: www.who.int/news-room/fact-sheets/detail/oral-health [Accessed 06.03.2020].

References

Centers for Disease Control and Prevention. 2020. *Oral Health*. Available at: www.cdc. gov/oralhealth/conditions/index.html#:~:text=Oral%20health%20refers%20to%20 the,)%20disease%2C%20and%20oral%20cancer [Accessed 05.11.2020].

Dalal, M., Clark, M., Quinonez, R. B. 2019. *Part 2 Pediatric Oral Health Fluoride Use Recommendations*. Available at: www.contemporarypediatrics.com/pediatrics/ pediatric-oral-health-fluoride-use-recommendations [Accessed 05.03.2020].

Dalgren, G., Whitehead, M. 1991. Policy and strategies to promote social equity in health. Background document to the WHO – Strategy paper for Europe. *Institute for Future Studies*. Available at: www.iffs.se/media/1326/20080109110739filmZ8UVQv2w QFShMRF6cuT.pdf [Accessed 05.12.2020].

Daly, B., Smith, K. 2015. Promoting good dental health in older people: role of the community nurse. *British Journal of Community Nursing*; 20(9), 431–436.

Eden, E., Akyildiz, M., Sönmez, I. 2019. Comparison of two school-based oral health education programs in 9-year-old children. *International Quarterly of Community Health Education*; 39(3), 189–196.

FDI World Dental Federation. 2020. *FDI's Definition of Oral Health*. Available at: www. fdiworlddental.org/oral-health/fdi-definition-of-oral-health [Accessed 06.03.2020].

Felton, S. H., Chapman, A. 2014. *Basic Guide to Oral Health Education and Promotion*. (2nd edn). Wiley Blackwell: Chichester.

Forward, C. 2014. Looking at resources for dental health promotion. *British Journal of School Nursing*; 9(6), 305–306.

Fukai, K., Ogawa, H., Hescot, P. 2017. Oral health for healthy longevity in an ageing society maintaining momentum and moving forward. *International Dental Journal*; 67, 3–6.

General Dental Council. 2020. *Oral Health Inequalities are Being Created and Exacerbated*. Available at: www.gdc-uk.org/standards-guidance/COVID-19/the-impacts-of-COVID-19/oral-health-inequalities [Accessed 12.03.2022].

Glick, M., Monteiro da Silva, O., Seeberger, G. K., et al. 2012. FDI Vision 2020. Shaping the future of oral health. *International Dental Journal*; 62, 278–291.

Godson, J., Csikar, J., White, S. 2018. Oral Health of children in England: a call to action! *Archives of Disease in Childhood*; 103(1), 5–10.

Godson, J., Seymour, D. 2019. Primary prevention and health promotion in oral health. In A. Emond (Ed.), *Health for All Children*. (5th edn). (pp. 147–159). Oxford University Press. Oxford:

Hakeberg, M., Wide, U. 2018. General and oral health problems among adults with focus on dentally anxious individuals. *International Dental Journal*; 65, 405–410.

Health & Social Care Information Centre. 2015. *Children's Dental Health Survey. Executive Summary: England, Wales and Northern Ireland, 2013*. Available at: https://files.digital. nhs.uk/publicationimport/pub17xxx/pub17137/cdhs2013-executive-summary.pdf [Accessed 12.03.2022].

Holmes, R., Porter, J., Vernazza, C., Tsakos, G., Ryan, R., Dennes, M. 2015. *Children's Dental Health Survey: Country Specific Report: England*. Available at: https://files.digital.nhs.uk/publicationimport/pub17xxx/pub17137/cdhs2013-england-report.pdf [Accessed 04.07.2020].

Infant & Toddler Forum. 2010. Protecting Toddlers from Tooth Decay. Available at: https://infantandtoddlerforum.org/toddlers-to-preschool/preventing-tooth-decay/ [Accessed: 10 Mar 2020].

Information Services Division. 2018. *National Dental Inspection Programme (NDIP) 2018*. Available at: www.scottishdental.org/wp-content/uploads/2018/10/2018-10-23-NDIP-Report.pdf [Accessed 04.07.2020].

Information Services Division. 2019a. *National Dental Inspection Programme (NDIP) 2019*. Available at: www.isdscotland.org/Health-Topics/Dental-Care/Publications/2019-10-22/2019-10-22-NDIP-Report.pdf [Accessed 04.07.2020].

Information Services Division. 2019b. *Scottish Adult Oral Health Survey 2016–2018*. Available at: www.scottishdental.org/wp-content/uploads/2019/04/2019-04-30-SAOHS-Report.pdf [Accessed 06.03.2020].

Integrated Care. 2018. *Happy Smiles Programme: Promoting the Oral Health of Pre-school Children*. Integrated Care, Health & Social Care Board: Derry/Londonderry.

Jacobsen, K. 2019. *Introduction to Global Health*. Jones & Bartlett Learning: Burlington.

National Institute for Health & Care Excellence (NICE). 2016. *Oral Health Promotion in the Community*. Available at: www.nice.org.uk/guidance/qs139/resources/oral-health-promotion-in-the-community-pdf-75545427440581 [Accessed 14.02.2020].

National Institute for Health & Care Excellence (NICE). 2020. *Making Every Contact Count*. Available at: https://stpsupport.nice.org.uk/mecc/index.html [Accessed 02.03.2020].

Porter, J., Holmes, R., Vernazza, C., Chadwock, B., Ryan, R., Dennes, M. 2015. *Children's Dental Health Survey 2013: Country Specific Report Wales*. Available at: https://files.digital.nhs.uk/publicationimport/pub17xxx/pub17137/cdhs2013-wales-report.pdf [Accessed 04.07.2020].

Public Health England. 2017a. *Delivering Better Oral Health: An Evidence-Based Toolkit for Prevention*. Public Health England: London.

Public Health England. 2017b. *Oral Health Improvement Programmes Commissioned By Local Authorities*. Public Health England: London.

Ravaghi, V., Hill, K., Ryan, R., Dennes, M. 2013. *Children's Dental Health Survey. Country Specific Report: Northern Ireland*. Available at: https://bda.org/news-centre/blog/Documents/CDHS2013-Northern-Ireland-Report.pdf [Accessed 06.03.2020].

Robinson, P. G., Marshman, Z. 2017. Dental public health. In R. Detels, M. Gulliford, Q. Abdool Karim, C. Chuan Tan (Eds), *Oxford Textbook of Global Public Health*. (pp. 1028–1045). Oxford University Press: Oxford.

Scottish Government. 2018. *Oral Health Improvement Plan*. Scottish Government: Oxford.

Shedlin, M. G., Birdsall, S. B., Northridge, M. E. 2018. Knowledge and behaviours related to oral health among underserved older adults. *Gerodontology*, 35(4), 339–349.

Steele, J., Treasure, E. T., O'Sullivan, I., Morris, J., Murray, J. J. 2011. *Executive Summary: Adult Dental Health Survey 2009*. The Health and Social Care Information Centre.

Voogd, C. 2014. Addressing tooth decay in children & young people. *British Journal of School Nursing*; 9(6): 276–281.

Warrilow, L., Dave, R., McDonald, S. 2019. Oral health promotion: Right person, right time prevention. *Journal of Health Visiting*; 7(8), 394–398.

Watt, R. G., Dly, B., Allison, P., et al. 2019. Ending the neglect of global oral health: time for radical action. *Lancet*; 394(10194), 261–272.

Weichselbaum, E., Buttriss, J. L. 2014. Diet, nutrition and schoolchildren: an update. *British Nutrition Foundation Nutrition Bulletin*; 39, 9–73.

Welsh Assembly Government. 2008. *Designed to Smile*. Available at: www.wales.nhs.uk/documents/WHC%282008%29008%2Epdf [Accessed 08.03.2020].

Welsh Government. 2017 *Re-focusing of the Designed to Smile Child Oral Health Improvement Programme*. Available at: https://gov.wales/sites/default/files/publications/2019-07/re-focussing-of-the-designed-to-smile-child-oral-health-improvement-programme.pdf [Accessed 25.02.2020].

World Health Organization. 1986. *Ottawa Charter for Health Promotion*. Available at: www.euro.who.int/__data/assets/pdf_file/0004/129532/Ottawa_Charter.pdf [Accessed 08.03.2020].

World Health Organization. 2015. *Tokyo Declaration on Dental Care and Oral Health for Healthy Longevity*. Available at: www.who.int/oral_health/tokyodeclaration_final.pdf?ua=1 [Accessed 06.03.2020].

World Health Organization. 2019a. *Oral Health Priority Action Areas*. Available at: www.who.int/oral_health/action/en/ [Accessed 11.11.2019].

World Health Organization. 2019b. *What is the Burden of Oral Disease?* Available at: www.who.int/oral_health/disease_burden/global/en/ [Accessed 11.11.2019].

World Health Organization. 2022. *Oral Health*. Available at: https://www.who.int/news-room/fact-sheets/detail/oral-health [Accessed 07.04.2022].

14

SEXUAL HEALTH IS PUBLIC HEALTH

DAVID EVANS

━━━━━━━━━ LEARNING OUTCOMES ━━━━━━━━━

By the end of this chapter you will be able to:

- Appreciate the importance of sexual health and wellbeing as an integral dimension of public health.
- Explore holistic definitions of sexual health, to improve your professional practice.
- Examine the need for proactively promoting the public's sexual health and wellbeing, challenging erotophobic prejudice and discrimination in service provision.
- Critique the impact of influences on legislative and policy guidance.
- Identify ways in which you can make a positive difference to public health sexual health and wellbeing.

Introduction

Sexual health *is* public health! A simple statement, but none the less true. Belfield et al. (2006, p. 17) state that sexual health is 'vital to overall health and wellbeing', an important point that health professionals aim to integrate into holistic client care (Nursing and Midwifery Council 2018). Any definition of holistic health, however, which does not include a full integration of sexual health and promotion of sexual wellbeing – equally, to all people, across the life course – is no more than lip-service to a philosophy, a tick-box exercise for 'activities of daily living'. This lip-service approach is contrary to genuine holism and equates to reductionism. Reductionistic healthcare treats physiological systems, not the person. Bold or controversial claims to make, or a call to public health action? This call to action will be explored in greater depth throughout this chapter.

This chapter supports practitioners in promoting a positive and respectful approach to sexuality, health and relationships. Equally, it raises awareness of definitions that can promote gender health, sexual health and wellbeing, supported by international human rights declarations, which are acknowledged as strategic imperatives within the wider, formal, public health agenda (Naidoo and Wills 2016).

A call-to-action is important for identifying ways in which a broader understanding of holistic health and wellbeing is fundamental, not just to each and every member of the public (i.e. humanity) but to the public health strategies, policies, laws and practices of their society, too. This call-to-action is for intentionally promoting the public's sexual health, gender health and wellbeing, including all aspects of reproductive and psychosexual health (Brough and Denman 2019).

Putting sexual health on the public health agenda

From the perspective of international public health policy, a notable shift across sexual (ill) health occurred in response to World War I. In the UK of 1914, and successive decades since, public health dimensions of sexual ill health – and what was perceived as a breakdown of hitherto social, class and moral orders – led to Parliament passing DORA, the Defence of the Realm Act 1914. This Act made sexual 'mores' (morality) sexual problems (e.g. conception outside of marriage, abortions, and, of course, illnesses i.e. sexual infections) formal public health concerns as never before. At that time, male homosexuality was a criminal offence in the UK and throughout the reach of the British Empire.

In that first quarter of the 20th century, sexual infections were referred to as 'venereal diseases', such as with the Venereal Disease Act 1917 (Steward and Wingfield 2016). Public health messages tended to be moralistic and judgemental. The practice of 'contact tracing and partner notification', common parlance in the era of COVID-19, had their origins in response to the growing incidence of 'VD' at the time of World War I.

The cultural, legal, psychopathologising and moralist agendas were strict and punitive on a wide range of sexual deeds and relations, some with resonance across parts of the world and their public health policies to this very day. For example, there were various forms of 'corrective' treatments such as psychopathological 'therapies', custodial incarcerations and commonplace traditional and 'back-street' quack remedies. These various 'treatments' were used in relation to poor sexual health outcomes and/or personal lifeways. Such 'corrective' treatments ranged from punitive action against people who had sex outside of marriage, especially sex that resulted in 'illegitimate' pregnancies (i.e. pregnancies conceived 'out of wedlock'). There were punitive actions against commercial sex workers (prostitutes) too, against same-sex relations (particularly male homosexuality), abortion and various non-reproductive sex acts. Non-reproductive sex acts included those purposefully avoiding conception (i.e. using contraception) and 'sex-for-one', such as solitary masturbation, frequently labelled 'Onanism' (Bockting and Coleman 2002). In relation to sexual 'ill health', elements of statutory public health legislation have shrouded sexual health promotion initiatives, as well as treatments and care provision, in stigma, invisibility, shame and guilt right into the third decade of the 21st century (Heath and White, 2002).

Public health facts today

Male masturbation can lead to a reduction of prostate cancer later in life (Aboul-Enein et al. 2016).

Live births outside of marriage and civil partnership in England and Wales reached 58.7% in 2017 (ONS, 2019).

Male sterilisation (vasectomy) is more than 99% effective, yet a poorly promoted method of contraception (NHS 2018, Everett, 2020).

Key concepts relating to sexual health for public health

In relation to promoting and protecting sexual rights, the World Health Organization (WHO) produced a definition of sexual health in 1975 which is still cited, popularly, today:

> Sexual health is the integration of the somatic, emotional, intellectual and social aspects of *sexual* being in ways that are positively enriching and that enhance personality, communication and love. (WHO 1975, emphasis added)

Since then the WHO has produced numerous definitions, as no one definition will be fit for purpose across all times, all places and for each and every society or individual within it (WHO 2002). Subsequent WHO definitions have been adapted to draw attention to local and regional concerns, as well as wider, transnational phenomena (WHO 2020). These public health policy definitions draw attention to people who are victims of abuse and sexual violence; those discriminated against and mistreated for minority sexual orientations and gender identities (SOGI); or those who suffer persecution simply because of their gender, orientation or practices. Later definitions highlight those living with stigmatised and/or chronic (sexual) health conditions, including infertility,

HIV infection and disease (especially AIDS), FGC/FGM (i.e. female genital cutting/mutilation) and those with attendant guilt associated with many such conditions and lifeways (Brough and Denman, 2019). This list is just the tip of the iceberg. WHO (2002) therefore encourages national and local communities to customise their own definitions, taking into consideration the profile of specific (local) needs and the demographics of their own diverse cultures and populations.

Action point

- If your organisation needed to draw up a definition of sexual health and wellbeing as part of its public health policy manifesto, what key terms would you consider 'essential' or even 'desirable' to go into it? Who would be included in this definition? Equally significant: who might be excluded or left out?
- You could have this conversation with your colleagues, sharing ideas to see how this exercise snowballs into a workable definition for your current practice setting, at this time and place. Remember, however, the WHO (2002) encourages definitions to be revised and updated, as often as necessary, not just written once and for all time.

Sexual pleasure – good for health

Several declarations of the World Association for Sexual Health (WAS) have been agreed-upon over the past few decades. They include the *Declaration of Sexual Health, Declaration of Sexual Rights* (WAS 2014) and now further declarations specifically promoting the relational aspects of sexuality and young people's sexual health and educational rights too. The international *Declaration on Sexual Pleasure* (WAS 2019) promotes sexual pleasure as an innate and inalienable right, for each and every individual.

These declarations, aspects of human rights, are a far cry from the moralising discourses against VD just over 100 years ago. It is crucial to remember that no matter how important these international public health declarations of rights may be, in reality, on the ground, in individual people's lives, far too often so many suffer because their rights are hidden or invisibilised and down-trodden by elements in the wider society in which they live (Collumbien et al. 2012).

Sex-negative or 'erotophobic' (Evans 2004) elements of cultures or societies often emanate from over-powerful, hegemonic, bullying dimensions of patriarchy, toxic masculinity and hetero-supremacy. Women, girls and all those who are held as different – who *queer* the cultural perception of masculinist supremacy – pay the price, be this through violence against them or lack of equality granted to their social, educational, legal and, especially, their healthcare needs, ultimately denying them individual respect and their human rights. Equally problematic are the intersecting cultural, institutional, inter-personal and intra-personal dimensions of erotophobia which come from other social forces, such as specific traditional cultures, age ranges, religions, locations or the impact of poverty, lack of learning capabilities and various personal or individual attributes.

Public health professionals (PHPs) have a duty and crucial role to play in challenging all forms of erotophobia, including homophobia, biphobia and transphobia, as well as the sexism and heterosexism which invisibilises a range of sexual matters across the public health arena. For example, PHPs are involved in commissioning and implementing policies, sourcing and conducting population research and advising people on ways which maximise their health and prevent ill health. This ill health may include sexually acquired infections (SAIs/STIs), particular conditions (e.g. infertility, erectile dysfunction) or life-changing situations (e.g. genital cancers).

If professionals themselves – students and registered practitioners – are erotophobic (or sexist, homo-, bi- or transphobic) to start with, then they may impose their own prejudices on the public health service they provide, through invisibilising people and specific sexual health needs. Invisibilisation of people and needs can happen in various PH initiatives or campaigns. For example, if a practitioner is heterosexist/homophobic and in a position of responsibility for commissioning public sexual health prevention campaigns, they may focus only on the issues or people whose morals or belief systems permit them to do, neglecting a genuine, proactive, health response for all others, especially lesbian, gay, bisexual, transpeople and others (LGBandT+) and matters detrimental to minority health (Government Equalities Office 2019). This lack of cultural competence around sexualities (Fish and Evans 2016) may be evidenced in a reproduction-only focus for campaigns, which lacks attention on the implications of sex for pleasure, and on the potential impact of condomless sex as a safer sex/infection control resource. A lack of cultural competence for all but heterosexual/reproductive people also invisibilises the root cause of poorer mental health for LGBandT+ people. Poorer mental health *sequelae* so often originates in societies that lack equal acceptance of LGBandT+ people, their sexual health matters and their cultural and relationship life-ways. Similarly, if a PHP has specific beliefs about abortion, or transpeople, or people with learning/physical disabilities and sex, or commercial sex workers, or child sexual exploitation (CSE), or pre-exposure prophylaxis (PrEP) against HIV – this list is endless – then without accurate personal and professional reflection by the individual PH practitioner to challenge their own world-view assumptions and knowledge-deficit, then the work they do may actually be sub-optimum from that which is genuinely required, all because of an imposition of *their* beliefs, *their* customs or traditions, on the work they are paid to do for the general public.

> **Consider** the restraining and facilitating forces that hinder/enable a sex-positive public health policy. This process is called a 'force field analysis', where the goal of the public health initiative can be written in the centre of a page, starting with the imperative 'to ....' do something, for example, 'To intentionally promote awareness of sexual pleasure and health needs of people, routinely hidden or discriminated against in traditional public health messages and campaigns'.

The goal of a force field analysis is to explore and overcome various 'restraining forces', that is, those which hinder public health efforts trying to maximise the aim. Equally important is to ensure that there are enough positive or 'facilitating forces' that will enable and ultimately enact the aim. This exploratory technique could be used with excellent benefit by teams of PHPs, exploring how they might conduct campaigns for advertising physical, mental and relational health benefits of pleasure in sex/sex for pleasure. Similarly, it might be a force field analysis on exploring how to route-out eroto-phobia and prejudice in public health services as well as specific campaigns. As a Queer Theory motif (*anon*) suggests, it is important not just to 'think outside the box, but think as though the box doesn't even exist!'.

Two other key concepts to explore with regard to sexual health for public health include wider understandings of sexuality, and an holistic approach to three key dimensions of sexual health (see section below) for promoting personal health and wellbeing.

Sexuality is …

According to Foucault (1978), sexuality is a relatively modern concept. It is more than some solitary dimension of a person's identity; more than something to be labelled simply as either one thing or another. It is important to consider multiple dimensions of this often-times binary labelled term 'sexuality', to avoid reducing people to being either 'straight' (heterosexual) on the one hand, or any of the many other identity labels for all people deemed 'not-straight' on the other. It should be noted that whilst many sexual identities – such as heterosexual, gay, lesbian, bisexual – rely on notions of orientation 'immutability' (Wintemute, 1995), that is, something given and unchangeable, as with a person's ethnicity or skin colour, the term 'queer' (often with a capital Q, when used in Queer Theory) is a critical theoretical rebellion against the need for putting people into any such labelled categories. Queer Theory originated as an active doing, a verb, for example 'to queer all heterosexualised spaces' (Evans 2011), rather than a noun, an identity or label – 'a queer' – although it is often used interchangeably.

Of course, with abbreviations such as LGBTI (or LGBandTI), the 'T' stands for transperson/transgender and as such is a gender identity not a sexual orientation; similarly so 'I' for intersex people. A '+' sign might indicate 'and all others' (Vincent 2016).

Evans (2017) suggests that the concept of 'sexuality', still a somewhat contested term across times and places, is beneficially considered from four inter-relating dimensions (see Figure 14.1): orientation, identity/expression, attractions and behaviours (sexual practices). This four-fold consideration of sexuality encompasses dimensions that not only agree with each other, but, more significantly, may *not* agree with each other. For example, a married couple in a country that criminalises male and female homosexuality are, without any need for consideration, perceived as straight (i.e. heterosexual). And yet this union might be a 'marriage of convenience', or a marriage for local law and custom's sake. No one needs to label the orientation of this couple as straight/heterosexual; it is a given. One or both parties, however, might actually have a different orientation to

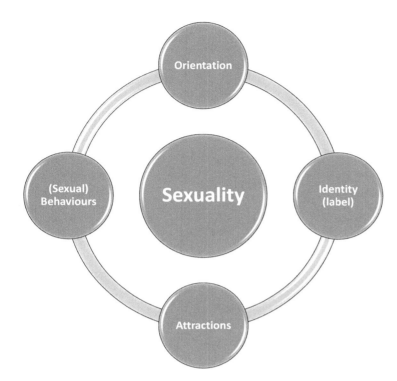

Figure 14.1 Four dimensions of sexuality (based on Evans 2017)

their perceived identity. Their orientation might be gay/lesbian, bisexual, heteroflexible, queer, questioning or a whole host of other non-heterosexual terms.

A person's sexuality is not reducible to an identity label; public health perspectives need to be cognisant of sexual behaviours (such as various sexual practices and relations) and associated risk factors. Hence the reason why MSM (Males who have Sex with other Males) refers to sexual acts or behaviours, whereas 'gay' and 'bisexual' are sexual identities. Self-acknowledged identities may be far more indicative of an orientation, and possibly a lifestyle, than a mere indication as to whether the person is sexually active or not (e.g. celibate or asexual). For example, a person may define themselves as gay, straight, lesbian or bisexual, but that says nothing about whether they are actually having sex, or what sort of sex they are having; whether sex is safer sex; protected; enjoyable; consenting and so on.

With sexuality an integral part of wider sexual health, a formal strategic approach for PHPs can be directed via three domains, as explained next.

A sexual health triptych – three key dimensions for public health

A 'triptych' usually refers to three panels of an integrated art production. Visually considering sexual health in three such panels, in the sexual health triptych (see Figure 14.2)

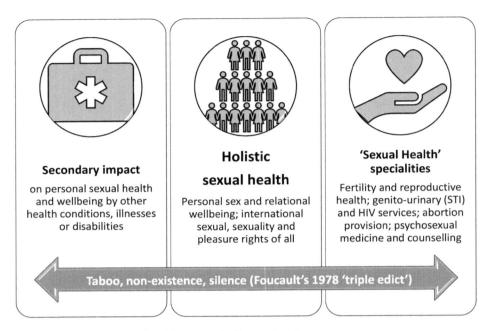

Figure 14.2 A sexual health triptych (Evans 2011)

Evans (2011) highlights, first, the central, 'holistic dimensions' of sexual health and wellbeing. The holistic dimensions apply to all individuals and incorporate the person's 'physical' (somatic), 'psychological' (mental), 'existential' (e.g. life-beliefs/spiritualty/religion/ethical standards and moral behaviours) aspects of being as well as their 'love and relationships' with self and others.

A second panel identifies ways in which so many other healthcare conditions, especially physical or mental illnesses or particular disabilities, can have a profound secondary impact on a person's sexual health and wellbeing. These secondary impact conditions may be detrimental to personal and sexual relationships, diminish an individual's sexual performance, inhibit positive esteem and wellbeing, or frustrate the outcome of various sexual preferences or choices.

> **Consider** how medications for certain conditions interfere with the successful functioning of methods of hormonal contraception; or when 1 in every 2 men with type 1 diabetes experiences erectile dysfunction (ED); or when people with low self-esteem care so little about themselves – or crave love and affection and are fearful of rejection – that they take sexual risks detrimental to their health and wellbeing.

The third element of the triptych model is focused on aspects of health traditionally catalogued under the umbrella term 'sexual health' or 'sexual and reproductive health' (SRH) (Royal College of Nursing 2019). 'Sexual health' more-often refers to associated problems of health, such as infections and conditions which are core to genito-urinary health-care practice; contraception and reproductive health; abortion care, and to psychosexual medicine and therapeutic counselling (Brough and Denman 2019).

As a somewhat neglected, hidden or taboo area of public health, sexual health is genuinely the com/passionate heart at the centre of the public's health. But notice how relatively few textbooks or journals have identifiable chapters or articles proactively rais-ing the profile of sexual health within the public health discipline. Too few texts address matters of sexual health, or enable practitioners to promote individual and societal equality, respect and wellbeing, including gender equality and sexual wellbeing, devoid of any form of discrimination (Mitchell et al. 2021).

From an epidemiological perspective, too, missing out sexual health from public health clearly counteracts the often-times preventable outcomes of condomless and unprotected sex. It is the intention, here, to demonstrate how sexual health is truly woven into the very fabric of public health, the political mission at the core of the PH speciality. Public health practice that adequately addresses sexual health and wellbeing can help maximise best outcomes 1) across primary prevention, that is, of the things that could go wrong; 2) across the promotion of holistic rights and wellbeing; and ultimately 3) help reduce the need for subsequent treatments and/or episodes of care.

Economic reality of good sexual public health reveals how it is far less expensive to prevent the unintended, as well as kinder on individuals. For example, the cost per capita for effective methods of contraception is a significant saving on any of the unwanted outcomes of unplanned conceptions (Hadley et al. 2018). Likewise, HPV (human papil-lomavirus) vaccination is reducing costs and impact on lives from genital warts as well as HPV-related cancers (cervical, oro-pharyngeal, penile and rectal). Free condoms and freely accessible pre-exposure prophylaxis (PrEP) against HIV are significantly less expen-sive and more desirable than a lifetime on antiretroviral medication for – currently, 37.9 million – people living with HIV (UNAIDS 2020).

PHPs are in an unparalleled position to positively influence sexual, reproductive and gender health: 1) holistically; 2) in areas of life impacted as secondary to other health conditions, as well as 3) specifically, across the range of sexual and reproductive health (RSH) specialities, too.

Empowering public health practitioners in the identification and facilitation of fundamental sexual health promoting behaviours

PHPs are accustomed to using scientific data resources and associated terminology for the study of population health (Oliffe and Greaves 2012, Green et al. 2019). These resources and terminology include the science of epidemiology; of counting personal level demo-graphics and applying these data to study the spread of disease, such as with epidemics and pandemics, across broad population densities (McClean et al. 2020).

PHPs are equally accustomed to investigating and reporting on the wider determi-nants of health and the impact on general population ill health phenomena, through primary and secondary prevention initiatives, in regard to communicable infections or risk-associated lifestyles and their *sequalae*. So many research-orientated resources are traditionally applied to particular cases across gendered health and sexual health (Oliffe and Greaves 2012). Typical examples to think of include the focus on unplanned teenage conceptions; HPV vaccination debates; intimate partner, gender or sexuality based violence; sex (gender)-related cancers and conditions; abortion; sexual infections and HIV. This list is not exhaustive, but significant to mention that many of these conditions are frequently hidden and marginalised, even in national public health strategies until they become too large to hide and result in being 'problematic'. Even when conditions become significant or 'problematic', national/international political will, public (and media) 'morals' or moralising, and lack of adequate funding often mean that a project ends up task-oriented (e.g. reduce numbers of XYZ) rather than being genuinely preventative, proactive, person-centred (holistic) and people-focused (Fowler, 2014).

Considerations for the facilitation of fundamental (safer) sexual health-promoting experiences include four messages often 'out-of-kilter' with wider public discourse and/or approval. First, **the ability to talk freely about all matters sexual**, especially to healthcare professionals, openly, without discrimination, shame or embarrassment. A prime example is the social or media furore or stigma about breastfeeding in public spaces, particularly in certain countries including the UK. Second, there is the matter of the **global unsustainability of humanity**, with one cause attributed to overpopulation. This problem emanates from the so-called procreative imperative – 'be fruitful, multiply, fill the earth and subdue it' – underpinning many religions, their approach to contraception, and the supremacy afforded to promoting reproductive heterosexual relations. The third consideration is the **hesitancy many healthcare professionals would have in *proactively* and intentionally promoting gender and sexual health**, including sexual pleasure (WAS, 2019) and wellbeing (Mitchell et al. 2021), and elements often left out of public discourses of 'sexual health' per se. By neglecting this key element of public health beneficence, professionals fail to promote this important aspect of life for a happier and healthier population. Finally, **so many non-heteronormative sexual practices and/or life-ways are considered by certain societies, religions and cultures to be abject** (i.e. dirty/filthy/shameful). The abjectification of matters sexual oftentimes renders the topic unspeakable, stigmatised, discredited and marked out as 'wrong'. To the extent that public health policies/policy makers are unable to challenge and overturn such negativities, then a fuller wealth of human sexual potential fails to be achieved or personally actualised.

Underpinning legislative and policy guidance: global and national perspectives

Over and above the influence and impact that various professional bodies and political unions can have, individual nurses and other healthcare professionals are oftentimes members of national or regional legislative authorities and governments. This, potentially, can have a positive bearing, especially for ensuring that inter-professional learning

and expertise are utilised, positively influencing sexual and gender health onto the public health agenda of a nation's health.

To add to the benefit of having PHPs in strategic positions of governance, the influence
of their specialist organisations collaborating together put them in a stronger position of
influence for public health partnerships, knowledge and resources. Other key influencers
include third sector/voluntary (charities) and direct-action organisations. These latter
embrace advocating for people living with HIV or AIDS; ending female genital mutilation; ending gender and sexuality-based violence; promoting safe abortion services;
advocating contraception and reproductive rights; sex workers and transgender people's
rights and sexuality rights organisations (ILGA 2020). There are many other institutions,
too, such as UNAIDS, International Planned Parenthood Federation, MSI (formerly Marie
Stopes International), the International AIDS Society and more.

Four essential difficulties against improving inter/national sexual and gendered public
health, however, can originate from:

1   Individual practitioners.
2   Practitioners' wider societies or cultures.
3   Multidimensional impacts of poverty.
4   A lack of funding adequate to need.

Poverty is especially maleficent to health when linked across other intersectional disadvantages, including disproportionate effects on age groups (the very young to the old),
ethnicities, geography and in those countries where a noticeable de-prioritisation of matters of sexual, reproductive or gender health and equality exist. In such circumstances,
promoting a positive awareness of all aspects of sex is compromised from within a public
health perspective.

International research highlights how many health care professionals still maintain
that they do not have the professional or personal knowledge, skills or attributes to
address sexual or gender health with their client populations. Neither do they have the
knowledge, skills or attributes to strategically address sexual health, in their capacity as
public health leaders, when in positions of influence (Wellings 2012). These problems
may stem from wider dimensions of sexual and gender health routinely missing from
pre-registration curricula (Cesnik and Zerbini 2017, Brown et al. 2021, Natzler and Evans
2021). Couple this personal and professional disadvantage with the shrouding of wider
aspects of sexuality and sexual health, in the individual professional's national or social
psyche, and it is no wonder that areas of sexual health and wellbeing are noticeably
absent from key public health strategies.

A lack of consistent funding, coupled with absence of public awareness of sexual
health matters, results in a socially deafening silence (Serrant-Green 2011). This silence
may be in regard to routine resources, such as freely available condoms, safer sex promotion campaigns, contraception and reproductive health provision, but also a silence
which goes much deeper. The silence can impact negatively on abortion legislation, provision and care; sexual abuse and rape; support services and refuge for those stigmatised

and shut out from their communities; and services for all those discriminated against on the grounds of invisibilised or marginalised status. For every one of these people, being silenced and missed out of public health initiatives – especially when they are not pro-actively targeted by PHPs – simply compounds their problems and further incentivises their oppression and neglect.

Conclusion

This chapter has highlighted opportunities where a formal public health recognition, across a range of matters sexual, may be invisibilised or wholly missing. The impact is deleterious to health and wellbeing. The role of public health services and professionals, is, of course, never solely reactionary, such as in exploring epidemiology to count what has gone wrong. Public health's promotion responsibilities are clearly grounded in being proactive, to champion the case for better health for all peoples, including their sexual health. That promotion responsibility could start by ensuring that students of public health have sexual health and sexuality matters specifically programmed into their cur-riculum and practice opportunities (Brown et al. 2021).

The paucity of entries in major public health textbooks and journals, intentionally promoting sexual health and wellbeing – including safer and pleasurable sexual experi-ences – requires a sufficient level of knowledge and training both in understanding and uncovering the issues, as well as being willing and able (confident and competent) to address them and challenge the professional's own assumptions or prejudices.

Collaboratively building on strategic declarations of the WHO, the World Association for Sexual Health (WAS), national programmes and individual healthcare professionals' own respect for sexual health in public health is a position that has been developed throughout this chapter. This position highlights the importance of the tripartite or trip-tych approach (Evans, 2011) to sexual health in public health, encompassing wider holis-tic dimensions of sexual health and wellbeing (Mitchell et al. 2021); elements of health secondary to, and impactful upon, sexual health and wellbeing, as well as the core specif-ics, under the umbrella term for sexual, reproductive and gender health. The challenge is for each PHP to be able to work towards ensuring these matters are clearly addressed and incorporated into the curriculum of students, as well as the policy and practice of their own organisation and in their wider national community.

Joining up the dots – how can you make a difference?

What further difference can you make? There are many ways in which PHPs can raise the profile of sexual health, directly – and indirectly. One indirect impact, out of many, is to join up the dots between various health and wellbeing campaigns; remember to factor-in the sexual health dimensions. For example, if a public health campaign is exploring how bullying of children often continues as discrimination into adulthood, it might examine how these phenomena can lead to isolation, low self-esteem, and a detrimental impact on poor mental health, increasing the risks of smoking, having condomless sex, increased alcohol consumption and substance abuse. Now, consider and highlight the impact of this scenario on an individual's sexual, reproductive or psychosexual wellbeing. This scenario is particularly relevant to all those stigmatised over their sexual orientation or identity, or those deemed not to fit in to a country's specific heteronormative model.

Remember: many consequences of poor sexual and gendered health are preventable, especially with strong, proactive, public health services and effective campaigns. All this takes adequate resourcing and the will to actively promote the positive benefits of sex and feeling good to talk about it in public health fora.

Consider the following questions

1. From the perspective of your own professional standpoint/field of practice/service area: what difference can you make to raise the profile of sexual health and wellbeing, as a public health matter?
2. What could prevent you from raising the profile or taking action on it, such as barriers or hindrances, or difficult gatekeepers that you need to manage?
3. What sources of enablement, strengths and opportunities can you maximise on, to achieve your aim of raising the profile of sexual health, as a public health matter, within your service?

Key terms

Erotophobia: Irrational fear of sex, including talking about sex/sexual health.
Onanism: Old-fashioned term for masturbation.
Sexual health
Sexual wellbeing
Sexual pleasure
Sexual rights

Further reading

Evans, D. T. 2013. Promoting sexual health and wellbeing: the role of the nurse. *Nursing Standard*; 28(10), 53–57. doi: 10.7748/ns2013.11.28.10.53.e7654

Mitchell, K. R., Lewis, R., O'Sullivan, L. F., Fortenberry, J. D. 2021. What is sexual wellbeing and why does it matter for public health? *Lancet Public Health*; 6, e608–13. Available at: https://doi.org/10.1016/ S2468-2667(21)00099-2 [Accessed 12.03.2022].

Wellings, K., Mitchell, K., Collumbien, M. (Eds). 2012. *Sexual Health – A Public Health Perspective*. McGraw-Hill: Maidenhead.

References

Aboul-Enein, B. H., Bernstein, J., Ross, M. W. 2016. Evidence for masturbation and prostate cancer risk: do we have a verdict? *Sexual Medicine Reviews*; 4(3), 229–234. Available at: www.sciencedirect.com/science/article/abs/pii/S2050052116000780 [Accessed 12.03.2022].

Belfield, T., Carter, Y., Matthews, P., Moss, C., Weyman, A. 2006. *The Handbook of Sexual Health in Primary Care*. FPA: London.

Bockting, W., Coleman, E. 2002. *Masturbation as a Means to Achieving Sexual Health*. The Haworth Press: New York.

Brough, P., Denman, M. (Eds). 2019. *Introduction to Psychosexual Medicine*. Fourth: London.

Brown, M., McCann, E., McCormick, F. 2021. *Making the Invisible Visible: The Inclusion of LGBTQ+ Health Needs and Concerns Within Nursing and Midwifery Pre-registration Programmes, Final Report. Queen's University Belfast/Trinity College Dublin*. Available at: www.qub.ac.uk/schools/SchoolofNursingandMidwifery/FileStore/Filetoupload, 1222743,en.pdf [Accessed 04.11.2021].

Cesnik, V. M., Zerbini, T. 2017. Sexuality education for health professionals: a literature review. *Estudos de Psicologia (Campinas)*; 34(1), 161–172. doi: 10.1590/1982-02752017000100016.

Collumbien, M., Datta, J., Davis, B., Wellings, K. 2012. Structural influences on sexual health. In K. Wellings, K. Mitchell, M. Collumbien (Eds), *Sexual Health – A Public Health Perspective*. (pp. 115–124). Open University Press, McGraw Hill: London.

Evans, D. T. 2004. Erotophobia. In J. Eadie (Ed.), *Sexuality – The Essential Glossary*. (p. 61). Arnold: London.

Evans, D. T. 2011. Sexual Health Matters: Learning for life. Mapping client need with professional sexual health education for nurses in England. EdD thesis (unpublished), University of Greenwich.

Evans, D. T. 2017. Sexualities. In *The Wiley-Blackwell Encyclopedia of Social Theory*. Wiley: Chichester. doi: 10.1215/9780822383451-009.

Everett, S. 2020. *Handbook of Contraception and Sexual Health*. Routledge: New York.

Fish, J., Evans, D. T. 2016. Guest editorial: promoting cultural competency in the nursing care of LGBT patients. *Journal of Research in Nursing*; 21(3), 159–162. doi: 10.1177/1744987116643232.

Foucault, M. 1978. *History of Sexuality – Volume 1: An Introduction*. Penguin: London.

Fowler, N. 2014. *AIDS Don't Die of Prejudice*. Biteback Publishing: London.

Government Equalities Office. 2019. *National LGBT Survey – Summary Report*. (p. 27). Government Equalities Office: London. Available at: www.gov.uk/government/organisations/government-equalities-office [Accessed 12.03.2022].

Green, J., Cross, R., Woodall, J., Tones, K. 2019. *Health Promotion Planning and Strategies*. Sage: London: Available at: https://study.sagepub.com/greentones4e [Accessed 12.03.2022].

Hadley, A., Ingham, R., Chandra-Mouli, V. 2018. *Teenage Pregnancy and Young Parenthood – Effective Policy and Practice*. Routledge: London. Available at: www.routledge.com/Teenage-Pregnancy-and-Young-Parenthood-Effective-Policy-and-Practice/Hadley/p/book/9781138699564 [Accessed 13.03.2022].

Heath, H., White, I. 2002. *The Challenge of Sexuality in Health Care*. Blackwell Science: Oxford.

ILGA. 2020. *Maps – Sexual Orientation Laws*. Available at: https://ilga.org/maps-sexual-orientation-laws [Accessed 28.06.2020].

McClean, S., Bray, I., de Viggiani, N., Bird, E., Pilkington, P. 2020. *Research Methods for Public Health*. Sage: London.

Mitchell, K. R., Lewis, R., O'Sullivan, L. F., Fortenberry, J. D. 2021. What is sexual wellbeing and why does it matter for public health? *Lancet Public Health*; 6, e608–13. https://doi.org/10.1016/ S2468-2667(21)00099-2

Naidoo, J., Wills, J. 2016. *Foundations for Health Promotion*. Elsevier: New York.

Natzler, M., Evans, D. T. 2021. *Student Relationships, Sex and Sexual Health Survey, HEPI Report 139*. Higher Education Policy Unit and Brook: London.

Nursing and Midwifery Council. 2018. *The Code: Professional Standards of Practice and Behaviour for Nurses, Midwives and Nursing Associates*. Nursing and Midwifery Council: London. Available at: www.nmc.org.uk/globalassets/sitedocuments/nmc-publications/nmc-code.pdf [Accessed 12.03.2022].

Office for National Statistics. 2019. *Conceptions in England and Wales, 2017, Statistical Bulletin*. (pp. 1–12). Office for National Statistics: London. doi: 10.1057/hsq.2009.8.

Oliffe, J. L., Greaves, L. (Eds). 2012. *Designing and Conducting Gender, Sex and Health Research*. Sage: London.

Royal College of Nursing. 2019. *Sexual Health Education Directory*. Available at: www.rcn.org.uk/clinical-topics/public-health/sexual-health/sexual-health-education-directory [Accessed 28.06.2020].

Serrant-Green, L. 2011. The sound of 'silence': a framework for researching sensitive issues or marginalised perspectives in health. *Journal of Research in Nursing*, 16(4), 347–360. Available at: https://journals.sagepub.com/doi/abs/10.1177/1744987110387741 [Accessed 12.03.2022].

Steward, J., Wingfield, N. M. 2016. Venereal diseases. In *International Encyclopedia of the First World War*. Freie Universität: Berlin. Available at: https://encyclopedia.1914-1918-online.net/article/venereal_diseases [Accessed 26.12.2019].

UNAIDS. 2020. *AIDS by the Numbers*. Available at: www.unaids.org/en [Accessed 28.06.2020].

Vincent, B. 2016. *Transgender Health: A Practitioner's Guide to Binary and Non-Binary Trans Patient Care*. Jessica Kingsley: London.

WAS. 2014. Declaration of Sexual Rights. *World Association for Sexual Health*, p. 2. www.worldsexology.org/wp-content/uploads/2013/08/declaration_of_sexual_rights_sep03_2014.pdf.

WAS. 2019. Declaration on Sexual Pleasure. *Mexico City World Congress of Sexual Health.* Available at: https://worldsexualhealth.net/wp-content/uploads/2019/10/2019_WAS_Declaration_on_Sexual_Pleasure.pdf [Accessed 12.03.2022].

Wellings, K. 2012. Communication and language. In K. Wellings, K. Mitchell, M. Collumbien (Eds), *Sexual Health – A Public Health Perspective.* (pp. 127–138). Open University Press, McGraw Hill: London.

Wintemute, R. 1995. *Sexual Orientation and Human Rights: The United States Constitution, the European Convention and the Canadian Charter.* Clarendon Press: London.

WHO (1975) Sexual and Reproductive Health and Research (SRH), 'Defining Sexual Health', cited at: https://www.who.int/teams/sexual-and-reproductive-health-and-research/key-areas-of-work/sexual-health/defining-sexual-health cited on 23/06/2022

World Health Organization. 2002. *Defining Sexual Health. Sexual Health Document Series, Report of a Technical Consultation on Sexual Health.* World Health Organization: Geneva. Available at: www.who.int/reproductivehealth/publications/sexual_health/defining_sexual_health.pdf [Accessed 12.03.2022].

World Health Organization. 2020. *Defining Sexual Health.* World Health Organization: Geneva. Available at: www.who.int/reproductivehealth/topics/sexual_health/sh_definitions/en/ [Accessed 28.06.2020].

Section 4:

SAFEGUARDING

15

SAFEGUARDING ADULTS, 21ST-CENTURY ISSUES

SUSAN GREENING AND PHILIP TREMEWAN

LEARNING OUTCOMES

By the end of this chapter you will be able to:

- Understand how and why the PREVENT agenda has developed.
- Understand the issues which affect vulnerable adults in our society making them possible targets for use in the modern slavery arena and understand the role of the practitioners in recognising and escalating concerns of human trafficking and modern slavery.
- Understand and recognise the principles of the Mental Capacity Act 2005 and their place in modern health care.
- Understand and appreciate why the Deprivation of Liberty Safeguards were introduced and their influence in safeguarding adults (in particular) and recognise how the new Liberty Protection Safeguards will move this agenda forward.

Introduction

There are specific areas of 21st century society that need a safeguarding overview. These include protection of individuals who can be open to religious and political factions who may involve them in terrorist activities and those who can be exploited for modern slavery. Both areas of safeguarding can have significant consequences for society and the individuals concerned and are illegal. These areas are the tenet of the police forces and border agencies primarily. Another area of concern is the protection of those vulnerable adults in society who require protection from being deprived of their liberty in relation to accommodation for ongoing care. The Mental Capacity Act 2005 is the statute that provides the appropriate legal framework and coupled with the Deprivation of Liberty Safeguards 2007 they both ensure that those people who are assessed as lacking capacity for ongoing care are protected in their best interests. This chapter explores how these areas are encapsulated in law and the processes involved.

The PREVENT agenda

The following section explores the government's PREVENT strategy which aims to reduce the likelihood of vulnerable people being drawn into terrorism. The narrative will discuss the National Health Service's responsibility in supporting the PREVENT initiative and considers whether the number of resources deployed into PREVENT by the health sector is proportionate. Finally, there is a wider discussion exploring if or how PREVENT is a safeguarding issue.

Over recent years there have been a significant number of terror attacks and atrocities on the UK mainland carried out by individuals or organisations holding extreme ideologies, for example:

- Nicky Reilly, the Exeter nail bomber was a failed suicide bomber who attempted to blow up a restaurant in 2008. He was jailed in 2009 and found dead in HMP Manchester in 2016. He was an 'easy target' for radicalisation, his mother told an inquest. At the hearing Reilly's mother said her son had Asperger's syndrome, was bullied and had self-harmed.
- Bilal Abdulla, 27, and 28-year-old engineer Kafeel Ahmed attempted to blow up a bomb at Glasgow Airport in 2007.
- Jo Cox MP was stabbed to death near Leeds in 2016 by a man with extreme right-wing ideology.
- The Manchester Arena bombing was a suicide bombing attack in Manchester, on 22 May 2017. A radical Islamist detonated a shrapnel-laden homemade bomb as people were leaving the Manchester Arena following a concert by the American singer Ariana Grande.
- Khalid Masood at Westminster Bridge on 22 March 2017. Six people died, including the attacker, and at least 50 people were injured after a terror attack near the

Houses of Parliament on 22 March. Evidence suggests that Masood was constantly targeted by an Islamist terror group.

- Shamima Begum was a south-east London schoolgirl who travelled to Syria to join so-called Islamic State. Ms Begum left the UK in 2015 as a 15-year-old and was found in a Syrian refugee camp after living under Islamic State rule for more than three years.

According to the UK Home Office (2019a) the purpose of PREVENT is to safeguard vulnerable people from becoming terrorists or supporting terrorism, by engaging with people who are vulnerable to radicalisation and protecting those who are being targeted by terrorist recruiters.

As part of the wider CONTEST strategy, PREVENT sits alongside other work that includes:

- *Pursue*: Stop terrorist attacks happening in the UK and overseas.
- *Protect*: Strengthen protection against a terrorist attack in the UK or overseas.
- *Prepare*: Mitigate the impact of a terrorist incident if it occurs.

PREVENT deals with all forms of terrorism, including Islamist and extreme right wing, and does not focus on any one community. PREVENT prioritises working in areas where there are risks of radicalisation and offers support predominantly through local community partnerships (Home Office 2019a). Through PREVENT, vulnerable individuals who are identified as at risk of radicalisation can be safeguarded and supported, while also enabling those already engaged in terrorism to disengage and rehabilitate (Home Office, 2019b).

The PREVENT duty came into force as part of the Counter-Terrorism and Security Act 2015 and ensures that specified authorities have due regard to the need to PREVENT people from being drawn into terrorism. It covers schools, colleges, universities, health, local authorities, police and prisons.

The responsibility of healthcare practitioners in supporting the PREVENT initiative

The Home Office (2019b) states that healthcare professionals will meet and treat people who may be vulnerable to being drawn into terrorism. Being drawn into terrorism includes not just violent extremism but also non-violent extremism, which can create an atmosphere conducive to terrorism and can popularise views which terrorists exploit.

According to the Home Office (2019b) the key challenge for the healthcare sector is to ensure that, where there are signs that someone has been or is being drawn into terrorism, the healthcare worker is trained to recognise those signs correctly and is aware of and can locate available support, including referral to CHANNEL where necessary. CHANNEL was first piloted in 2007 and rolled out across England and Wales in April 2012. CHANNEL is a programme which focuses on providing support at an early stage to people who are identified as being vulnerable to being drawn into terrorism (Home Office 2019c). The programme uses a multi-agency approach to protect vulnerable people by:

- Identifying individuals at risk.
- Assessing the nature and extent of that risk.
- Developing the most appropriate support plan for the individuals concerned.

CHANNEL is about ensuring that vulnerable children and adults of any faith, ethnicity or background receive support before their vulnerabilities are exploited by those that would want them to embrace terrorism, and before they become involved in criminal terrorist activity (Home Office 2019c). The Home Office (2019b) suggests that preventing someone from being drawn into terrorism is substantially comparable to safeguarding in other areas, including child abuse or domestic violence. NHS England has incorporated PREVENT into its safeguarding arrangements so that PREVENT awareness and other relevant training is delivered to all staff who provide services to NHS patients.

In response to the terrorist attacks in 2017 the Deputy Chief Nursing Officer for England highlighted that prevention and safeguarding are familiar concepts in the NHS, well understood in relation to health and wellbeing (NHS England 2017a). However, she also reiterated that prevention is also about keeping people protected from harm and it is the duty of NHS staff to ensure they identify and support vulnerable people who could be tempted down the path of extremism, whether that is radical Islamism or poisonous far-right hatred (NHS England 2017a).

Since 2015 the Home Office has been recording the number of PREVENT referrals across England and Wales made by relevant agencies and organisations. In the year ending March 2019, a total of 5,738 individuals were referred to PREVENT (Home Office 2019d). This is the lowest number of referrals since comparable data is available. The education sector accounted for the highest number of referrals (33%) and as in previous years most individuals were male (87%) and the majority of referrals were for people aged 20 years or under (58%) (Home Office 2019d). The same figures collected by the Home Office (2019d) demonstrated that the Police (29%) and Local Authorities across England and Wales (11%) made a higher number of referrals than the National Health Service (10%).

Section 26 of the Counter-Terrorism and Security Act 2015 is better known as the 'PREVENT duty'. The PREVENT duty placed a legal responsibility on health and social care agencies including the NHS to have 'due regard to the need to PREVENT people from being drawn into terrorism'. According to Heath-Kelly and Strausz (2017) employees receive training to recognise the signs of radicalisation and are encouraged to report any concerns about radicalisation to their line managers or safeguarding team. This is clearly an area of concern for Heath-Kelly and Strausz, who suggest that the UK has never before trained its educators, medics and social care professionals to detect those who might become involved in terrorism. They continue by suggesting that the UK has made the public sector responsible for reporting extremist views or conduct under the rubric of safeguarding (Heath-Kelly and Strausz 2017). The intention is that NHS staff trained in the PREVENT duty will recognise potential extreme ideology before they become involved in criminal activity and refer on accordingly. In PREVENT guidance produced by NHS England (2017a) this redirection is situated within the 'pre-criminal space'. According to Goldberg et al. (2017) this is not a recognised term in criminology, social science or the healthcare professions, yet it appeared in NHS training before being cascaded down into local Trust documentation.

Despite NHS England's strong focus on raising the profile of the PREVENT programme and establishing comprehensive training packages for all front-line staff across the NHS, questions remain as to whether this demonstrates a positive return on this investment. Of the 5,738 individuals referred to PREVENT during 2018/19, 1,320 were discussed at a local CHANNEL panel and 561 were adopted as a CHANNEL case (Home Office 2019d). The Home Office figures indicate that referrals to PREVENT from health organisations amount to 10% of the overall total, suggesting that only 56 cases referred by the NHS during 2018/19 were formally adopted as a CHANNEL case.

In 2017 NHS England published the *PREVENT Training and Competencies Framework*. The framework was developed in order to meet the PREVENT duty and to encourage a consistent approach to training and competency development in respect of PREVENT. It provides clarity on the level of training required for healthcare workers through identifying staff groups that require basic PREVENT awareness and those who are required to attend the Workshop to Raise Awareness of PREVENT (WRAP).

In 2015 the Home Office produced a resource which was used to train NHS staff to spot the signs of radicalisation and make referrals if staff notice that 'someone may be becoming involved in or supporting terrorism'. The document supported NHS provider organisations, NHS Commissioners and organisations providing services on behalf of the NHS to meet contractual obligations in relation to safeguarding training, as set out in Clause 32 of the *NHS Standard Contract* (NHS England 2017b).

Scrutiny of the training and data compliance across NHS Trusts in England is monitored on a quarterly basis by NHS Digital and Clinical Commissioning Groups (CCGs) (NHS Digital 2019). The aim of the data collection is to demonstrate how NHS providers are delivering the key elements of the duty. These include identified PREVENT leads, delivery of awareness training, the level of referrals made and the engagement with relevant partnership forums that coordinate the PREVENT strategy at local and regional levels. It should assist NHS providers in identifying potential areas for development and give CCGs an assurance framework on which they monitor their commissioned providers' delivery of the PREVENT strategy (NHS Digital 2019).

PREVENT agenda within healthcare

From the information discussed above there is strong evidence to support the claim that the NHS has invested heavily in raising the profile of the PREVENT duty and the subsequent options that allow staff to escalate their concerns. The Department of Health presents the PREVENT duty as a patient safeguarding measure, which entails no extra responsibilities on behalf of clinical and non-clinical staff (Department of Health 2011). Safeguarding processes are designed to protect those with care and support needs from abuse. They are a necessary societal protection for those with reduced individual capacity or agency (Heath-Kelly and Strausz 2017). High-profile events reflected nationally and various pieces of legislation have resulted in formalising safeguarding processes across the UK. The Children Act 1989 formalised the UK's child protection procedures and put them on a statutory footing (Mandelstam 2009).

A view supported by Heath-Kelly and Strausz (2017) suggests that the extension of children's safeguarding measures to adults has been more problematic because the desire to protect those adults at risk of harm, abuse and neglect must be balanced against a wider commitment to the freedom of adults in general. The Department of Health (2011) guidance is also divided between recognising the increased risk of radicalisation of people with care and support needs and the generalised risk of all patients, visitors and staff to radicalisation.

From the research carried out by Heath-Kelly and Strausz (2017) it is suggested that in healthcare, unlike education, safeguarding is associated with protective intervention upon adults with 'care and support needs' in line with legislation contained in the Care Act 2015. At this point the practice of the PREVENT duty as a safeguarding matter becomes somewhat ambiguous. Heath-Kelly and Strausz (2017) summarise this dilemma by suggesting that 'when radicalisation is presented as risk to people with care and support needs, radicalisation is framed as a type of abuse. However, when radicalisation is presented as a condition which could affect anyone, it loses its association with care and support needs and is framed as a societal and security risk.'

From the position adopted by the Home Office and NHS England it is clear that the PREVENT duty remains high on the political agenda. Continued terrorist attacks on the UK mainland ensures that awareness of radicalisation across the whole of society can reduce future risk of harm to individuals who go about their normal day-to-day lives. There is, however, a wider debate to be had challenging the existing philosophy that the PREVENT agenda sits within the safeguarding threshold. There is little doubt that vulnerable people have been targeted for radicalisation, but the challenge remains as to whether the considerable investment by the NHS in raising the profile of PREVENT is justifiable given the mediocre return.

Modern slavery overview and history

According to history, British involvement in slavery is over 2,000 years old. Cicero noted in about 54 BC that the 'British' enslaved by Julius Caesar 'were too ignorant to fetch fancy prices in the market' (Trevelyan, 1912). Domestic slavery also existed in Britain: serfs were bought and sold with the estate on which they had to work for a fixed number of days a year without payment; they could only marry with their lord's consent, could not leave the estate and had few legal rights (Sherwood 2007). During the 16th–19th centuries Britons were also enslaved by the Barbary pirates where they would be used as galley slaves on ships sailing the Mediterranean Sea (Vitkus 2001).

In 1789 William Wilberforce gave a famous speech on abolition of slavery before the House of Commons. This led to the enactment of the Abolition of the Slave Trade Act 1807, prohibiting the slave trade in the British colonies as well as making it illegal to carry slaves in British ships (OpenLearn 2020). Britain forbade slavery across the British

Empire in 1833 following the enactment of the Slavery Abolition Act 1833. The adoption of this legislation granted freedom to all slaves in Britain and made slavery illegal (OpenLearn 2020).

In a foreword written for a Local Government Association (LGA) publication on tackling modern slavery, Councillor Simon Blackburn (LGA 2017) claimed that it was a shocking fact that while most people consider the slave trade to have ended when slavery was abolished in 1833, there are more slaves today than ever before in human history. Figures from the International Labour Organization (ILO) suggest that there are more than 21 million held in forced labour and modern slavery across the world. They have previously estimated that forced labour is generating criminal profits of approximately US$150 billion a year (ILO 2014).

According to the ILO (2014) the phrase 'modern slavery' has emerged as a catch-all for forced labour, human trafficking, forced sexual exploitation and some of the worst forms of child labour. The ILO also argue there is no question that slavery, in all its forms, is unacceptable and must be eradicated. However, not all children exposed to hazardous work are 'slaves', and not all labour that is not compensated with a fair wage is necessarily forced (ILO 2014).

The ILO's Forced Labour Convention, 1930 (No. 29) defines forced labour as: 'All work or service which is exacted from any person under the menace of any penalty and for which the said person has not offered himself voluntarily' (ILO C.29, Art. 1). Forced labour includes practices such as slavery and those similar to slavery, debt bondage and serfdom as defined in other international instruments, such as the League of Nations' 1926 Slavery Convention and the United Nations' 1956 Supplementary Convention on the Abolition of Slavery, the Slave Trade, and Institutions and Practices Similar to Slavery.

Human trafficking is the recruitment and movement of people – often by means such as coercion, deception and abuse of vulnerability. Trafficking in human beings is a crime, which has a strong human rights dimension. It involves the recruitment of the victim and their transportation to another state or within the same state for the purposes of exploitation (OpenLearn 2020). Human trafficking now falls within the UK's Modern Slavery Act 2015. The Act addresses both human trafficking and slavery, defining slavery as knowingly holding a person in slavery or servitude or knowingly requiring a person to perform forced or compulsory labour.

As stated above, modern slavery is an umbrella term encompassing human trafficking, slavery servitude and forced labour. According to Unseen (2020) someone is in slavery if they are:

- Forced to work through mental or physical threat.
- Owned or controlled by an 'employer', usually through mental or physical abuse or the threat of abuse.
- Dehumanised, treated as a commodity or bought and sold as 'property'.
- Physically constrained or have restrictions placed on their freedom.

According to the LGA (2017) there are a number of different types of exploitation that victims of modern slavery may be subjected to, and victims may experience more than one type of exploitation at the same time. The most common forms of exploitation are:

- **Sexual and labour exploitation**: Victims may be forced into prostitution or pornography. A victim is made to work with little or no pay and their passports may be confiscated. They are often made to live in terrible conditions and under constant threat.
- **Domestic servitude**: Victims work in a household where they may be ill-treated, forced to live under unbearable conditions or forced to work for little or no pay (Home Office 2016).
- **Forced criminality and county lines exploitation**: 'County lines' is the police term for urban gangs supplying drugs to suburban areas and towns using dedicated mobile phone lines. Gangs establish a base in the market location, typically by taking over the homes of local vulnerable adults in a practice referred to as 'cuckooing' (LGA, 2017).

The role of the NHS in responding to human trafficking

According to a report commissioned by the Department of Health (2015), under the Modern Slavery Act 2015 various health bodies, including NHS Foundation Trusts, have a duty to cooperate with the Independent Anti-Slavery Commissioner. Trafficked people experience a range of health risks prior to, during and following their trafficking experiences (Zimmerman et al. 2011). For example, studies suggest that trafficked people experience high levels of physical and sexual violence and have significant physical, sexual and mental health needs (Oram et al. 2012).

In England and Wales, NHS professionals are encouraged to notify the Home Office via the National Referral Mechanism (NRM) when they come into contact with a patient they suspect has experienced human trafficking or modern slavery (Department of Health 2015). Yet according to this report little is known about whether NHS professionals encounter trafficked people. However, by 2019 the profile of modern slavery and human trafficking is seen firmly as a priority area for NHS England. In their *Safeguarding Annual Update 2018/19*, NHS England (2019a) recognise the need to raise the profile of modern slavery across the healthcare system and to ensure that health is represented in regional and local anti-slavery partnerships.

The safeguarding of vulnerable people has always been a key part of the NHS, and victims of modern slavery are just that. Caring for these individuals that are almost invisible to society requires concerted effort from all healthcare providers. Every staff member at the NHS has a part to play in the identification and consequently the prevention of modern slavery. It is, according to Dearnley (2019), a big ask because vulnerable individuals might be distressed and distrustful, but it is important to remember that these are victims and therefore the NHS has a moral duty to help in any way that it can.

Safeguarding adults who lack capacity to make their own decisions

In the UK there is a massive change in the elderly demographic of the population. Essentially, an increase in the number of surviving centenarians since the 1960s from 300 to 6,000 in 2004 and a projected increase to over 6,000 in 2036 (ERSC 2007). Recent figures from the Office for National Statistics (2017) indicate that the trend towards an older population is increasing and spreading to more urban areas. With advancing age and illness inextricably linked within Western society it should be no surprise that internationally any illness which increases health care needs in this group will have some priority for care and research providers (Leishman 2008, Luengo-Fernandez et al. 2010). Figures in 2009 state that 36 million people worldwide suffered from dementia. This is projected to reach 115 million by 2050 (Poppe et al. 2013). Macaden (2016) reported even more alarming figures: 74.7 million in 2015 and by 2050 that is projected to rise to 135.1 million. Dementia is now a priority for the members that make up the G8 committee: Japan, USA, Russia, Italy, Germany, UK, Canada and France.

These changes have now been recognised by the developing countries. Almost two-thirds of people admitted to hospital are aged over 65 years of age (Cornwell et al. 2012) and 50% of these have some cognitive impairment (Royal College of Psychiatrists 2005). Higgins (2013) reinforces the evidence presented at all levels stating that 80% of people living in care homes also have dementia or a significant cognitive impairment. These residents often, due to their frailty, are admitted into hospital for ongoing care and treatment and it has been recognised that their mental capacity is affected adversely by the admission (Age UK 2014). The world's population is ageing and with it the burden on the NHS is palpable and identifiable. That is not to say that age and lack of capacity are always present in decision making. There are other factors that can affect a person's ability to make decisions: serious ill health, acquired brain injury, a learning disability. Statistics are, however, revealing that age/dementia/capacity (or lack of it) are a major concern in today's health care landscape. Dementia is increasing due to an ageing population, family history (possible genetic effect) and physical causes – the heart–head link (Alzheimer's Society 2015).

The Diagnostic and Statistical Manual of Mental Disorders (DSM-5) (American Psychiatric Association 2013) has re-categorised the criteria for dementia in order to recognise the facets of neuro-cognitive disorder which indicate evidence of significant cognitive decline. It uses a comparison in performance levels in learning and memory, language, executive function, attention, social cognition and perceptual motor ability. These deficits in cognition are assessed to interfere with independence in everyday living and are not better described by another disorder and do not occur just as part of delirium.

It is a fact that many individuals who are admitted to hospital are assessed as being unable to make decisions with regard to their care and treatment due to the conditions outlined above. Capacity is time- and decision-specific, which can make assessment more problematical especially if the person's capacity fluctuates; also individuals may have capacity for some things but not others. The Mental Capacity Act 2005 (MCA 2005) promotes the view that practitioners need to accept and embrace the principles of the act. These are a basic tenet for person-centred care and a core consideration in relation to informed consent. The MCA 2005 clearly aims to empower those people who lack capacity to be protected by a legal process. It embodies the principles of rights of the Human Rights Act 1998, in particular **Articles 5 and 8** and interactions between the statutes were brought to the forefront following the European Court ruling of HL v UK (Brown et al. 2009). These Articles are essentially the right of a person to have liberty and security. This includes the right not to be arbitrarily deprived of their liberty. **Article 8** supports this by respecting a person's personal autonomy. The MCA 2005 became 'live' in April 2007, and it placed on statutory authorities a legal obligation to ensure that anyone who lacks capacity to decide or act for themselves are supported to do so and if someone else has to act for them that all decisions are made in their best interests. This applies to all individuals aged 16 years and over in hospital and registered care settings. Consent to treatment and the principles of the MCA are intertwined in their philosophy. Consent to treatment must be informed or the treatment must be considered in the patient's best interests. It is important to note that Section 5 of the MCA Code of Practice (CoP) 2007 (Department for Constitutional Affairs 2007) does not give people caring for patients who lack capacity the power to make decisions on their behalf, however, it offers protection from liability so they can act in connection with the person's care or treatment (Department for Constitutional Affairs 2007, p. 94). The MCA is described as a 'visionary piece of legislation for its time' (House of Lords 2014). It is intended to provide those who lack capacity with a 'step change' and give them potential for a better life which involves their wishes and feelings to be at the centre of decision making.

The principles of the MCA 2005

Principle 1: Assume a person has capacity unless proved otherwise.
Principle 2: Do not treat people as incapable of making a decision unless all practicable steps have been tried to help them.
Principle 3: A person should not be treated as incapable of making a decision because their decision may seem unwise.
Principle 4: Always do things or, take decisions for people without capacity, in their best interests.
Principle 5: Before doing something to someone or making a decision on their behalf, consider whether the outcome could be achieved in a less-restrictive way.

The MCA 2005 uses those principles put forward by the European Convention on Human Rights in 1950 that emphasise a person's autonomy to make decisions based on information and their ability to weigh up this information so that they can live a full and active life. Set up to protect human rights in member countries, the UK has adopted these principles. Harding (2012) has explored the 'right to autonomy' for people with dementia. She states that often the law can come into conflict with principles and guidelines, and this was emphasised when the MCA (Amendment) Bill was presented to the UK Government in March 2017. In her conclusion Harding (2012) states that people with dementia do not fit neatly into legal boxes due to their position on the periphery of capacity and incapacity and the laws pertaining to the Mental Health Act or the MCA. Using an ethical framework will allow for a person's personhood to be considered and to consider their autonomy. Dimond (2007) reiterates this problem of defining capacity within the decision-making paradigm.

Deprivation of Liberty Safeguards (soon to become Liberty Protection Safeguards)

The Deprivation of Liberty Safeguards (DoLS) form part of the Mental Capacity Act 2005. These safeguards apply in respect of people who lack capacity specifically to consent to treatment or care in either a hospital or care home that, in their own best interests, can only be provided in circumstances that result in a deprivation of liberty and where it is not appropriate to detain under the Mental Health Act that time. It is essentially used for patients in hospital who have an impairment of the mind or brain (e.g. dementia) but who are in hospital for other forms of treatment such as surgery or infections. It can be used for mental health patients who lack capacity but do not need to be detained. The safeguards came into force on 1 April 2009 in England and in Wales. They apply to people aged 18 years and over. They are covered by a Code of Practice from the Ministry of Justice (2008).

The DoLS include a number of assessments to be carried out by at least two independent assessors. These assessments ensure that the person is over 18 years of age, they lack capacity for care and treatment, and to be accommodated in the care setting in their best interests they are not eligible to be detained (do not meet the criteria) under the MHA 1983, and consideration is given to any advance decisions and to any Lasting Power of Attorney decisions. Traditionally these assessments have been carried out by trained Best Interests Assessors (BIAs) and psychiatrists registered under Section 12 of the MHA 1983. The MCA 2005 introduced the new Independent Mental Capacity Advocacy (IMCA) Service to assist individuals who had no support with regards to decision making. The Code of Practice states:

> The purpose of the IMCA service is to help particularly vulnerable people who lack capacity to make important decisions about serious medical treatment [...] who have no family or friends that it would be appropriate to consult with.
> (Ministry of Justice 2008, p. 178)

Initially only patients in hospital who were trying to leave or objecting to treatment were the subject of DoLS scrutiny; however, in a landmark decision made in the House of Lords, affectionately known as Cheshire West [2014], the number of referrals increased dramatically – in one health board from 45 to 445 to 973 in one year. This led to health boards and local authorities being unable to manage the workload, and it was soon evident that using the current system was 'overly complex and excessively bureaucratic' according to the Law Commission Review set up to look at this (Law Commission 2017).

DoLS was assessed as not fit for purpose (Ruck Keene and Dobson 2015). The review has been completed and on 16 May 2019 The Mental Capacity (Amendment) Act 2019 received the Royal Assent. The Liberty Protection Safeguards will apply to England and Wales only. Scotland and Northern Ireland have their own process. The current comparison between the two schemes DoLS and LPS can be found in Table 15.1.

Initial timescales for the implementation of LPS were initially set for 1 October 2020 following the completion of the Parliamentary process. This was delayed due to the impact of the COVID-19 pandemic. The amended timescale for implementation was then scheduled for April 2022, however, this is now unachievable due to the need for consultation on the new codes of practice and procedural parliamentary overview. Partners in health and social care are still working towards an implementation in 2022, and there are now documents out for consultation with a timescale of implementation set for October 2022. This includes codes of practice proposals for both England and Wales. Whatever the outcome there will be a scheme in place to protect those individuals aged 16+ in relation to those care decisions that require support and safeguards against unlawfully depriving them of their liberty to provide health and social care and the agencies responsible for providing that care.

Table 15.1 Consideration of the perceived differences between the current DoLS system and the new LPS proposals

Deprivation of Liberty Safeguards	Liberty Protection Safeguards
People aged 18+	People aged 16+
Applies to hospitals and registered care settings	Any setting – person's own home, sheltered housing, extra care facilities, shared lives placements etc.
6 assessments	3 assessments and using current care planning processes
Emphasis on best interests	Emphasis on what is necessary and proportionate to prevent harm
Urgent authorisation – 7 days	Interim authorisation for up to 28 days
Independent Best Interests Assessors (BIAs) – assess and go	Approved Mental Capacity Practitioners (AMCPs) (likely to carry caseloads and have a more strengthened role similar to Approved Mental Health Practitioners)
Blanket approach – everyone who lacks capacity	Those who need it
Supervisory body (Wales)	Responsible body
Timescales up to 12 months and then re-assessment – no renewals	Timescales up to 12 months, renewal for 1 year and then 3 years
Relevant person representative	Appropriate person – extends the role of the IMCA
BIAs employed by health boards and local authority	AMCP numbers should be confirmed by the LA as sufficient to meet the need of the client population
Section 12 – Doctors complete eligibility assessments	No longer required
Waiting list remains high in most areas	LPS hopes to reduce this

Conclusion

It is clear that there remains the need for inter-agency and multi-professional input across the PREVENT and Modern Slavery Agenda. This approach has yielded results and its constant review is essential for this to continue. The introduction of the Liberty Protection Safeguards to replace the bureaucracy of the current Deprivation of Liberty Safeguards will ensure a widening of the protection for vulnerable people who need to have decisions made in their best interests. It will also streamline assessments and make decision making clearer from the start of the process. This can only increase the protection for those who need it and in various settings making the assessment of mental capacity for decision making a fundamental tenet for providing care.

Consider the following questions

1. Does the PREVENT agenda offer a proportionate response?
2. What is the role of the practitioner within the PREVENT agenda?
3. Does the PREVENT duty belong within healthcare and is it a safeguarding matter?
4. What is mental capacity and why is lack of mental capacity an issue?
5. What affect will replacing DoLS with LPS have for individuals who lack capacity to make decisions with regard to their accommodation for care and treatment?

Key terms

PREVENT – is about safeguarding individuals from being drawn into terrorism ensuring that those who are vulnerable to such extremist narratives can be identified and supported at an early stage.

Human Trafficking – A person is trafficked if they are brought to, or moved around, a country by others who threaten, frighten, hurt and force them to do work or other things that they don't want to do (WG 2019 Modern Slavery: Guidance for professionals)

Mental Capacity – Mental capacity is the ability to make one's own decisions. It is time and decision specific. It can be affected by mental health, physical health – stroke, brain injury or by degenerative conditions – dementia and even old age cognitive decline.

Modern Slavery (as per chapter 14) - the enforcement of labour on an individual which includes trapping and controlling of the victim. Modern slavery includes sexual exploitation and labour exploitation.

Dementia – 'a devastating illness that is more than just memory loss. It is a life limiting brain disease that impacts upon every level of an individual's physical, cognitive, emotional and social functioning.' (Palmer 2009:4 in report for Older People's Commissioner for Wales)

Deprivation of Liberty Safeguards (DoLS) – is the procedure prescribed in law when it is necessary to deprive someone of their liberty. This can be a resident or patient who lacks the capacity to give consent with regards to their accommodation for care and treatment. It is intended to keep them from harm. DoLS applies to adults aged over 18 years of age.

Liberty Protection Safeguards (LPS) – is the proposed procedure in law to replace the Deprivation of Liberty Safeguards. They are proposed to provide a clearer system for authorising a deprivation of liberty for people age over 16 years of age.

CONTEST – is the UK's counter terrorism strategy. It aims to reduce the risk from terrorism so people can live freely and without fear.

CHANNEL – an early intervention multi-agency process designed to safeguard vulnerable people from being drawn into violent extremist or terrorist behaviour. It works in the same way as existing safeguarding partnerships.

Best Interests Assessor – A professional trained to undertake assessments under the Mental Deprivation of Liberty Safeguards. Under law this is currently a Registered Nurse, Occupational Therapist, Social Worker or Psychologist.

Local Government Association – represents the interests of local government and promotes local democracy in Wales.

Further reading

Dearnley, R. 2019 *Preventing Modern Slavery: The Role of the NHS*. Available at: www.england.nhs.uk/blog/preventing-modern-slavery-the-role-of-the-nhs/ [Accessed 12.02.2020].

Department of Health. 2011. *Building Partnerships, Staying Safe: The Health Sector Contribution to HM's Government Prevent Strategy: Guidance for Healthcare Workers*. p. 3. HM Government: London.

House of Lords. 2014. *Mental Capacity Act 2005: Post-legislative Scrutiny, Select Committee on the MCA 2005, Report of Session 2013*, 14. The Stationery Office: London.

Law Commission. 2017. *Mental Capacity Act and Deprivation of Liberty Safeguards*, Law Commission No 372. The Stationery Office: London.

Ministry of Justice. 2008. *Mental Capacity Act 2005 Deprivation of Liberty Safeguards. Code of Practice to Supplement the Main Mental Capacity Act Code of Practice*. The Stationery Office: London.

NHS England. 2017. *Prevent Training and Competencies Framework*. NHS England: Leeds.

References

Age UK. 2014. *Implementing John's Campaign*. Age UK: London.

Alzheimer's Society. 2015. *Living and Dying with Dementia in Wales: Barriers to Care*. Marie Curie Cancer Care: London.

American Psychiatric Association. 2013. *Diagnostic and Statistical Manual of Mental Disorders* (5th edn) (DSM-5). American Psychiatric Association: Arlington, VA.

Brown, R., Barber P., Martin, D. 2009. *The Mental Capacity Act 2005: A Guide for Practice*. (2nd edn). Sage: London.

Cornwell, J., Sonola, L., Levenson, R., Poteliakhoff, E. 2012. *Continuity of Care for Older Hospital Patients: A Call for Action*. The King's Fund: London.

Dearnley, R. 2019. *Preventing Modern Slavery: The Role of the NHS*. Available at: www.england.nhs.uk/blog/preventing-modern-slavery-the-role-of-the-nhs/ [Accessed 12.02.2020].

Department for Constitutional Affairs. 2007. *Mental Capacity Act 2005 Code of Practice*. The Stationery Office: London.

Department of Health. 2011. *Building Partnerships, Staying Safe; The Health Sector Contribution to HM's Government Prevent Strategy: Guidance for Healthcare Workers*. (p.3). HM Government: London.

Department of Health. 2015. *Protect: Provider Responses Treatment and Care for Trafficked People: Final Report for the Department of Health Policy Research Programme*. Department of Health: London.

Dimond, B. 2007. Mental capacity and decision-making: defining capacity. *British Journal of Nursing*; 16, 18.

ERSC. 2007. *Ageing in the UK*. Available at: www.ersc.ac.uk/ESRCmtoCentre/facts/index.8.asps [Accessed 20.01.2020].

Goldberg, D., Jadhav, S., Younis, T. (2017) Prevent: what is pre-criminal space? *BJPsych Bulletin*; Aug 41(4), 208–211.

Harding, R. 2012. Legal constructions of dementia: discourses of autonomy at the margins of capacity. *Journal of Social Welfare and Family Law*; 34(4), 425–442.

Heath-Kelly, C., Strausz, E. 2017. *Counter-terrorism in the NHS Evaluating Prevent Duty Safeguarding in the NHS*. University of Warwick: Coventry.

Higgins, P. 2013. Meeting the relational needs of residents with dementia. *Nursing Older People*; 25(9), 25–29.

Home Office. 2015. *Workshop to Raise Awareness of Prevent, Workshop Script*. (p. 1). HM Government: London.

Home Office. 2016. *Victims of Modern Slavery – Frontline Staff Guidance*. HMSO: London.

Home Office. 2019a. *Factsheet: Prevent and Channel*. Home Office: London. Available at: https://homeofficemedia.blog.gov.uk/2019/11/05/factsheet-prevent-and-channel/ [Accessed 09.01.2020].

Home Office. 2019b. *Statutory Guidance: Revised Prevent Duty Guidance for England and Wales*. Available at: www.gov.uk/government/publications/prevent-duty-guidance/revised-prevent-duty-guidance-for-england-and-wales [Accessed 09.01.2020].

Home Office. 2019c. *Channel and Prevent Multi-agency Panel (PMAP) Guidance*. Home Office: London. Available at: www.gov.uk/government/publications/channel-guidance [Accessed 09.01.2020].

Home Office. 2019d. *Individuals Referred to and Supported through the Prevent Programme, England and Wales, April 2018 to March 2019*. HMSO: London.

House of Lords. 2014. *Mental Capacity Act 2005: Post-legislative Scrutiny, Select Committee on the MCA 2005, Report of Session 2013*. The Stationery Office: London.

International Labour Organization. 1930. *Forced Labour Convention, 1930 (No. 29)*. Available at: www.ilo.org/dyn/normlex/en/f?p=NORMLEXPUB:12100:0::NO::P12100_ ILO_CODE:C029 [Accessed 24.03.2022].

International Labour Organization. 2014. *Profits and Poverty: The Economics of Forced Labour*. ILO: Geneva.

Law Commission. 2017. *Mental Capacity Act and Deprivation of Liberty Safeguards,* Law Commission No 372. The Stationery Office: London.

Leishman, J. L. 2008. Death, dying and end-of-life care. *Quality in Ageing*; 9(4), 36–43.

Local Government Association. 2017. *Tackling Modern Slavery: A Council Guide*. LGA: London. Available at: www.local.gov.uk/sites/default/files/documents/22.12_Modern_ slavery_WEB%202.pdf [Accessed 12.03.2022].

Luengo-Fernandez, R., Leal, J., Gray, A. 2010. *Dementia 2010: The Prevalence, Economic Cost and Research Funding of Dementia Compared with Other Major Diseases*. Alzheimer's Research Trust: London. Available at: www.alzheimersresearchuk.org/wp-content/ uploads/2015/01/Dementia2010Full.pdf [Accessed 12.03.2022].

Macaden, L. 2016. Being dementia smart (BDS) – a dementia nurse education journey in Scotland. *International Journal of Nurse Education*; 13(1), 1–9.

Mandelstam, M. 2009. *Safeguarding Vulnerable Adults and the Law*. Jessica Kingsley: London.

Ministry of Justice. 2008. *Mental Capacity Act 2005 Deprivation of Liberty Safeguards. Code of Practice to Supplement the Main Mental Capacity Act Code of Practice*. The Stationery Office: London.

NHS Digital. 2019. *Prevent*. Available at: https://digital.nhs.uk/data-and-information/data- collections-and-data-sets/data-collections/prevent#guidance [Accessed 20.01.2020].

NHS England. 2017a. *Prevent Training and Competencies Framework*. NHS England: Leeds.

NHS England. 2017b. *2016/17 NHS Standard Contract*. Available at: www.england.nhs.uk/ nhs-standard-contract/16-17/ [Accessed 20.01.2020].

NHS England. 2019a. *Safeguarding Annual Update 2018/2019*. Available at: https://www. norfolksafeguardingadultsboard.info/about-us/latest-news/nhs-england-safeguarding- annual-update-20182019/ [Accessed 24/03/2022].

NHS England. 2019b. *Preventing Modern Slavery: The Role of the NHS*. Available at: www. england.nhs.uk/blog/preventing-modern-slavery-the-role-of-the-nhs/ [Accessed 12.02.2020].

Office for National Statistics. 2017. *Overview of the UK Population: July 2017*. Office for National Statistics: London.

OpenLearn. 2020. *Modern Slavery*. Available at: www.open.edu/openlearn/people-politic s-law/the-law/modern-slavery/content-section-1.1.1 [Accessed 06.02.2020].

Oram, S., Stockl, H., Busza, J., Howard, L.M., Zimmerman, C. 2012. Prevalence of risk and violence and the physical, mental and sexual health problems associated with human trafficking: systematic review. *PLos Med.*; 9(5), e1001224.

Poppe, M., Burleigh, S., Banerjee, S. 2013. Qualitative Evaluation of Advance Care Planning in Early Dementia (ACP-ED). *PLoS One*; 8(4), e60412.

Royal College of Psychiatrists. 2005. *Who Cares Wins: Guidelines for the Development of Mental Health Liaison Services for Older People*. Royal College of Psychiatrists: London.

Ruck Keene, A., Dobson, C. 2015. *Deprivation of Liberty in the Hospital Setting*. Essex Chambers: London.

Sherwood, M. 2007. Britain, slavery and the trade in enslaved Africans. *History in Focus*. Available at: https://archives.history.ac.uk/history-in-focus/Slavery/articles/sherwood.html [Accessed 06.02.20].

Trevelyan, G. M. 1912. *History of England*. Longmans, Green: London.

United Nations. 1926. *Slavery Convention*. Available at: https://www.ohchr.org/en/instruments-mechanisms/instruments/slavery-convention [Accessed 24.03.2022].

United Nations. 1956. *Supplementary Convention on the Abolition of Slavery, the Slave Trade, and Institutions and Practices Similar to Slavery*. Available at: https://treaties.un.org/pages/ViewDetailsIII.aspx?src=TREATY&mtdsg_no=XVIII-4&chapter=18&Temp=mtdsg3&clang=_en [Accessed 24.03.2022].

Unseen. 2020. *What is Modern Slavery?* Available at: www.unseenuk.org/modern-slavery/modern-slavery [Accessed 11.02.2020].

Vitkus, D. J. 2001. *Piracy, Slavery and Redemption: Barbary Captivity Narratives from Early Modern England*. Columbus University Press: New York.

www.england.nhs.uk/wp-content/uploads/2019/04/safeguarding-annual-update-18-19.pdf (accessed 12/02/2020) NHS Digital, Safeguarding Aduts England 2018 – 19 (accessed 12/02/2020).

www.gov.uk/government/publications/prevent-duty-guidance Published 12 March 2015, updated 1 April 2021

Zimmerman, C., Hossain, M., Watts, C. 2011. Human trafficking and health: a conceptual model to inform policy, intervention and research. *Social Science & Medicine*; 73(2), 327–335.

16

SAFEGUARDING CHILDREN AND YOUNG PEOPLE

MICHELLE MOSELEY

━━━━━━━━━━━━━ LEARNING OUTCOMES ━━━━━━━━━━━━━

By the end of this chapter you will be able to:

- Explore what constitutes significant harm to a child/young person (CYP).
- Consider the accumulation of risk factors associated with abuse.
- Understand the importance of an authoritative approach when safeguarding children and young people, placing the child at the centre of safeguarding practice.
- Comprehend the importance of safeguarding supervision.

Introduction

Practitioners in health and social care require evidence-based knowledge associated with safeguarding principles to enable them to assess safeguarding risk in a child/young person (CYP). The age-range of a child is 0–18 years and exposure to risk throughout childhood is potentially harmful to their physical, psychological/emotional, behavioural and social development. It is often quoted that child protection is everyone's responsibility and safeguarding encompasses the prevention of child abuse as well as the protection of CYP. Therefore, practitioners must have an awareness of risk factor impact and maintain the child as a focus of their safeguarding practice. The aim of this chapter is to raise awareness of risk factor escalation as well as exploring the concept of an ecological approach in assessing risk. The impact of adverse childhood experiences links to risk escalation theory and will be considered as well as how to take an authoritative stance when working with families where protection of the child is paramount. There is a need, first, to consider the principles of safeguarding to set the context of this safeguarding section of the book as well as this chapter.

The principles of safeguarding

The six principles of safeguarding were first established by the Department of Health in 2011 but are now embedded in the Care Act 2014. They include:

1   *Empowerment*: Individuals need to be supported to make informed decisions.
2   *Prevention*: Action needs to be taken before any harm occurs.
3   *Proportionality*: Any action needs to be proportionate to the risk.
4   *Protection*: Those with the greatest of need require support, protection and representation.
5   *Partnership*: Partnership working is essential across all agencies and disciplines when aiming to identify, report and reduce risk.
6   *Accountability*: All professionals are accountable for their own action/practice within their practice which includes the safeguarding of individuals. (SCIE 2020)

Table 16.1   UK-wide safeguarding legislation

Children Act 1989/2004
UN Convention on the Rights of the Child (UNCRC) (UNICEF 1989)
Wales – Social Services and Well-being Wales Act (2014), Children (Abolition of Defence of Reasonable Punishment) (Wales) Act 2020
Scotland – Children and Young People Scotland Act (2014), Adult Support and Protection (Scotland) Act 2007 (for 16–18-year-olds)
England – Working Together to Safeguard Children. A guide to interagency working to safeguard and promote the welfare of children (HM Government 2018)
Ireland – Cooperating to safeguard children and young people in Northern Ireland (Department of Health 2017)

The above principles are underpinned within legislation and guidance across the UK. These key principles span safeguarding legislation, policy and guidance. They are applicable within the safeguarding adult agenda but are transferrable to CYP safeguarding practice. From a CYP perspective consent for referral is not necessary if a child is considered at risk of significant harm (this applies to section 47 of the Children Act 1989). Consent is required for a child in need of referral in England (Section 17 of the Children Act 1989) or a care and support plan in Wales (Social Services and Well-being (Wales) Act 2014). Legislation and policy vary across the UK home nations (Table 16.1), but the principles of safeguarding across the UK are the same. Two key principles in the safeguarding of CYP are that safeguarding and protection of CYP is everyone's responsibility as well as taking a child-centred/children's rights (UNCRC 1989) approach to practice. The CYP voice is essential and a child-centred approach to practice must include being cognisant of their rights. Their views, wishes and feelings need to be sought wherever appropriate, whilst respecting individuality, culture and beliefs (Wales Safeguarding Procedures 2019).

Understanding risk factors – an ecological approach to safeguarding

An ecological approach to assessing what constitutes risk for CYP offers a broader, holistic perspective to safeguarding practice. Various terminology defining 'child abuse' is used across the literature. It is commonly coupled with the word 'neglect', or the term 'child maltreatment' is often used. Within this chapter the terms will be interchanged based on the evidence explored. The World Health Organization (WHO 2021) define child abuse as:

> Violence against children includes all forms of violence against people under 18 years old. For infants and younger children, violence mainly involves child maltreatment (i.e. physical, sexual, and emotional abuse and neglect) at the hands of parents and other authority figures. Boys and girls are at equal risk of physical and emotional abuse and neglect, and girls are at greater risk of sexual abuse. As children reach adolescence, peer violence and intimate partner violence, in addition to child maltreatment, become highly prevalent.

The WHO suggest that violence against children is preventable and response to violence requires a multi-system approach which prevents, assesses risk as well as consideration of any protective factors present. This is recognised in the application of Bronfenbrenner's (1979) ecological model considering the relationship between the four levels within it. The model was later adapted by Belsky in 1980 and the four levels represented are: individual, family/relationship, community and society depicted in Figure 16.1.

Wales is the only country in the world to have a Future Generations Commissioner and legislation, namely the Well-being of Future Generations (Wales) Act 2015. This sets out public health drivers to enhance the population prosperity and experience in health,

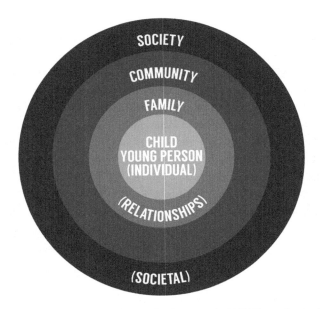

Figure 16.1   Author's adaptation of Bronfenbrenner's (1979) ecological model

education and environmental matters which link to the WHO Sustainable Development Goals (SDGs). These also relate to the social determinants of health set out by Dahlgren and Whitehead (1991) as well as aligning to the domains of Bronfenbrenner's (1979) ecological model. CYP deserve the best start in life, but this is sometimes hampered and influenced by their early childhood experiences which potentially can damage their future physical, mental health and developmental potential.

In 2016 the WHO published their 'Inspire' strategy for ending violence against children (WHO 2016, and see Table 16.2). This links to the recommended ecological stance taken by agencies but also relates to the wider determinants of health. It demonstrates the importance of involvement by policy makers to ensure that children's safety is paramount and the influence from that macro level (global), underpinning safeguarding policy at meso (national) and micro (local) levels. The aim of the strategy is to strengthen partnerships across all levels including governments, agencies and society, placing the focus on delivery of services and placing the child at the centre, with the aim of every child meeting their full potential. It is underpinned by the United Nations Convention

Table 16.2   The 'Inspire' acronym (WHO 2016)

Implementation and enforcement of laws
Norms and values
Safe environments
Parent and caregiver support
Income and economic strengthening
Response and support services
Education and life skills

on the Rights of the Child (UNICEF 1989) as well as the SDGs (UN 2019) which includes a wide range of global public health targets with target 16.2 of the SDG's referring to the safeguarding of children which advocates to:

> end abuse, exploitation, trafficking, and all forms of violence against torture of children. (United Nations 2019)

The aspirations of 'Inspire' link the macro, meso and micro levels of safeguarding practice placing CYP and their family at the centre and as the priority in safeguarding policy development. This is essential in allowing them to meet their full potential with their basic needs being met. For some families the impact of the wider determinants on health, family, community and society (Belsky 1980, Bronfenbrenner 1979) greatly impact on those basic needs being met.

An ecological approach to safeguarding is a well-known concept and associated with child protection practice and assessment in the UK today (Figure 16.2). Vygotsky (1978) and Bronfenbrenner (1979) developed learning theories which explored how individual learning is affected by family, friends, the community/culture, and society in which they live. In particular Bronfenbrenner's (1979) ecological model of child development recognised that child development progresses based on the interactions they receive from its family and surrounding environment. This concept (Figure 16.1) links to the assessment framework triangle (with the child depicted at the centre and it addresses through its

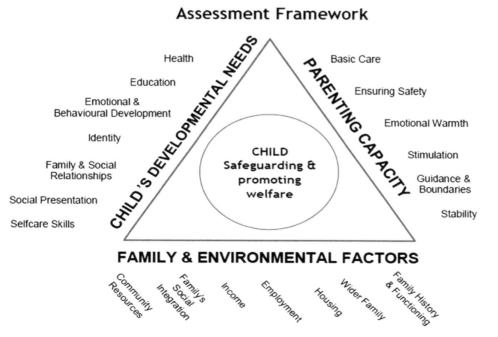

Figure 16.2 Assessment framework triangle (Department of Health 2000)

domains, the impact of the carer's parenting capacity, the environmental factors and the child's developmental needs.

The seminal work of Bronfenbrenner (1979) and Belsky (1980) underpins the assessment framework (DoH 2000) and determined that individuals develop within the complexity of social systems which interact and influence each other and includes:

- The characteristics of **the individual**. (What increases the risk of maltreatment of the child?)
- The **micro-system** explores the **relationships** within the **family**. (What increases the risk of maltreatment which is family related?)
- The **exo-system** examines community contexts. (What is it about the community that increases risk of child maltreatment?)
- The **macro-system** includes the cultural beliefs and values of society. (What is it about **society** that increases risk of child maltreatment?)

When applying Bronfenbrenner's (1979) model in assessing risk it will involve examining the CYP characteristics (physical, emotional, psychological, behavioural). At this level the CYP characteristics can affect their development. Exploration of the complexity associated with family size, family relationships/dynamic, support and protective factors is essential. Consideration will need to be given to family stability as this can directly affect the CYP as well as parenting capacity which directly influences the way in which parents/carers care for and prioritise their children (Figures 16.1 and 16.2). From a community level the support the community provides needs to be factored in. For example, are there community factors which would impact the CYP safety and wellbeing placing them at risk of further significant harm? Risk factors from a societal level can also impact the safety and wellbeing of CYP. These factors could include safeguarding and public health legislation as well as cultural and religious beliefs.

Assessing risk in the safeguarding of CYP is complex. The interacting levels of the ecological model with the child at the centre allows practitioners to explore a preventative and proactive approach to their safeguarding practice. It is essential for practitioners to be aware of what constitutes significant harm, and how adverse childhood experiences and escalation of risk has a significant impact on the CYP future wellbeing outcomes. Traditionally, risk is generally associated with familial risk factors within the home environment. The concept of 'contextual safeguarding' is related to the risk(s) that CYP are exposed to outside of the family home (Appleton et al. 2021). For example, at community or societal levels and be out of the control/protection of the parent/carer/family, exposing the CYP to significant harm.

Categories of abuse

Harm refers to the 'impairment of physical or mental health … and the impairment of physical intellectual, emotional, social or behavioural development (including that suffered from seeing or hearing another person suffer ill treatment)' (Wales Safeguarding

Procedures 2019). Types of harm include physical, emotional/psychological, sexual, neglect and financial. Financial abuse is less prevalent within childhood but can have an impact within some of the other categories. Other types of harm include:

- Child sexual exploitation (CSE)
- Criminal exploitation/county lines
- Radicalisation
- Modern slavery
- Trafficking
- Honour-based violence
- Female genital mutilation (FGM)

There is not a statutory definition of what constitutes significant harm. The Children Act 1989 states that practitioners need to consider how and when harm becomes significant by comparing the CYP's health and development to that of another CYP of the same age and stage of development. In determining what constitutes significant harm, a detailed assessment of risk and risk accumulation is required. This includes acknowledgement of the impact of adverse childhood experiences (ACEs) and taking a trauma-informed approach to practice.

Trauma-informed approach to safeguarding practice

A trauma-informed approach to safeguarding practice involves practitioners changing their conversation with CYP and their families and instead of stating or thinking 'What is wrong with you?' to one that considers 'What has happened to you?'. The Wave Trust (2021) defines trauma-informed care as a 'strengths-based framework which recognises the complex nature and effects of trauma and promotes resilience and healing.' Trauma as an external event can have a long-term impact on individuals with trauma being experienced and interpreted differently. Therefore, practitioners need to understand the context of certain behaviours/traits/perceptions of the CYP and families they are working with. The Wave Trust (2021, see Figure 16.3) have identified that all practitioners need to have a basic awareness (realisation) of trauma-informed care and its impact; this allows for a trauma-informed approach to be applied to practice. They suggest five key principles which are identified within Figure 16.3: safety, trust, choice, collaboration and empowerment. These key principles are arguably fundamental in building any therapeutic relationship with families, especially within the safeguarding arena. Therefore, identification, recognition and potential universal screening of trauma (Wave Trust 2021) as well as the impact of ACEs is suggested when establishing an early intervention and prevention plan for families (Hardcastle and Bellis 2019). Mothers who were part of the Hardcastle and Bellis research agree/strongly agreed that a practitioner with knowledge of ACEs improved the help and support provided as the practitioner (health visitor) understood the experiences of parents during their childhood.

Epigenetics and adverse childhood experiences (ACEs)

Epigenetics explains how early experiences can have a lifelong impact and relates to the research around ACEs. Epigenetics is a new area within scientific research which explores how extrinsic experiences can affect children and the impact on their gene expression. Inherited genes provide information that guide development (height, temperament). When children experience certain risk factors during development, this can alter 'the epigenetic markers that govern gene expression they can change whether and how genes release the information they carry' (Center on the Developing Child 2021). Therefore, the epigenome (chemical marker) is affected by positive as well as negative experiences and reinforces how sensitive young brains are when exposed to stressors and risk. Best practice would be supporting relationships with children that are nurturing, demonstrating positive attachment and reducing stress(ors) to enable the development of healthy, strong brains. Any epigenetic alteration will influence future healthy development as well as resilience factors. This reinforces the early identification of ACEs to empower and promote future healthy relationships and preventing potential significant harm.

ACEs have been described as traumatic events that affect children while growing up, such as suffering child maltreatment or living in a household affected by domestic

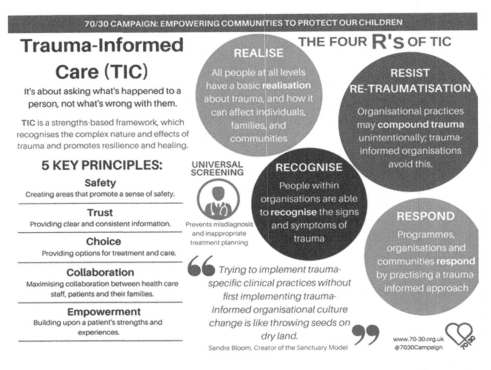

Figure 16.3 Trauma-informed care (reproduced with kind permission of the Wave Trust 2021)

violence/abuse, substance misuse or mental ill health (Bellis et al. 2016). There is no universal definition, but the impact of early adverse experiences is well recognised and identified by Felitti et al. in the late nineties (1998). The Center on the Developing Child at Harvard University produces extensive research on the impact of toxic stress, poor attachment and neglect on the developing brain. Their research clearly underpins the theory associated with how early foundations and experiences shape childhood and beyond. Public Health Wales has provided insight into what constitutes an ACE (see Table 16.3) and Sabates and Dex (2015) have explored the cumulative impact of risk factors through the life course. The ACEs listed in Table 16.3 when combined with other societal extrinsic factors such as poverty and poor housing as well as lack of local service provision can have a major impact on the health and development of CYP. Therefore, the accumulation of risk has been identified as most damaging and is identified within many serious case reviews/child practice reviews where complex and multiple risk factors prevail with subsequent negative outcomes for CYP (Brandon et al. 2008, 2009, 2012, Sabates and Dex 2015).

Assessment of risk

There are several risk assessments/tools to guide practitioners in their day-to-day practice in assessing the wellbeing of CYP. Some examples are:

Family Resilience Assessment Instrument and Tool (FRAIT) (Wallace et al. 2017): This tool developed in Wales aids evidence-based decision making in health visiting practice, planning future interventions based on family resilience and need.

Various toolkits to assess neglect: For example, the 'graded care profile' is designed for use with social workers to measure quality of physical care, safety, and love/esteem provided by families by using a scale to assess neglect. This was devised by Srivastava and Polnay (1997) and forms the basis of adapted graded care profile tools published by local authorities within safeguarding boards across the UK.

Day in the life of a child: Developed by Jan Horwath in 2007, this is also incorporated into UK-wide safeguarding board neglect assessment toolkits. This tool focuses the practitioner on the daily activity of a CYP in their given situation. It allows the practitioner to explore and assess what it is like for CYP on waking, during morning, afternoon and night and whatever activities would be associated with their daily

Table 16.3   Adverse childhood experiences (Bellis et al. 2016)

Verbal abuse	Mental illness
Physical abuse	Alcohol misuse
Sexual abuse	Parental separation
Domestic violence	Drug use
Incarceration	

family routines. It allows the practitioner to think about what it is like for that CYP in their given situation. It is a powerful tool to use in practice and brings practitioner focus back to the CYP. This is informed by speaking to the parent/caregiver or by speaking to and observing the CYP.

Signs of safety: This tool was created in the 1990s by Andrew Turnell (social worker/family therapist) and Steve Edwards (child protection practitioner) (Turnell and Edwards 1997). The model can be and is being applied in child protection work across the world. It uses techniques associated with solution-focused brief therapy. This is a technique where parents/carers' future is explored by practitioners with the aim of resolving an issue or problem, identifying strengths and goals to improve their outcomes and achieve their goals. It can be used on a one-to-one basis with families, in the construction of child protection referrals, within child protection meetings as well as offering structure and discussion points within safeguarding children supervision. Its principles are embedded in building constructive working relationships and partnerships between professionals as well as with parents/carers/CYP promoting an honest approach (Baginsky et al. 2020). It also advocates positive multi-agency working where critical thinking and reflection can be enhanced, as well as advocating that the CYP experience is the focus and at the centre of any intervention. The original tool consists of four domains (key danger/harm factors, complicating factors, positive factors, and grey areas). The tool has been adapted and is evolving and now includes three areas/domains: What are we worried about? (Previous harm, key dangers, future harm), What is working well? (Positive factors, strengths, current safety), What needs to happen? (Safety goals, what is next for future safety?) (Baginsky et al. 2020).

Authoritative practice in safeguarding children and young people

Assessing risk and identification of safeguarding concerns is a complex and challenging process for practitioners. An authoritative stance in safeguarding practice is recommended by Sidebotham (2013) based on the principles of authoritative parenting described by the seminal work of Baumrind (1967), which is concerned with being caring but having control of a situation, setting appropriate boundaries, developing loving and nurturing relationships but with high expectations to promote effective discipline. Sidebotham uses the terminology of 'authoritative child protection practice' referred to in the serious case review findings of Lord Laming in 2009 following the death of Peter Connelly. Lord Laming states that the mother's parenting was passively accepted by the professionals involved. Carers can disguise compliance, be hostile and uncooperative, manipulative and successfully evade practitioners' attempts to assess the 'true' situation. Most recently this has been further exacerbated by the COVID-19 pandemic where practitioners have been unable to undertake home visits and resorted to 'virtual' platforms to access families which has hampered effective safeguarding practice. Sidebotham (2013, p. 2) reinforces Laming's recommendation of authoritative child protection and suggests three domains (authority, empathy, humility) deemed 'aspirational' elements of child protection practice:

Authority: Based on knowledge, skills, experience, competence in safeguarding practice and confidence.

Empathy: This relates to the voice of the CYP. The CYP must be at the centre of safeguarding practice with recognition of experiences and their rights. A children's rights, ACE and a trauma-informed approach is recommended. Consideration must be given to what is is like for the CYP living in their given situation as referred to by Howarth (2007) within the 'Day in the life of a child' model. The CYP needs to be recognised in the context of their family situation. Authoritative practice therefore has high expectations of parents to meet the child's basic needs, enable potential, support them to deliver those expectations and be confident and able to challenge them and advocate for them and the CYP when they are unable to.

Humility: A positive quality, a self-awareness trait which aids practitioners to explore any practice or educational limitations, building their knowledge base and experience to enhance their safeguarding practice. This links to the promotion of multi-agency/multi-disciplinary working and the realisation that each agency could hold a different segment of information in relation to a family. A single agency cannot protect and hold on to their information, it must be shared if there is a risk to the safeguarding of an individual. This applies to adult safeguarding as well as CYP and has been criticised in previous serious case reviews/child practice reviews. Partnership working across agencies is key in supporting CYP and their families. Humility within safeguarding also promotes the need for reflective practice and supervision.

Safeguarding supervision

Safeguarding children supervision is essential for practitioners working within the remit of safeguarding children (Public Health Wales 2017, Warren 2018). High-profile serious case reviews have highlighted a lack of or ineffective safeguarding supervision for practitioners (Laming 2003, 2009, Ofsted 2010). It has been identified that effective supervision is essential for frontline practitioners to aid positive outcomes for vulnerable CYP and their families. Safeguarding supervision allows support to be provided with an aim to develop effective practitioners who can critically think and analyse complex situations (Public Health Wales 2017). Supervision allows the practitioner to confront and discuss the emotional strain of their workload within their safeguarding children caseloads (Brandon et al. 2005, 2008, Smikle 2018, Warren 2018, Moseley 2020).

Clinical supervision has been defined as a process where staff work together to discuss practice issues including professional, organisational and personal issues leading to mutually agreed objectives (Morrison 2008). Safeguarding supervision offers a formal process of support; Botham (2013) and the Ofsted (2010) Munro review state that it allows dedicated time for discussion about children who are causing concern to the practitioner. It has the potential to reduce risks associated with child protection/safeguarding issues if undertaken effectively (Warren 2018). The supervision process has to be meaningful allowing practitioners to have an analytical view on the complex cases they deal with, sometimes on a day-to-day basis. A task-oriented approach to supervision is ill advised by Smikle (2018).

Some practitioners access supervision monthly (social workers), every 4–6 months (health visitors, school nurses) and more frequently if requested by the practitioner. Safeguarding supervision can be undertaken on a one-to-one basis or within a group (within disciplines, multi-disciplinary, multi-agency). As in social work, it is considered an integral part of public health nursing practice (Appleton and Peckover 2015, Powell 2016). Safeguarding supervision is complex and includes emotional support, practical support, identifying training needs, as well as trouble-shooting issues within complex child protection cases and vulnerable family situations. Frontline practitioners manage large, heavy caseloads that require support from a practitioner experienced and trained in delivering supervision, and with knowledge of the supervisees' roles and responsibilities (Gibbs 2009, Hall 2007, Morrison 2008, Wallbank 2010, Wallbank and Wonnacott 2015, Warren 2018). Safeguarding supervision requires supporting the professional to think critically and 'feel restored' and is effective when critical reflection is combined with a 'restorative approach' (Wallbank and Wonnacott 2015). Regular, structured supervision using an appropriate model focuses the practitioner on the current experience with the family, reflecting on concerns, analysing the information shared and creating a plan of action. The supervisor requires the necessary skills to facilitate an effective supervisory session (Warren 2018), taking an authoritative stance to enhance the session. Experience in safeguarding supervision, training and leadership qualities are required. The application of an authoratative leadership approach within safeguarding supervision would be beneficial to enable and promote the development of professional curiousity and critical analysis/reflection, to aid professional judgement, professional challenge and focus on the CYP at the centre of the practitioners safegaurding practice.

Conclusion

This chapter set out to explore what constitutes significant harm in CYP. A general overview has been provided around the key concepts of safeguarding and the safeguarding agenda globally and from a UK perspective. The ecological model is well recognised when assessing risk in CYP with consideration of the impact of the wider determinants of health underpinned by legislation, the UNCRC SDG's which led to discussion on assessment of risk, risk accumulation and ACEs. The importance of an authoritative approach when safeguarding CYP is recommended, placing the child at the centre of safeguarding practice. Exposure to safeguarding issues in practice can prove challenging and a critically reflective, competent, confident practitioner will offer the most effective support to CYP. Access to safeguarding supervision is essential and should be prioritised.

CONSIDER THE FOLLOWING QUESTIONS

1. Do you consider the wider determinants of health along with the ecological model when assessing risk in CYP? Consider how they inter-relate with the ecological model and how they impact on CYP wellbeing potential from a safeguarding perspective.
2. Do you apply a trauma-informed approach to your safeguarding practice?
3. Apply the three areas of authoritative leadership to your practice: authority, empathy, humility. Are you able to recognise these traits in your safeguarding practice?
4. Do you access and prioritise safeguarding supervision? Think about how and why it is effective and necessary.

Key terms

Adverse childhood experiences (ACEs): Traumatic events experienced by children which include domestic violence/abuse, substance misuse, verbal abuse, physical abuse, sexual abuse, mental illness, parental separation and incarceration.

Child sexual exploitation: A form of child sexual abuse where an 'exchange' occurs.

Children and young people (CYP): Children aged 0–18 years.

Criminal exploitation/county lines: The involvement of children under the age of 18 in criminal activity. This could include moving drugs or money for themselves or others and will involve violence and/or threats of violence against the individual or others linked to the individual.

Determinants of health: Factors that determine health and wellbeing.

Epigenetics: The exploration of how extrinsic factors affect gene expression and explores how early experiences can have a lifelong impact on individuals.

Female genital mutilation (FGM): This involves all procedures that partially remove/remove the external female genitalia as well as causing injury to the female genitalia which is not on medical grounds.

Honour-based violence: This involves abuse and/or violence which can lead to murder and is undertaken by individuals attempting to protect the reputation of their family or community.

Modern slavery: The enforcement of labour on an individual which includes trapping and controlling of the victim. Modern slavery includes sexual exploitation and labour exploitation.

Radicalisation: This occurs when children have access to or are exposed to or coerced into receiving information that is deemed radical or extreme. Radicalisation when the child or young person then supports, comes to believe and becomes involved in 'extremist ideologies' leading to acts of terrorism and therefore is deemed 'harm' (NSPCC 2021).

Safeguarding: Prevention of abuse as well as protection.

Sustainable Development Goals (SDGs): Endorsed by the United Nations General Assembly and the World Health Organization, they aim to promote worldwide partnership in a response to global health matters. There are 17 in total.

Trafficking: Child trafficking involves the recruitment, movement, 'harbouring or receipt' and transferring of children. Abuse could be in the form of 'sexual exploitation, criminal exploitation, forced labour, domestic servitude, slavery, financial exploitation, illegal adoption or removal of organs (Wales Safeguarding Procedures 2019).

Further reading

Association of Child Protection Professionals. Available at: www.childprotection professionals.org.uk/ [Accessed 12.03.2022].

Harvard Center on the Developing Child. Available at: https://developingchild.harvard. edu/ [Accessed 12.03.2022].

NSPCC. 2020. *How Safe Are Our Children? An Overview of Data on Abuse of Adolescents.* Available at: https://learning.nspcc.org.uk/media/2287/how-safe-are-our-children-2020.pdf [Accessed 12.03.2022].

Royal College of Nursing. 2019. *Safeguarding Children and Young People: Roles and Competencies for Healthcare Staff.* (4th edn). Available at: www.rcn.org.uk/-/media/royal-college-of-nursing/documents/publications/2019/january/007-366.pdf?la=en [Accessed 12.03.2022].

United Nations. n.d. *Violence Against Children.* Available at: https://sdgs.un.org/topics/violence-against-children [Accessed 12.03.2022].

References

Adult Support and Protection (Scotland) Act. 2007. Available at: www.legislation.gov.uk/asp/2007/10/contents [Accessed 03.01.2021].

Appleton, J. V., Harrison, J., Mumbry-Croft, K. 2021. Safeguarding children: a public health imperative. In S.Cowley, K. Whittaker (Eds), *Community Public Health in Policy and Practice.* Elsevier: Poland.

Appleton, J. V., Peckover, S. 2015. *Protecting Children and Young People: Child Protection, Public Health and Nursing.* Dunedin Academic Press: Edinburgh.

Baginsky, M., Hickman, B., Moriarty, J., Manthorpe, J. 2020. Working with signs of safety: parents' perception of change. *Child and Family Social Work;* 25, 154–164.

Baumrind, D. 1967. Effects of authoritative control on child behavior. *Child Development;* 37(4), 887–907.

Bellis, M. A, Ashton, K., Hughes, K., Ford, K., Bishop, J., Paranjothy, S. 2016. *Adverse Childhood Experiences and their Impact on Health Harming Behaviours in the Welsh Adult Population. Alcohol Use, Drug Use, Violence, Sexual Behaviour, Incarceration, Smoking and Poor Diet.* Public Health Wales: Cardiff.

Belsky, J. 1980. Child maltreatment: an ecological integration. *American Psychologist;* 35(4), 320–335.

Botham, J. 2013. What constitutes safeguarding children supervision for health visitors and school nurses. *Community Practitioner;* 86(3).

Brandon, M., Bailey, S., Belderson, P., Gardner, R., Sidebotham, P., Dodsworth, J., Warren, C., Black, J. 2009. *Understanding Serious Case Reviews. A Biennial Analysis of Serious Case Reviews, 2005–2007*. Department for Children, Schools and Families: London.

Brandon, M., Belderson, P., Warren, C., Howe, D., Gardner, R., Dodsworth, J., Black, J. 2008. *Analysing Child Deaths and Serious Injury through Abuse and Neglect: What Can We Learn? A Biennial Analysis of Serious Case Reviews 2003–2005*. University of East Anglia DcSF: Norwich.

Brandon, M., Dodsworth, J., Rumball, D. 2005. Serious case reviews: learning to use expertise. *Child Abuse Review*; 14(3), 160–176.

Brandon, M., Sidebotham, P., Bailey, S., Belderson, P., Hawley, C., Ellis, C., Megson, M. 2012. *New Learning from Serious Case Reviews: a 2-Year Report for 2009–2011*. Department for Education: London.

Bronfenbrenner, U. 1979. *The Ecology of Human Development: Experiments by Nature and Design*. Harvard University Press: Cambridge, MA.

Care Act 2014. Available at: www.legislation.gov.uk/ukpga/2014/23/contents/enacted [Accessed 03.01.21].

Center on the Developing Child. 2021. *Epigenetics and Child Development: How Children's Experiences Affect Their Genes*. Harvard University: New York. Available at: What is Epigenetics? The Answer to the Nature vs. Nurture Debate (harvard.edu) [Accessed 10.01.2021].

Children (Abolition of Defence of Reasonable Punishment) (Wales) Act 2020. Available at: https://www.legislation.gov.uk/anaw/2020/3 [Accessed 24.03.2022].

Children Act 1989. Available at: www.legislation.gov.uk/ukpga/1989/41/contents [Accessed 03.01.21].

Children Act 2004. Available at: www.legislation.gov.uk/ukpga/2004/31/contents [Accessed 03.01.21].

Children and Young People (Scotland) Act 2014. Available at: www.legislation.gov.uk/asp/2014/8/contents [Accessed 03.01.2021].

Dahlgren, G., Whitehead, M. 1991. *Policies and Strategies to Promote Social Equity in Health*. Stockholm Institute for Future Studies: Stockholm.

Department of Health. 2017. *Co-operating to Safeguard Children and Young People in Northern Ireland*. Available at: www.health-ni.gov.uk/publications/co-operating-safeguard-children-and-young-people-northern-ireland [Accessed 03.01.2021].

Department of Health. 2020. *Framework for the Assesment of Children in Need and their Families*. Available at: https://bettercarenetwork.org/sites/default/files/Framework%20for%20the%20Assessment%20of%20Children%20in%20Need%20and%20Their%20Families%20-%20Guidance%20Notes%20and%20Glossary.pdf [Accessed 18.04.2022].

Felitti, V. J., Anda, R. F., Nordenburg, D., Williamson, D. F., Spitz, A. M., Edwards, V., Koss, M. P., Marks, J. S. 1998. Relationship of childhood abuse and household dysfunction to many of the leading causes of death in adults: the Adverse Childhood Experiences (ACE) Study. *American Journal of Preventive Medicine*; 14(4), 245–258.

Gibbs, J. 2009. Changing the cultural story in child protection: learning from the insider's experience. *Child and Family Social Work*; 14(3), 289–299.

Hall, C. 2007. Health visitor's and school health nurses' perspectives on child protection supervision. *Community Practitioner*, 80(10), 26–31.

Hardcastle, K., Bellis, M. A. 2019. *Asking About Adverse Childhood Experiences in Health Visiting. Findings From a Pilot Study.* Public Health Wales: Cardiff.

HM Government. 2018. *Working Together to Safeguard Children. A Guide to Interagency Working to Safeguard and Promote the Welfare of Children.* The Stationery Office: London.

Horwath, J. 2007. *The Neglected Child: Identification and Assessment.* Palgrave: London.

Lord Laming. 2003. *The Victoria Climbié Inquiry.* London: The Stationery Office.

Lord Laming. 2009. *The Protection of Children in England: A Progress Report.* The Stationery Office: London.

Morrison, T. 2008. *Staff Supervision Care in Social Care.* (3rd edn). Pavilion: Brighton.

Moseley, M. 2020. An evaluation of group supervision in health visiting practice. *Primary Healthcare*; 32(1). Available at: https://journals.rcni.com/primary-health-care/evidence-and-practice/an-evaluation-of-group-safeguarding-supervision-in-health-visiting-practice-phc.2020.e1611/abs [Accessed 21.07.21].

NSPCC. 2021. *Radicalisation.* Available at: https://learning.nspcc.org.uk/safeguarding-child-protection/radicalisation [Accessed 21.12.2021].

Ofsted. 2010. *The Munro Review of Child Protection. Interim Report: The Child's Journey.* Ofsted: London.

Powell, C. 2016. *Safeguarding and Child Protection for Nurses, Midwives, and Health Visitors.* Open University Press: Maidenhead.

Public Health Wales. 2017. *All Wales Safeguarding Supervision Policy.* Public Health Wales: Cardiff.

Sabates, R., Dex, S. 2015. *Multiple Risk Factors in Young Children's Development.* Institute of Education, University of London: London.

Sidebotham, P. 2013. Authoritative child protection. *Child Abuse Review*; 22(1), 1–4.

Smikle, M. 2018. Safeguarding children: providing nursing staff with supervision. *Nursing Times*; 114(12), 36–40. Available at: www.nursingtimes.net/roles/childrens-nurses/safeguarding-children-providing-nursing-staff-with-supervision-19-11-2018/ [Accessed 18.03.2020].

Social Care Institute for Excellence (SCIE). 2020. *What are the Six Principles of Safeguarding?* Available at: www.scie.org.uk/safeguarding/adults/introduction/six-principles [Accessed 03.01.2021].

Social Services and Well-being (Wales) Act 2014. Available at: www.legislation.gov.uk/anaw/2014/4/contents [Accessed 03.02.2021].

Srivastava, O. P., Polnay, L. 1997. Field trial of graded care profile (GCP) scale: a new measure of care. *Archives of Disease in Childhood*; 76, 337–340.

Turnell, A., Edwards, S. 1997. Aspiring to partnership: the signs of safety approach to child protection. *Child Abuse Review*; 6, 179–190.

UNICEF. 1989. *United Nations Convention on the Rights of the Child.* Available at: www.unicef.org.uk/what-we-do/un-convention-child-rights/ [Accessed 28.05.2021].

United Nations. 2019. *Sustainable Development Goals*. Available at: https://sdgs.un.org/goals [Accessed 03.02.2021].

Vygotsky, L. 1978. *Mind and Society: The Development of Higher Mental Processes*. Harvard University Press: Cambridge.

Wales Safeguarding Procedures. 2019. Available at: www.safeguarding.wales [Accessed 03.01.2021].

Wallace, C., Dale, F., Jones, G., O'Kane, J., Thomas, M., Wilson, L., Pontin, D. 2017. *Health and Care Research Wales*. Available at: www.frait.wales/ [Accessed 12.03.2022].

Wallbank, S. 2010. Effectiveness of individual clinical supervision for midwives and doctors in stress reduction: findings from a pilot study. *Evidence-based Midwifery*; 8(2), 65.

Wallbank, S., Wonnacott, J. 2015. The integrated model of restorative supervision for use within safeguarding. *Community Practitioner*; 88(5), 41–45.

Warren, L. 2018. Role of leadership behaviours in safeguarding supervision: a literature review. *Primary Health Care*; 28(1), 31–36.

Wave Trust. 2021. *Childhood Trauma and Trauma Informed Care*. Available at: www.wavetrust.org/childhood-trauma-trauma-informed-care [Accessed 12.03.2021].

Welsh Government. 2015. *Well-being of Future Generations Act. The Essentials*. Welsh Government: Cardiff.

World Health Organization. 2016. *INSPIRE. Even Strategies for Ending Violence against Children*. Available at: https://www.who.int/publications/i/item/inspire-seven-strategies-for-ending-violence-against-children [Accessed 18.04.2022].

World Health Organization. 2021. *Violence Against Children*. Available at: www.who.int/health-topics/violence-against-children#tab=tab_1 [Accessed 12.02.2021].

17

DOMESTIC ABUSE

CAROLINE BRADBURY-JONES AND DANA SAMMUT

LEARNING OUTCOMES

By the end of this chapter you will be able to:

- Understand the ways domestic abuse can manifest, together with the dynamics under-pinning abusive relationships and the pervasiveness of this phenomenon.
- Relate knowledge of domestic abuse to current legislation and policy in the UK.
- Identify the role of health and social care practitioners in recognising, addressing and escalating concerns about domestic abuse using evidence-based knowledge and tools.

Introduction

Domestic abuse is a multifaceted issue with complex dynamics at its core. Due to its 'hidden' nature we may never know the true extent of this phenomenon, but a growing body of literature has provided a foundation for professional practice which is sensitive to the needs of vulnerable service users. This chapter provides an overview of domestic abuse, covering its prevalence, impact, latest legislation and policy in the UK, and the role health and social care practitioners have in addressing this important issue. Our focus is on adults' experiences of abuse; for an overview of domestic abuse and its impact on children, we make recommendations for further reading at the end of the chapter.

What is domestic abuse?

'Domestic abuse' is an umbrella term describing harmful or threatening behaviours that occur between individuals who are or have previously been in an intimate relationship, family members, and those with family-type relationships (e.g. carers) (Women's Aid 2019a).

Domestic abuse can take a number of forms including:

- Coercive control
- Physical
- Sexual
- Psychological/emotional
- Financial/economic
- Harassment and stalking
- Online and digital
- Domestic elder abuse

Domestic abuse is rarely a 'one-off' incident and is usually underpinned by a pattern of controlling or manipulative behaviour. The term also encompasses so-called 'honour' violence, forced marriage and female genital mutilation/cutting (FGM/C). However, these specific forms of abuse are covered in Chapter 15 and will not be discussed in detail here. Individuals of any age, gender and sexuality can experience domestic abuse, although certain groups are statistically more likely to be affected, and in specific ways. This will be discussed in more detail later in the chapter.

Prevalence of domestic abuse

Most forms of domestic abuse are unlikely to occur in isolation. Many of the types of abuse listed above are interrelated and co-occur to produce aggregated effects; for example, restricting a person's access to finances or monitoring someone's online activity both represent forms of control and will inevitably involve a degree of intimidation or threat.

International data from the World Health Organization (WHO) (García-Moreno et al. 2005) and the Pan American Health Organization (Bott et al. 2012) similarly show that women who experience emotional abuse or controlling behaviours from their intimate partners are significantly more likely to report physical or sexual violence.

Globally, estimates suggest that 30% of all women who have been in a relationship report having experienced physical and/or sexual violence by an intimate partner (WHO 2017). These data do not include the wider forms of domestic abuse, meaning that actual numbers are likely to be much higher. Across England and Wales, data from the Office for National Statistics (ONS) show that in the year ending March 2019, 7.5% of women and 3.8% of men reported experiencing domestic abuse (ONS, 2019a). These data are obtained via the Crime Survey for England and Wales (CSEW), which uses a broader definition of domestic abuse, encompassing emotional and financial abuse as well as stalking, but notably its developers acknowledge that it does not fully capture experiences of coercive control. New survey questions to more comprehensively measure the prevalence of coercive control are currently being developed (ONS, 2019b). Moreover, the CSEW does not collect data on honour violence, forced marriage or FGM/C, again meaning that these forms of abuse are not captured by the above statistics. Domestic abuse statistics also cannot account for the many cases that are never recognised or reported. Reasons for underreporting are various and complex, including (but not limited to):

- Fear of retaliation from abuser(s).
- Concerns about losing custody of children.
- Shame or embarrassment.
- Lack of confidence in professional responses.
- Risk of homelessness or deportation.
- Denial, low self-esteem, or not recognising the abuse. (HMIC 2015, Women's Aid 2019b)

Legislation and policy

Coinciding with the global rise in feminist activism, the phenomenon of domestic abuse started gaining attention in the UK during the 1970s. Up until this time violence between intimate partners had generally been considered a 'normal' (yet private) occurrence. In 1971 what is considered to be the first ever women's shelter was founded in London by Erin Pizzey. Groups such as Women's Aid, a national charity founded in 1974, were to become pivotal in campaigning for the safety of abused women. In 1973 the term 'domestic violence' was reportedly used for the first time in the UK to describe violence occurring in the home by MP Jack Ashley. In his address to Parliament, Mr Ashley's speech focused on violence perpetrated by husbands against their wives, calling upon cabinet ministers to safeguard the interests of 'battered wives' (Parliament, House of Commons 1973). Over the years, terminology and definitions have evolved to reflect our developing understanding of the phenomenon. 'Wife battering' was phased out in recognition of the fact that non-married intimate partners can also experience domestic abuse, and 'intimate partner violence' (IPV) has become more widely used. While the terms 'domestic abuse' and 'domestic violence' are often used interchangeably, many people favour the former, arguing that the word 'violence' emphasises the physical nature of abuse when in reality this often plays only a small part in abusive relationships. This argument is illustrated by the following quotation by forensic social worker Evan Stark:

> [T]he women in my practice have repeatedly made clear that what is done to them is less important than what their partners have prevented them from doing for themselves by appropriating their resources; undermining their social support; subverting their rights to privacy, self-respect, and autonomy; and depriving them of substantive equality. (Stark 2009, p. 13)

Stark introduced the term 'coercive control' to describe the controlling behaviour which exists at the core of most abusive relationships (see Table 17.1). Due to its 'invisibility' coercive control can easily go unrecognised, even by the individuals who experience it daily. This can make it especially difficult for 'outsiders', including law enforcement and health and social care professionals, to recognise coercive control. In fact it wasn't until 2015 that UK law recognised 'controlling or coercive behaviour in an intimate or family relationship' as a specific offence (Serious Crime Act 2015, c. 7, Section 76).

In April 2021 – four years after the Bill was first announced – the Domestic Abuse Act became law. The Act introduces a statutory definition of domestic abuse, covering a range of violent and non-violent harms, as well as a number of health, social and criminal justice reforms to prioritise survivors. Prior to becoming law, some groups were critical of the Bill's overwhelming focus on criminal justice:

> It is important to remember that official statistics show that just one in five victims will ever talk to the police about domestic abuse. With a law that focuses largely on crime, policing and the courts, we will miss most survivors, who will turn to other public services for help. (Lucy Hadley, Campaign and Public Affairs Officer for Women's Aid. UK Parliament 2019, p. 2)

Table 17.1 Cross-Government definition of controlling and coercive behaviour (Home Office 2015, p. 3)

Controlling behaviour	A range of acts designed to make a person subordinate and/or dependent by isolating them from sources of support, exploiting their resources and capacities for personal gain, depriving them of the means needed for independence, resistance and escape and regulating their everyday behaviour.
Coercive behaviour	A continuing act or a pattern of acts of assault, threats, humiliation and intimidation or other abuse that is used to harm, punish or frighten their victim.

N.B. These are not legal definitions. For legal definitions, see Serious Crime Act 2015, c. 7, Section 76.

Following campaigning efforts from survivors and activists, changes were made to the new Act to address these gaps. However, Hadley's point is an important one to highlight. As noted earlier, domestic abuse remains underreported for a number of reasons. Attrition is also high in domestic abuse cases, meaning that many reports do not result in a criminal conviction (CPS 2018). Beyond these issues, many abused individuals do not recognise their experiences as being abusive. This may be the result of psychological manipulation by abusers, denial of severity (particularly if physical violence is absent) or diminished self-worth. In some cases it may be that individuals have experienced abuse for so long that they cannot remember living without it. Some authors have referred to the process of acknowledging one's abuse and taking steps to seek support as 'asserting one's candidacy'; in other words, the individual both realises and accepts that they are a deserving candidate for support (Dixon-Woods et al. 2006). In view of the many barriers preventing abused individuals from disclosing their experiences, health and social care workers are taking on an increasingly important role in identifying domestic abuse in day-to-day practice.

The dynamics of abuse

There have been innumerable debates in the academic literature regarding the gendered nature of domestic abuse. There is little basis to argue that women are not disproportionately affected, with national and international statistics almost universally supporting this conclusion. As noted earlier, data from the ONS (2019a) suggest that in the year ending March 2019, women across England and Wales were almost twice as likely than men to experience domestic abuse. However, statistics in isolation often paint an unreliable picture, and context is important.

Some authors have argued that men and women are equally violent in intimate relationships (e.g. Straus, 2010). The issue at the heart of this conflict is often one of conceptualisation, whereby domestic abuse is largely equated to incidental physical and verbal assault, resulting in studies which are methodologically flawed in their approach to measuring 'domestic abuse' (in reality, capturing only a fraction of the phenomenon). Many of these studies use the Conflict Tactics Scale (CTS), which has been widely criticised for omitting coercive tactics in intimate relationships and failing to capture information about the context of violence (see Dobash and Dobash, 2004). Qualitative research indicates that men are more likely to initiate violence and to use more severe violence against their partners, with women more often acting in self-defence (Downs et al. 2007). As a result, injury rates are significantly higher in cases of violence perpetrated by men against women (Walby and Allen, 2004). Many authors refer to this as 'gender asymmetry', meaning that men and women use violence differently and suffer different outcomes as a result (see Hester 2013, Johnson 2006). This is another shortcoming of the CTS, which focuses only on incidents of conflict without consideration for the consequences, therein implying that all violent episodes are equivalent. Much of the research which concludes that violence is gender symmetrical also fails to account for coercive and controlling behaviours. Many studies have found that women are more likely to be fearful of violent intimate partners than men (Hester 2013). This is not an arbitrary factor in this discussion: as Nixon and Humphreys summarise, 'fear is one method of control, and the threat or fear of violence can be an important means of establishing an imbalance of power and control in a relationship' (2010, p. 146).

Arguing that domestic abuse is not a 'unitary phenomenon', Johnson (2006) identified four different contexts in which violence occurs: (1) 'intimate terrorism', characterised by unilateral violence and control; (2) 'violent resistance', where violence is bilateral but only one partner exhibits controlling behaviour; (3) 'situational couple violence', where violence exists but neither partner is controlling; and (4) 'mutual violent control', characterised by bilateral violent and controlling behaviour. Intimate terrorism – which Hester (2013, p. 633) refers to as the 'archetypal' form of abuse – is disproportionately perpetrated by men and results in the most severe level of injury (Hester 2013, Johnson 2006). Johnson makes a clear argument for distinguishing between each form of violence when conducting research into the broad phenomenon of 'domestic abuse', and his arguments provide a very solid basis for explaining discrepancies in the degree of gender (a)symmetry found across the literature.

Domestic abuse by women against men

While we have argued for the case of gender asymmetry in domestic abuse, we do not deny or diminish the reality of female-perpetrated abuse. As a result of the gendered approach taken by many researchers and policymakers, female-on-male domestic abuse is underexplored and often under-recognised. A critical literature review by Perryman and Appleton (2016) supports these conclusions, with the authors asserting that a lack of literature and policy focus on abuse against men has increased the 'invisibility' of abused men to health and social care services. Men are known to be more reluctant than women to disclose their abuse or seek help, with some authors attributing this to the different social expectations of men, traditional views of masculinity, status perception and feelings of shame (Perryman and Appleton 2016). As a result, statistics are likely to underestimate the true prevalence and impact of domestic abuse on men, an issue which is compounded by the fact that the majority of tools designed to facilitate professionals' detection of abuse are tailored towards women (see Arkins et al. 2016).

Domestic abuse in the LGBT+ (lesbian, gay, bisexual, transgender) population

Recent research from Stonewall and YouGov (Bachmann and Gooch 2018) found that 11% of the LGBT+ population had experienced domestic abuse by a partner within the last year. This increased to 12% for bisexual men, 13% for bisexual women, and 17% for transgender and non-binary individuals. As with opposite-sex abuse, the issue is likely under-reported, although reasons for non-reporting may be more complex in LGBT+ populations, with additional barriers including fear of homophobia or transphobia from professional services, or threats of 'outing' from abusers (McNamara and Ng 2016). Research also indicates that LGBT+ individuals have more complex needs at the point of accessing services, including higher rates of mental ill health and recent history of drug and alcohol misuse (SafeLives, 2018).

Intersectionality

Anyone can be affected by domestic abuse, regardless of age, ethnicity, disability or socio-economic status. However, as already highlighted, research shows that certain groups are more likely to be affected and in certain ways. The concept of 'intersectionality', coined by civil rights activist Kimberlé Crenshaw in 1989, describes and analyses the ways in which multiple inequalities overlap and combine to create an 'intersectional experience [which] is greater than the sum [of its components]' (Crenshaw 1989, p. 140). The intersecting relationship between domestic abuse and social categorisations such as class and ethnicity (among others) is complex and, as with most complex issues, subject to much debate. We will not explore these debates in great detail here, but instead illustrate some of the ways in which intersectional inequalities can manifest.

Figure 17.1 depicts a simple representation of how inequalities might intersect for individuals experiencing domestic abuse.

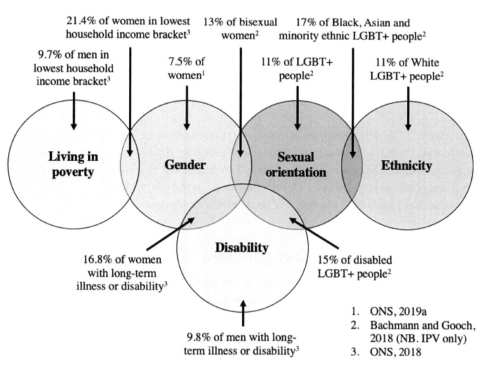

Figure 17.1 Illustration of intersecting inequalities in relation to domestic abuse (Note: Percentages refer to UK prevalence of domestic abuse among specified groups).

In reality, the combined intersections of different inequalities cannot be captured so neatly, and attempts to quantitatively summarise or predict individuals' experiences of domestic abuse will inevitably oversimplify and homogenise those experiences. As Crenshaw argued in her original paper (1989), the intersectional experience should not be equated to the sum of each inequality. Nixon and Humphreys (2010) similarly point out the dangers of essentialism; that is, the grouping together of individuals with a shared identity and assuming a 'sameness' among them.

The Case Study below illustrates a more nuanced approach to understanding intersectionality.

Case study: Amaira

Amaira is a 29-year-old Indian woman who recently moved to Birmingham with her husband Ravinder. Amaira cannot speak fluent English and has struggled to find work for this reason. Ravinder has discouraged Amaira's efforts to start English classes at their local library, falsely telling her that they cannot afford the course. He often teases Amaira for being financially reliant on him, while also asserting that once she becomes pregnant she will be too 'fragile' to work. She has no money of her own and only limited access to the household finances, with Ravinder insisting that she account for anything she spends. Ravinder also monitors Amaira's online activity, arguing that this is his right since he pays the bills. Amaira has thought of leaving Ravinder but fears the responses of her parents and extended family in India, knowing that they disapprove of divorce. She feels lonely and isolated, having no one to confide in and no awareness of the sources of support available to her in the UK.

Consider which forms of domestic abuse Amaira is experiencing and make a list of potential sources of support available to her. It might be helpful to discuss your ideas with a friend or colleague.

In Figure 17.2 we present an alternative representation of how inequalities might manifest and intersect for Amaira. While not depicted by the illustration, it is possible to see patterns of causality among the identity categories. For example, Amaira's language and unemployment intersect to amplify her social isolation, which in turn is likely to perpetuate her inability to identify her abuse and seek support.

Health and social care responses

From a public health point of view, early detection and response to domestic abuse is of paramount importance, yet research continues to show that health professionals are reluctant to discuss the issue with their patients (Beynon et al. 2012, Taylor et al. 2013). We know that people experiencing abuse are more likely to disclose if asked directly (Feder et al. 2011), and importantly, that abuse survivors *want* professionals to raise the issue (Bradbury-Jones et al. 2014). Frequently cited reasons for professionals' non-asking include lack of confidence and fear of causing offence. Worryingly, some studies have

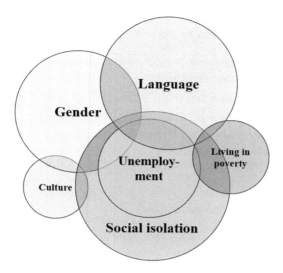

Figure 17.2 Illustration of intersecting inequalities in relation to case study (Amaira)

found that a minority of health (e.g. Taylor et al. 2013) and social work (e.g. Black et al. 2010) professionals continue to endorse negative myths surrounding domestic abuse, including that individuals who refuse to leave abusive relationships are complicit in their own abuse. Overall, however, lack of knowledge seems to be one of the most significant factors perpetuating the issue of non-asking among helping professionals, with many indicating that they would not know how to respond to a disclosure. We recently undertook a literature review to identify which learning strategies are most effective for health and social care students, focusing on the subject of violence against women, and one of our findings was that learning should be practice-focused (Sammut et al. 2019). To incorporate this principle here, we introduce the mnemonic SAFE & SOUND (Figure 17.3) to facilitate the sensitive encouragement of abuse disclosure.

Asking

In 2008, routine enquiry of domestic abuse was introduced in NHS Scotland, following the issue of the *Gender-Based Violence Action Plan*, and applied to all professionals working in selected priority settings (including A&E, maternity, sexual and reproductive health services) (Scottish Government, 2008). The Action Plan distinguished between 'routine' and 'selective' enquiry as follows:

Routine Enquiry: Involves asking *all* people presenting to a service direct questions in relation to abuse. This can be at a particular point in their use of a service, or on all occasions at which they present.
Selective Enquiry: Refers to direct/indirect questions to *some* people with whom there may be some suspicion of abuse, or who meet certain criteria indicating

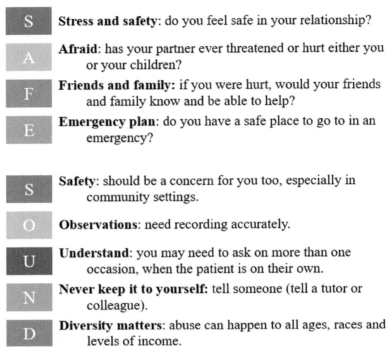

Stress and safety: do you feel safe in your relationship?

Afraid: has your partner ever threatened or hurt either you or your children?

Friends and family: if you were hurt, would your friends and family know and be able to help?

Emergency plan: do you have a safe place to go to in an emergency?

Safety: should be a concern for you too, especially in community settings.

Observations: need recording accurately.

Understand: you may need to ask on more than one occasion, when the patient is on their own.

Never keep it to yourself: tell someone (tell a tutor or colleague).

Diversity matters: abuse can happen to all ages, races and levels of income.

Figure 17.3 The SAFE & SOUND mnemonic

> additional vulnerability to such abuse e.g. homeless women, or women with mental health problems. (Scottish Government 2008, p. 10)

The National Institute for Health and Care Excellence (NICE 2014) public health guideline on domestic violence and abuse [PH50] now extends the recommendation of routine enquiry in priority areas to the rest of the UK, although the guideline acknowledges that there is insufficient evidence to recommend routine enquiry in *all* healthcare settings. This is not to say that professionals working in non-priority areas should avoid asking patients about domestic abuse, but rather that selective enquiry (guided by professional judgement) should be undertaken.

The practicalities of asking about domestic abuse are not always straightforward. The first thing for professionals to consider is safety: conversations need to take place somewhere private, without the (potential) perpetrator(s) present or within earshot. Official interpreters should be used for non-English speakers wherever possible and use of family members should *always* be avoided. Evidence from SafeLives (2018) also highlights the harmfulness of making inaccurate assumptions about individuals' sexuality or gender identity. Professionals are encouraged to be aware of their use of pronouns and to use gender-neutral language (e.g. partner or ex-partner).

Professionals may be reluctant to ask about domestic abuse out of fear that they will need to breach confidentiality during the reporting process. Again, the principles of consent and information sharing are not uncomplicated, particularly in high-risk cases and where children are involved. Many national guidelines and local policies advise that professional judgement should be used to decide whether referrals should be made without patient consent. However, this will be a daunting prospect for those who have had no training or exposure to domestic abuse in practice. SafeLives, in partnership with the Association of Chief Police Officers, developed the Dash risk checklist to help frontline professionals to identify 'high risk' cases of domestic abuse, stalking and honour violence (SafeLives 2015). While not intended to replace professional judgement, the Dash risk checklist, together with accompanying guidance on its use, provides a comprehensive and practice-oriented summary of factors to consider when assessing the severity of abuse.

Responding

In high-risk cases, health and social care professionals may face the difficult decision of having to refer to specialist agencies (e.g. multiagency risk assessment conferences, or MARACs) without the patient's consent. This must be done in accordance with Caldicott principles, which state that information can be shared without an adult's consent if serious harm or crime might be prevented (Department of Health 2012).

In all cases, regardless of risk level and subsequent outcomes, it is important that all professionals respond to disclosures of abuse with sensitivity. Above all else, professionals should validate each individual's concerns and make it clear that they are not to blame. As discussed earlier, acknowledging one's abuse and taking steps to seek help is a challenging process and often involves a number of uncertainties ('What kind of help do I need?' 'What if my abuser finds out?' 'What if I'm not taken seriously?'). Questioning an individual's credibility during a time of such heightened vulnerability can be hugely damaging and will likely inhibit future attempts to seek help. Similarly, professionals must bear in mind that not all individuals will be prepared to leave their abuser; in these cases, the professional's response should be no less sympathetic, and under no circumstances should patients be unduly pressurised to leave their abuser. Women in particular are at a heightened risk of lethal violence during the post-separation period (Campbell et al. 2007) in addition to new emotional, social and financial constraints, as well as threats of danger to any children involved (Humphreys and Thiara 2003). Instead, professionals might start by simply asking how they can be of help, allowing the patient to guide the conversation and determine the type of support they feel they need.

Conclusion

This chapter has outlined a number of key issues surrounding domestic abuse. We have described the various ways in which domestic abuse can manifest and introduced the concept of intersectionality, highlighting that although domestic abuse can affect people of all genders, cultures and socioeconomic backgrounds, certain groups are disproportionately affected and often in specific ways. Finally, we have discussed the important role of health and social workers in recognising domestic abuse and facilitating safe disclosure. We have emphasised the importance of approaching this issue sensitively and with an awareness of the many barriers and challenges individuals face when they choose to share information with professionals.

CONSIDER THE FOLLOWING QUESTIONS

1. For many people the term 'domestic abuse' conjures an image of physical violence. Looking at the terms on page 276, how might each form of abuse manifest differently? It may help to write these down and then refer to our summaries below.
2. What are the potential signs and markers of domestic abuse? Remember that there is a lot more to domestic abuse than physical violence; the signs will not always be apparent.
3. Using the SAFE & SOUND mnemonic (Figure 17.3) consider the steps you might take to ensure a 'safe space' for disclosure in practice. This could include hospital inpatient settings, an outpatient department or community settings. Think of the language you might use, remembering that your patient may not recognise that they are experiencing abuse.
4. Imagine you are on a community placement and encounter a service user with advanced dementia whom you suspect is experiencing abuse. Can you think of any challenges in this scenario and what steps you might take to overcome them? Thinking back to the SAFE & SOUND mnemonic: which steps would require a different approach and which would remain the same?

Key terms

Coercive control: A pattern of behaviour intended to make a person feel subordinate, isolated, fearful and otherwise dependent on the abuser. Coercive control is usually subtle and exists at the core of most abusive relationships.

Domestic elder abuse: Older people can be vulnerable to most forms of domestic abuse, particularly when they are dependent on another person to meet their basic needs. When abuse of an older person is perpetrated by a family member or family-type carer, regardless of setting, this is domestic elder abuse.

Financial/economic abuse: Using finances as a means of controlling or restricting a person's freedom. This can include limiting a person's access to family finances or preventing them from undertaking paid work.

Harassment and stalking: A pattern of behaviour involving the giving of unwanted attention to a person, often in a way that causes intentional fear, anxiety or alarm.

Online and digital abuse: Using technology to intimidate, bully or harass a person. This type of abuse can also include the use of technology to monitor or restrict someone's behaviour;

for example, demanding access to a person's social media accounts or using GPS technology to keep track of a person's movements.

Physical abuse: Involving physical aggression, use of force or restraint, either to inflict physical harm or to withhold access to resources.

Psychological/emotional abuse: Including, but not limited to, gaslighting, blackmail, use of intimidation, and intentional exploitation of vulnerabilities.

Sexual abuse: Forced sexual contact or activity, including rape, or use of sex as a tool to manipulate another person; for example, via coercion or blackmail.

Further reading

For an accessible introduction to gender-based violence with an international focus, see our e-learning resource:

Bradbury-Jones, C., Billings, H., Hegarty, K., Hinsliff-Smith, K., Kishchenko, S., McFeely, C., McGarry, J., Sammut, D., Sheridan, J. 2019. *Gender-based Violence: A Resource to Support Students in Health and Social Care*. Available at: www.nottingham.ac.uk/helmopen/index.php/rlos/keyword/544 [Accessed 12.03.2022].

For a practice-oriented overview of domestic abuse and children:

Bradbury-Jones, C., Morris, A., Sammut, D., Humphreys, C. 2020. Domestic violence and abuse and children: principles of practitioner responses. In P. Ali, J. McGarry (Eds), *Domestic Violence in Health Contexts: A Guide for Healthcare Professions*. Springer.

For comprehensive guidance on responding to domestic abuse:

Department of Health. 2017. *Guidance: Domestic Abuse: A Resource for Health Professionals*. Available at: www.gov.uk/government/publications/domestic-abuse-a-resource-for-health-professionals [Accessed 12.03.2022].

For a list of resources to facilitate severity assessment in cases of domestic abuse, including multi-lingual versions of the Dash risk checklist:

SafeLives. 2019. *Resources for Identifying the Risk Victims Face*. Available at: www.safelives.org.uk/practice-support/resources-identifying-risk-victims-face [Accessed 12.03.2022].

For information and resources relating to MARACs:

SafeLives. 2019. *Resources for People Referring*. Available at: http://safelives.org.uk/practice-support/resources-marac-meetings/resources-people-referring [Accessed 12.03.2022].

References

Arkins, B., Begley, C., Higgins, A. 2016. Measures for screening for intimate partner violence: a systematic review. *Journal of Psychiatric and Mental Health Nursing*; 23(3–4), 217–235.

Bachmann, C. L., Gooch, B. 2018. *LGBT in Britain: Home and Communities*. Available at: www.stonewall.org.uk/sites/default/files/lgbt_in_britain_home_and_communities.pdf [Accessed 28.01.2020].

Beynon, C. E., Gutmanis, I. A., Tutty, L. M., Wathen, C. N., MacMillan, H. L. 2012. Why physicians and nurses ask (or don't) about partner violence: a qualitative analysis. *BMC Public Health*; 12.

Black, B. M., Weisz, A. N., Bennett, L. W. 2010. Graduating social work students' perspectives on domestic violence. *Affilia: Journal of Women and Social Work*; 25(2), 173–184.

Bott, S., Guedes, A., Goodwin, M., Adams Mendoza, J. 2012. *Violence Against Women in Latin America and the Caribbean: A Comparative Analysis of Population-based Data from 12 Countries.* PAHO: Washington, DC. Available at: www.paho.org/hq/dmd ocuments/2014/Violence1.24-WEB-25-febrero-2014.pdf [Accessed 20.01.2020].

Bradbury-Jones, C., Taylor, J., Kroll, T., Duncan, F. 2014. Domestic abuse awareness and recognition among primary healthcare professionals and abused women: a qualitative investigation. *Journal of Clinical Nursing*; 23(21–22), 3057–3068.

Campbell, J. C., Glass, N., Sharps, P. W., Laughon, K., Bloom, T. 2007. Intimate partner homicide: review and implications of research and policy. *Trauma, Violence & Abuse*; 8(3), 246–260.

Crenshaw, K. 1989. Demarginalizing the intersection of race and sex: black feminist critique of antidiscrimination doctrine, feminist theory and antiracist politics. *University of Chicago Legal Forum*; 139–168.

Crown Prosecution Service (CPS). 2018. *Violence Against Women and Girls Report 2017–2018.* Available at: www.cps.gov.uk/sites/default/files/documents/publications/cps-vawg-report-2018.pdf [Accessed 20.01.2020].

Department of Health. 2012. *'Striking the Balance': Practical Guidance on the Application of Caldicott Guardian Principles to Domestic Violence and MARACs (Multi Agency Risk Assessment Conferences).* Available at: https://assets.publishing.service.gov.uk/government/uploads/system/uploads/attachment_data/file/215064/dh_133594.pdf [Accessed 30.01.2020].

Dixon-Woods, M., Cavers, D., Agarwal, S., Annandale, E., Arthur, A., Harvey, J., Hsu, R., Katbamna, S., Olsen, R., Smith, L., Riley, R., Sutton, A. J. 2006. Conducting a critical interpretive synthesis of the literature on access to healthcare by vulnerable groups. *BMC Medical Research Methodology*; 6(35).

Dobash, R. P., Dobash, R. E. 2004. Women's violence to men in intimate relationships working on a puzzle. *The British Journal of Criminology*; 44(3), 324–349.

Domestic Abuse Act 2021. Available at www.legislation.gov.uk/ukpga/2021/17/contents/enacted [Accessed 25.03.2022].

Downs, W. R., Rindels, B., Atkinson, C. 2007. Women's use of physical and nonphysical self-defense strategies during incidents of partner violence. *Violence Against Women*; 13(1), 28–45.

Feder, G., Davies, R. A., Baird, K., Dunne, D., Eldridge, S., Griffiths, C., Gregory, A., Howell, A., Johnson, M., Ramsay, J., Rutterford, C., Sharp, D. 2011. Identification and referral to improve safety (IRIS) of women experiencing domestic violence with a primary care training and support programme: a cluster randomised controlled trial. *The Lancet*; 378(9805), 1788–1795.

García-Moreno, C., Jansen, H. A. F. M., Ellsberg, M., Heise, L., Watts, C. 2005. *WHO Multi-Country Study on Women's Health and Domestic Violence Against Women: Initial Results on Prevalence, Health Outcomes and Women's Responses.* World Health Organization: Geneva. Available at: www.who.int/reproductivehealth/publications/violence/24159358X/en/ [Accessed 20.01.2020].

Her Majesty's Inspectorate of Constabulary (HMIC). 2015. *Increasingly Everyone's Business: A Progress Report on the Police Response to Domestic Abuse.* Available at: www.justiceinspectorates.gov.uk/hmicfrs/wp-content/uploads/increasingly-everyones-business-domestic-abuse-progress-report.pdf [Accessed 20.01.2020].

Hester, M. 2013. Who does what to whom? Gender and domestic violence perpetrators in English police records. *European Journal of Criminology*; 10(5), 623–637.

Home Office. 2015. *Controlling or Coercive Behaviour in an Intimate or Family Relationship Statutory Guidance Framework.* Available at: https://assets.publishing.service.gov.uk/government/uploads/system/uploads/attachment_data/file/482528/Controlling_or_coercive_behaviour_-_statutory_guidance.pdf#page=17 [Accessed 19.01.2020].

Humphreys, C., Thiara, R. K. 2003. Neither justice nor protection: women's experiences of post-separation violence. *Journal of Social Welfare and Family Law*; 25(3), 195–214.

Johnson, M. P. 2006. Conflict and control gender symmetry and asymmetry in domestic violence. *Violence Against Women*; 12(11), 1003–1018.

McNamara, M., Ng, H. 2016. Best practices in LGBT care: a guide for primary care physicians. *Cleveland Clinic Journal of Medicine*; 83(7), 531–541.

National Institute for Health and Care Excellence (NICE). 2014. *Domestic Violence and Abuse: Multi-Agency Working. Public Health Guideline [PH50].* Available at: www.nice.org.uk/guidance/ph50 [Accessed 30.01.2020].

Nixon, J., Humphreys, C. 2010. Marshalling the evidence: using intersectionality in the domestic violence frame. *Social Politics*; 17(2), 137–158.

Office for National Statistics. 2018. *Domestic Abuse: Findings from the Crime Survey for England and Wales: Year Ending March 2018.* Available at: www.ons.gov.uk/peoplepopulationandcommunity/crimeandjustice/articles/domesticabusefindingsfromthecrimesurveyforenglandandwales/yearendingmarch2018 [Accessed 29.01.2020].

Office for National Statistics. 2019a. *Domestic Abuse Prevalence and Trends, England and Wales: Year Ending March 2019.* Available at: www.ons.gov.uk/peoplepopulationandcommunity/crimeandjustice/articles/domesticabuseprevalenceandtrendsenglandandwales/yearendingmarch2019 [Accessed 29.01.2020].

Office for National Statistics. 2019b. *Developing a Measure of Controlling or Coercive Behaviour.* Available at: www.ons.gov.uk/peoplepopulationandcommunity/crimeandjustice/articles/developingameasureofcontrollingorcoercivebehaviour/2019-04-18 [Accessed 20.01.2020].

Parliament, House of Commons. 1973. *Battered Wives (HC Deb 16 July 1973 vol 860 cc218–28).* Available at: https://api.parliament.uk/historic-hansard/commons/1973/jul/16/battered-wives [Accessed 18.01.2020].

Perryman, S. M., Appleton, J. 2016. Male victims of domestic abuse: implications for health visiting practice. *Journal of Research in Nursing*, 21(5–6), 386–414.

SafeLives. 2015. *SafeLives Dash Risk Checklist for the Identification of High Risk Cases of Domestic Abuse, Stalking and 'Honour'-based Violence*. Available at: www.safelives.org.uk/sites/default/files/resources/Dash%20for%20IDVAs%20FINAL_0.pdf [Accessed 30.01.2020].

SafeLives. 2018. *Free To Be Safe: LGBT+ People Experiencing Domestic Abuse*. Available at: www.safelives.org.uk/sites/default/files/resources/Free%20to%20be%20safe%20web.pdf [Accessed 28.01.2020].

Sammut, D., Kuruppu, J., Hegarty, K., Bradbury-Jones, C. 2019. Which violence against women educational strategies are effective for prequalifying health-care students? A systematic review. *Trauma, Violence & Abuse* [published online]. Available at: https://pubmed.ncbi.nlm.nih.gov/31122182/ [Accessed 12.03.2022].

Scottish Government. 2008. *Chief Executive Letter 41: Gender-Based Violence Action Plan*. Available at: www.sehd.scot.nhs.uk/mels/CEL2008_41.pdf [Accessed 30.01.2020].

Serious Crime Act 2015, c. 7. Available at: www.legislation.gov.uk/ukpga/2015/9/contents [Accessed 19.01.2020].

Stark, E. (2009) *Coercive Control: How Men Entrap Women in Personal Life*. Oxford University Press: Oxford.

Straus, M. A. (2010) Thirty years of denying the evidence on gender symmetry in partner violence: implications for prevention and treatment. *Partner Abuse*; 1(3), 332–362.

Taylor, J., Bradbury-Jones, C., Kroll, T., Duncan, F. 2013. Health professionals' beliefs about domestic abuse and the issue of disclosure: a critical incident technique study. *Health and Social Care in the Community*; 21(5), 489–499.

UK Parliament. (2019). *Joint Committee on the Draft Domestic Abuse Bill. Oral Evidence: Draft Domestic Abuse Bill, HC 2075. Tuesday 2 April 2019*. Available at: http://data.parliament.uk/writtenevidence/committeeevidence.svc/evidencedocument/draft-domestic-abuse-bill-committee/draft-domestic-abuse-bill/oral/99005.pdf [Accessed 19.01.2020].

Walby, S., Allen, J. 2004. *Domestic Violence, Sexual Assault and Stalking: Findings from the British Crime Survey*. Home Office Research Study 276. Home Office: London.

Women's Aid. 2019a. *What is Domestic Abuse?* Available at: www.womensaid.org.uk/information-support/what-is-domestic-abuse/ [Accessed 18.01.2020].

Women's Aid. 2019b. *Why Don't Women Leave Abusive Relationships?* Available at: www.womensaid.org.uk/information-support/what-is-domestic-abuse/women-leave/ [Accessed 21.01.2020].

World Health Organization. 2017. *Violence Against Women*. Available at: www.who.int/news-room/fact-sheets/detail/violence-against-women [Accessed 20.01.2020].

18

HONOUR-BASED VIOLENCE – A PUBLIC HEALTH ISSUE: PROTECTION, PROMOTION AND PROVISION OF SERVICES

JOANNE MCEWAN AND MICHELLE MOSELEY

—————————————— LEARNING OUTCOMES ——————————————

By the end of this chapter you will be able to:

- Define honour-based violence/abuse (HBV) offering definitions of 'forced marriage' and female genital mutilation (FGM) whilst exploring its impact on health.
- Signposted to recognise practitioners will be guided on how to recognise signs and triggers of HBV and refer to the relevant agencies associated with supporting individuals subjected to this form of abuse.
- Recognise the global context of FGM will be explored with a focus on the UK with reference to key public health themes including communication, health inequalities, policy and legislation, analysis of the data, and behaviour change.
- Re-enforce the response of practitioners where HBV is suspected is contrary to usual safeguarding practice.

Introduction

The concept of honour-based violence (HBV) has become seemingly more prevalent in later years due to its exposure within the media, in particular honour killings (Gill et al. 2012). The term 'honour-based violence' and 'honour-based abuse' will be used interchangeably within this chapter due to variance of terminology within the literature. HBV as all types of abuse has been prevalent throughout the globe for centuries. HBV can be defined as a type of violence perpetrated against women or men. There are four aspects of HBV (Brandon and Hafez 2008):

- Forced marriage (FM)
- Domestic violence
- Honour killings
- Female genital mutilation (FGM)

Three of these aspects will be covered in this chapter, namely forced marriage, honour killings and FGM; Chapter 17 is dedicated to domestic abuse. Although it is important to recognise domestic abuse associated with honour, can be undertaken by close family members (children, siblings, parents, parents in law, extended family members) to protect the 'perceived' honour bestowed on the family as well as its reputation (Helba et al. 2014).

HBV

The Crown Prosecution Service (CPS) define HBV as a breach of a person's human rights:

> HBV is a collection of practices, which are used to control behaviour within families or other social groups to protect perceived cultural and religious beliefs and/or honour. Such violence can occur when perpetrators perceive that a relative has shamed the family and/or community by breaking their honour code. It is a violation of human rights and may be a form of domestic and/or sexual violence.
> There is no, and cannot be, honour or justification for abusing the human rights of others. (CPS 2020)

As practitioners, it is imperative to try to grasp the concept of honour and to do this we need to consider what faith, culture, religion and belief means to us personally and professionally as well as exploring what honour is and its place in society. When attempting to define each of these terms a plethora of descriptions and definitions based on personal and professional experiences, expertise and exposure to honour-based issues will come into play. The concept of a breach of 'honour' is centuries old.

'Faith' can relate to trust, belief, a belief without any proof or faith in a certain religion/concept. 'Religion' can refer to a specific faith and worship within a religion, whilst 'belief' could refer to a certain level of trust or having 'faith' whereas 'honour' can relate to pride, status and power. Honour has many meanings across cultures and communities.

It is very powerful throughout many communities and deemed more important than the law which it supersedes. It is reported that over 5,000 women and girls are murdered each year worldwide in the name of 'honour'. The murders often go unpunished, prevention and disclosure is difficult due to the very nature of abuse, and honour killings have been evidenced in at least 26 countries. There are many words associated with honour which include 'Ird' (Arab countries), 'Namus' (Pakistan, Turkey, Kurdistan and Iran), 'Zina and Izzat' (mainly South Asia). 'Izzat' is one of the most common words associated with Honour and has no single meaning and relates to a 'learnt' set of very complex rules. It is followed to protect the family name and position within the community/society. It is a silent code of behavioural practice, introduced at birth, is deep-seated within the community and more important than a person's human rights, liberty and security. Honour can be damaged by:

- Disobeying parents.
- Displaying certain behaviour (wearing certain clothes, behaving differently, displaying a disrespectful attitude).
- Having sex or a relationship prior to marriage.
- Drug or alcohol use.
- Gossip (this could involve rumours generated about a family). (Brandon and Hafez 2008)

Karma Nirvana (2021) also refer to:

- Expressing sexuality.
- Being in a relationship with someone who is not accepted by your family.
- Pregnancy before marriage or outside of a marriage.
- Abortion.
- A change of religion or faith.
- Not accepting/refusing an arranged marriage.
- Choosing your own career, not approved by the family/community.
- Disclosing abuse to an 'outsider'.

Any of the above are deemed immoral acts, but the main issue is these immoral acts becoming public with the consequence of bringing shame or dishonour on the family. This could hamper future family relationships, building businesses, providing stability and a sense of worth, social standing and superiority within a community (Brandon and Hamez 2008, Helba et al. 2014). Families therefore will go to extreme lengths to maintain and preserve their family honour. Honour-based crimes include blackmail, acid attacks, blood feuds, domestic abuse, forced marriage, FGM and honour killings. It is essential to place the numbers of victims of HBV in some context, demonstrated in Table 18.1.

The statistics depicted in Table 18.1 highlight some of the challenges to those individuals affected by HBV. Some are individuals with no access to public funding; this further complicates their situation and therefore asking for help is normally a last resort in trying

Table 18.1   The reality of HBV – the statistics

SafeLives (2017) report:
- Almost one-quarter of victims at risk of 'honour'-based abuse are not eligible for public funds such as tax credits,or housing support; this is called 'no recourse to public funds'.
- Of those seen at the Forced Marriage Unit, 15% are under 16 years of age.
- 57% of HBV victims visiting their GP over a 12-month period; of these, there were only 6% of referrals to specialist services.
- 43% of HBV victims remain in a relationship with the perpetrator, compared to victims of domestic abuse where 29% are reported to stay.

Karma Nirvana (2021) report the following calls to their Honour-based Abuse Helpline in 2019:
- 12,107 calls received (70% were related to victim support).
- There were 597 migrants (40 men, 540 women); 25% of these had no recourse to public funds.
- 1,931 women accessed helpline support; 600 had children who were exposed to and impacted by honour-based abuse.

to escape their situation. Before reaching out for support it is thought that victims of HBV remain in their situation for at least two years before seeking help (SafeLives 2017). Many return and accept their fate, which could lead to death.

Diana Nammi, Executive Director of the Iranian and Kurdish Women's Rights Organisation (IKWRO 2017) stated:

> So many crimes are never reported because the perpetrators are the victim's own families and/or community members, who often have convinced them that going to the police is shameful and they fear retribution.

The situations of individuals leading to HBV are complex and not specific to any particular culture or religion. HBV is seen and has been seen across society as a whole. There is no 'honour' in abuse and 'where culture or tradition are used to exert power or control over others, this can only be a misuse of that culture (SafeLives 2017).

Honour killings

From a global perspective there are approximately 5,000 individuals murdered each year due to HBV (Eshareturi et al. 2014). It has been estimated that 10–12 women are killed in honour-based incidents within the UK yearly, which equates to approximately 1 per month (Brandon and Hamez 2008). Of course the numbers are an estimation, as it is thought that numbers exceed those recorded due the very nature of the abuse and how it is hidden, and these figures are inaccurate due to the lack of reliable data. A freedom of information request to the police within the UK identified that just over 11,000 cases relating to so-called HBV were recorded from 2010–2014 with the Forced Marriage Unit supporting 1,400 individuals in 2016 (SafeLives 2017). In 2019/2020 there were 2,024 offences relating to HBV. Police recorded 74 of these were associated with FGM, 140 to forced marriage and 1,810 were other 'HBV tagged' offences (Home Office 2020). The data presented covers 30 forces across England and Wales and 78% were HBV related.

The numbers of HBV have increased in 2020/21 with a total of 2,725 HBV-related offences. There were 78 victims who experienced FGM, 125 experienced forced marriage with the remaining 2,725 victims related to 'other' HBV offences (Home Office 2022).

There have been high-profile cases of honour killings identified within the media (Table 18.2).

Forced marriage

Marriage should be entered into only with the free and full consent of the intending spouses. (United Nations Universal Declaration of Human Rights 1948)

Arranged marriages are commonplace within many communities; it is when the arrangement becomes forced that it breaches UK law and human rights. An arranged marriage occurs when families of both spouses take the lead in arranging the marriage. It is a traditional event based on compatibility, *consent* and *choice*. It occurs frequently within communities and the choice of whether to accept the arrangement remains with the betrothed. It becomes forced when the parents choose a partner regardless of the individuals' feelings/opinion. Forced marriage can and will occur within those communities underpinned by 'honour, pride and shame' (Brandon and Hamez 2008). Girls, boys, women and men can be pressurised into a forced marriage; if refused, extreme violence and murder can occur as identified in the deaths of the above individuals subjected to HBV (Table 18.2).

Evidence suggests that forced marriage is primarily against women. Most of the cases reported involve women and girls aged between 11 and 40 years. There is evidence to suggest 15% of those affected by HBV are male and, in some cases, victims do not know they are subject to a forced marriage as they are brought up to believe this is the 'norm' (Brandon and Hamez 2008, SafeLives 2017). The reasons behind forced marriage relate to 'honour' with the added motivation of developing strong family ties; dowries are commonplace and therefore potential financial gain. The aim of forced marriage is also to prevent marriage outside of the community from an ethnic, cultural or religious group, caste perspective as well as ensuring the order in which siblings marry, the eldest first (Brandon and Hamez 2008). Other reasons include enforcing an individual to marry who is LGBTQ+ to hide their sexuality as well as searching for a partner to look after the individual who may have a disability (Safeguarding Hub 2020).

Table 18.2   High profile cases of HBV

SafeLives (2017) state that victims of honour-based violence are seven times more likely to have a number of perpetrators rather than one which is common in other cases of domestic abuse. Here are some high-profile cases of Honour killing:
Heshu Yones, age 16 murdered in 2002
Shafilea Ahmed, age 17, murdered in 2003
Banaz Mahmod, age 20, murdered in 2006
Celine Dookrhan, age 19, murdered in 2017

The UK government set up the Forced Marriage Unit in 2005 offering advice to victims of forced marriage and in 2007 legislation was developed to support victims of forced marriage: the Forced Marriage (Civil Protection) Act 2007. Karma Nirvana (2021) report that in the UK in 2019, 350 victims were threatened with forced marriage. There was an 83% increase in forced marriage protection orders. During the COVID-19 pandemic there has been a 355% increase in calls to the HBV helpline, and a 347% rise in emails received. There was a 36% rise in contacts from pregnant women and a 17% rise in contacts from migrant women. The Forced Marriage Unit saw 1,355 cases of forced marriage in 2019. Of these, 1,080 were female, 363 were aged 18 years and under, 29 were LGBTQ+, 39 were repatriated and 81% had an overseas involvement. These are complex issues and with an ongoing global pandemic victims will feel stranded in their situations. Practitioners need to recognise the signs of HBV as they may have just one chance to act.

Female genital mutilation (FGM): definition and global perspectives

The United Nations International Children's Emergency Fund (UNICEF 2013) estimates that FGM affects 200,000 million females in the world, with 3 million women and girls a year at risk of FGM. FGM has been documented in 30 countries mainly in Africa, some parts of Asia and Southeast Asia. It is approximated that there are over half a million FGM survivors living in the EU (Van Baelen et al. 2016). The World Health Organization (WHO) defines FGM as all procedures that involve the partial or total removal of the external part of the female genitalia or other injury to the female organs for non-medical reasons (WHO 2021, see also Table 18.3).

FGM is performed on girls of different ages, varying between cultures, from babies to 16-year-olds (and sometimes older) (UNICEF 2013). Commonly held beliefs underpinning the practice of FGM include ensuring chastity, beliefs about hygiene, that it enhances male sexual pleasure, or as a religious or cultural identity requirement. FGM is a crude and informal practice often performed by traditional cutters who have minimal understanding of human anatomy, and in some countries by medical professionals (UNICEF 2013). The classifications are approximations and cannot fully describe the extent of physical trauma. Immediate complications include haemorrhage and death. Later complications include chronic pain, difficulties passing urine, infections, painful intercourse, complications in childbirth, post-traumatic stress disorder, anxiety, infertility and death (Royal College of Obstetrics and Gynaecology 2015). In the UK, FGM

Table 18.3 FGM classifications

Type I: removal or damage to the clitoral glands or clitoral hood
Type II: removal or damage to the clitoris and inner lips
Type III: also known as infibulation and is the narrowing of the vaginal opening to create a seal, by sewing the inner and outer lips together leaving a tiny hole to urinate, menstruate and have penetrative intercourse; may or may not involve removal of clitoris/clitoral hood or gland
Type IV: all other procedures including stretching the labia, piercing, scraping or burning.

statistics are presented as estimates which are derived from census data that includes country of birth data, informed from the household studies above. Therefore, it was estimated that 137,000 women and girls in England and Wales were affected by FGM in 2011 (MacFarlane and Dorkenoo 2015).

Policy and legislation

FGM is a safeguarding issue. Public health requires protecting children from harm. FGM has been illegal since the Prohibition of Female Circumcision Act 1985, followed by the Female Genital Mutilation Act 2003 in England, Wales and Northern Ireland, and the Prohibition of Female Genital Mutilation (Scotland) Act 2005. By 2012 there was fierce criticism that the UK had failed to secure any prosecutions and was accused of political correctness and failing in protecting children from Black and Minority Ethnic backgrounds (Dias et al. 2014). In 2014 the *Female Genital Mutilation Declaration* (HM Government 2014), the *Intercollegiate Recommendations* (RCM et al. 2013) and the Home Affairs Select Committee's case for a national action plan (2014) were launched. This coincided with the FGM Summit (BBC News 2014) at which the UK government vowed to end FGM in a generation. Existing FGM legislation in England and Wales was amended with the Serious Crime Act 2015, making it a legal duty for all registered professionals to report a first-hand disclosure of FGM in under 18-year-olds to the police called the Mandatory Reporting Duty (MRD) (Department of Health n.d., HM Government 2015). Additionally, in 2015 an FGM enhanced dataset was introduced requiring primary, community and acute health trusts to submit quarterly data returns on patients with FGM to NHS Digital (Department of Health 2015). Identifiable information, including name and date of birth, submitted to NHS Digital to enable data validation is then anonymised. Submission to the FGM dataset does not require the patient's consent, although clinicians retain fair processing responsibility. Opting out requires the patient's written application after submission (NHS Digital 2018).

Communicating about FGM

Bernhardt (2004) states that public health communication should comprise of relevant, accurate, accessible and understandable messages that are strategically delivered to the intended audience and evaluated to improve the public's health. Communicating about FGM at both system and individual levels can pose potential challenges. Tackling this important public health issue requires communication that meets the needs of both affected communities and professionals, involving partnerships with communities and agencies to develop understanding (Dixon et al. 2021).

The role of language and terminology

'Female genital mutilation (FGM)' is the internationally agreed term encompassing the overall harm to healthy genital tissue (WHO 2021). The word 'mutilation' replaced 'circumcision' or 'excision' to emphasise the extent of injury (African General Assembly 2005). Some campaign groups prefer 'FGM/C' due to the sensitivity around 'mutilation', and other groups disagree that their practice is FGM; for example, a study of African women in England who experienced labial elongation (type IV) stated that they did not align their cultural practice with FGM (Ariyo et al. 2016). While 'FGM' is generally the accepted term, health communication with individuals and communities affected by FGM should incorporate mutually agreed wording. Best practice is to refer to 'affected communities' rather than 'practising communities' (Baillot et al. 2014, Hemming 2011). Women from communities affected by FGM describe how insensitive language and lack of knowledge led to them feeling stigmatised (Johnsdotter 2009, Karlson et al. 2019). Thoughtful wording, sensitivity and using interpreter services when required are essential for developing a shared understanding of care needs. Failure to provide access to interpreters exacerbates social inequalities.

Building relationships to communicate about FGM

Effective public health communication about FGM can facilitate collaborative relationships between professionals and FGM-affected communities. Understanding cultural norms and FGM complications can enable health care workers to enquire about symptoms which the patient may have accepted as normal, thereby increasing their access to care (Dixon et al. 2021). Studies demonstrate that women from FGM-affected communities experience relationships with health professionals as unequal, experiencing cultural vulnerability (Karlson et al. 2019, Pirie 2015). Evans et al. (2019) call for 'cultural safety' based on trust to facilitate a clinical service mutually negotiated to suit their needs. Public health professionals have a role to play in engaging communities to negotiate services around FGM protection, health promotion and FGM care provision. Whether the public health role is commissioning, designing or delivering health care, this requires open dialogue and sensitive, honest communication with communities.

Impact of the legislation

Doctors expressed concerns that the duty to report to the police would put the doctor–patient relationship at risk (Mather and Rymer 2015) and that the duties stood out from procedures for other forms of child abuse. In a realism synthesis of 92 papers from primary care Dixon et al. (2021) stated that the MRD could deter women from seeking care, affect the therapeutic relationship and reduce trust in health professionals. The legislation was also compounded with lack of training and knowledge on FGM. Studies also stated the duty to collect personally identifiable information was an obstacle to raising FGM in consultations with the women doubting the confidentiality (Dixon et al. 2021). Such views were echoed by Creighton (2019) who said that legislation was disproportionate and should be reconsidered. This sparked a debate in the response to the Creighton *British Medical Journal* editorial (Albert 2019, Dixon et al. 2019, Kelly 2019).

There have been mixed responses to the legislative changes from FGM-affected communities. Integrate, a Bristol-based charity, successfully spurred young women and men to raise awareness about FGM, working with safeguarding partners and forging the Bristol Model aimed at collaboration, empowerment and safeguarding (Bristol Against Violence and Abuse 2015). Prominent activists welcomed the changes, stating they were long overdue and would help protect girls. Qualitative studies with FGM-affected communities in Oxford, Bristol and London identified dismay and perceptions of stigma in response to the legislation (Karlson et al. 2019, Pirie 2015, Plugge et al. 2018). This included reporting experiences of suspicion and shame when seeking care from midwives, GPs and health visitors, and repeated questioning about FGM was experienced as re-traumatising (Karlson et al. 2019). Community members considered that the intense focus on safeguarding in Bristol was evident among teachers, social workers and the police who had insufficient knowledge of FGM and demonstrated bias (Karlson et al. 2019). All three communities studied reported wanting to end FGM, calling for a collaborative approach to policy making.

Tackling FGM in the UK

A range of community approaches to changing behaviour have emerged. Examples include the Sisters Circle, developed by the African Advocacy Foundation providing a safe space where women can talk about 'any' issue of concern (Khalifa and Brown 2016), community mobilisation, advocacy and leadership programmes developed by FORWARD (2020). The impact of these approaches has been measured by engagement rather than change in practice.

FGM is an act of violence against women and girls, and in children is child abuse. FGM is illegal in the UK. Evidence on how many girls and women in the UK are living with FGM or how many girls are taken abroad to be cut is scant. There are suggestions that FGM is not as prevalent as previously estimated. Professionals are duty-bound to fulfil their safeguarding obligations to protect girls. Awareness among professionals is increasing, which is welcome, but communication between professionals and community members needs to be delivered effectively and sensitively, including explaining why FGM is being discussed, and avoiding repeated questioning. This also applies to public health professionals when they are strategically engaging with communities. More research is required to understand how to support FGM-affected communities living in the UK to disengage with the practice.

Disclosure response

When an individual discloses that they are at risk of any form of HBV or if a practitioner suspects HBV they need to act immediately as this may be the one chance they have to support them to prevent further abuse. The past decade has seen an increase in awareness of HBV across agencies. There remains to be a lack of accurate data reflecting the true impact of all aspects of HBV due to its hidden nature. There needs to be a call to action across all frontline agencies working with families and within communities where a cultural awareness needs to be fostered in an attempt to support, prevent and protect victims. Multi-agency training with the development of local policy and guidance is recommended. Therefore, when disclosure occurs the response is different from the perspective of *not* involving the family. The individual affected needs to be seen in a secure private environment, on their own. It is essential not to turn them away; do not say you will visit them at home, do not approach family members, the community or local interpreters, use an external interpretation service. Do not attempt to mediate with the family and if under 18 years, this is a child protection issue and the local authority and police will need to be called. Seek advice from safeguarding leads if necessary.

In summary:

- If an individual is at risk of immediate harm and wants to leave the household, contact the police in light of immediate danger.
- If they feel they are not in immediate danger, provide advice and support with resources (helpline numbers) if it is safe to do so.
- If the individual is unsure if they want to leave the household, gain consent for referral to a supporting agency. Offer access to a phone, offer to call for them, provide relevant contact numbers.
- If the individual wants no action, offer to speak to them again if they wish (unless it is a child protection issue in which case action will need to be taken in referral to other agencies).
- If there is any doubt, seek advice from a safeguarding lead.

A change in culture within professions is just one step of preventing HBV. A step has to be taken to raise awareness within the communities where HBV is most prevalent, including schools, to break this cycle of HBV and protect future generations within our communities.

Table 18.4 Support contacts

Karma Nirvana:
Telephone 0800 5999 247
Monday – Friday 9am – 5pm.
Email: info@karmanirvana.org.uk

Forced Marriage Unit:
Telephone: 020 7008 0151
From overseas: +44 (0)20 7008 0151
Monday to Friday, 9am to 5pm
Out of hours: 020 7008 1500 (ask for the Global Response Centre)
Email: fmu@fcdo.gov.uk

Conclusion

This chapter has offered a general overview of what constitutes honour-based violence. The definition and concept of HBV was explored and signs of forced marriage, FGM and honour killing. This will allow practitioners to recognise potential signs and triggers of HBV and refer to the relevant agencies associated with supporting individuals subjected to this form of abuse.

The response of practitioners where HBV is suspected is contrary to usual safeguarding practice. Practitioners need to seek advice from a safeguarding lead where HBV is suspected. The concept of 'honour' is difficult to define but literature, HBV organisations as well as activists reiterate that 'honour' being used to enforce power and control over an individual disguised within culture or tradition is inappropriate and abusive.

Consider the following questions

1. Examine the meanings of faith, culture, religion and belief. Do they relate to honour? If so, how? How would you define and explain the term 'honour'?
2. Review the cases of those affected by honour killings listed in Table 18.2. Review the history and behaviours of them, as well as the behaviour of the family and members involved. Are there any common themes?
3. In your role, what does effective dialogue on FGM look like when working with different members of FGM-affected communities?
4. Considering the social determinants of health, how do we prioritise FGM in a public health context?
5. How should FGM data be collected and analysed to critically represent the risk of FGM and health care provision?
6. In your local context, how do we approach behaviour change on FGM and how should we evaluate it?

Key terms

Honour-based violence – a type of violence perpetrated against women or men which has four aspects. These are forced marriage (FM), domestic violence (DV), honour killings and female genital mutilation (FGM). *'HBV is a collection of practices, which are used to control behaviour within families or other social groups to protect perceived cultural and religious beliefs and/or honour. Such violence can occur when perpetrators perceive that a relative has shamed the family and/or community by breaking their honour code. It is a violation of human rights and may be a form of domestic and/or sexual violence. There is no, and cannot be, honour or justification for abusing the human rights of others'* (CPS 2020).

Female Genital Mutilation – The World Health Organization (WHO) defines FGM as all procedures that involve the partial or total removal of the external part of the female genitalia or other injury to the female organs for non-medical reasons (WHO 2018).

Arranged Marriage - Arranged marriages are commonplace within many communities it is when the arrangement becomes forced it breaches UK law and human rights. An arranged marriage occurs when families of both spouses take the lead in arranging the marriage. It is a traditional event based on compatibility, consent and choice.

Forced Marriage - Girls, boys, women and men can be pressurised into a forced marriage, if refused, extreme violence and murder can occur as identified in the deaths of the above victims subjected to HBV.

Honour killing - Honour based crimes include blackmail, acid attacks, blood feuds, domestic abuse, forced marriage, FGM and honour killings. Families will go to extreme lengths to maintain and preserve their family honour even homicide.

Further reading

Behavioural Insights Team. 2020. *Publications*. Available at: www.bi.team/our-work/publications/ [Accessed 12.03.2022].

Centre for Behaviour Change. 2022. *Harnessing Cross-disciplinary Expertise to Address Social, Health and Environmental Challenges*. University College: London. Available at: www.ucl.ac.uk/behaviour-change/ [Accessed 12.03.2022].

Halo Project. n.d. *The Forced Marriage Unit*. Available at: www.haloproject.org.uk/forced-marriage-unit-W21page-31 [Accessed 12.03.2022].

Karma Nirvana. n.d. *Working to End Honour-based Abuse in the UK*. Available at: https://karmanirvana.org.uk/ [Accessed 12.03.2022].

NHS Oxford Health. n.d. *Let's Talk FGM: Enabling Conversations on FGM - Helping NHS Health Professionals Sensitively Discuss Female Genital Mutilation*. Available at: www.letstalkfgm.nhs.uk [Accessed 12.03.2022].

Safeguarding Hub. 2018. *Forced Marriage – Signs and Tactics*. Available at: https://safeguardinghub.co.uk/forced-marriage-signs-and-tactics/ [Accessed 12.03.2022].

SafeLives. 2017. *Victims of 'Honour-based' Abuse Seven Times More Likely to Have Multiple Perpetrators than Other Victims of Domestic Abuse*. Available at: https://safelives.org.uk/honour-based-violence-and-domestic-abuse [Accessed 12.03.2022].

References

African General Assembly. 2005. *Declaration on the Terminology of FGM (IAC)*. Available at: www.28toomany.org/static/media/uploads/Thematic%20Research%20and%20Resources/Terminology/bamako_declaration_on_the_terminology_fgm__6th_iac_general_assembly_4_-_7_april_2005.pd [Accessed 28.01.2020].

Albert, J. 2019. Editorial: Tackling female genital mutilation in the UK. *BMJ*; 364. Available at: www.bmj.com/content/364/bmj.l15/rapid-responses [Accessed 31.01.2020].

Ariyo, D., Ssali, R., Nambuya, B., Olurin, F. 2016. An AFRUCA Community Research Project. *Voices of the Community: Exploring Type IV (Labia Elongation) Female Genital Mutilation in the African Community across Greater Manchester*. Available at: www.afruca. org/wp-content/uploads/2016/11/Final-Labia-Elongation-FGM-Report.pdf [Accessed 30.01.2020].

Baillot, H., Murray, N., Connelly, E. 2014. *Tackling FGM in Scotland: A Scottish Model of Intervention*. Scottish Refugee Council: Edinburgh. Available at: www. scottishrefugeecouncil.org.uk/wp-content/uploads/2019/10/Tackling-Female-Genital-Mutilation-in-Scotland-A-Scottish-model-of-intervention.pdf [Accessed 30.01.2020].

BBC News. 2014. *FGM Summit: Cameron Calls for End 'in this Generation'*. 22 July. Available at: www.bbc.co.uk/news/uk-28412179 [Accessed 30.01.2020].

Bernhardt, J. 2004. Editorial: communication at the core of public health. *American Journal of Public Health*; 94, 12. Available at: www.ncbi.nlm.nih.gov/pmc/articles/PMC1448586/pdf/0942051.pdf [Accessed 30.01.2020].

Brandon, J., Hafez, S. 2008. *Crimes of the Community. HBV in the UK*. Centre for Social Cohesion: London.

Bristol Against Violence and Abuse. 2015. *The Bristol Model*. Available at: www.bava.org. uk/wp-content/uploads/The-Bristol-Model.pdf [Accessed 29.01.2020].

Creighton, S. 2019. Editorial: Tackling FGM in the UK. *British Medical Journal*; 364: 115. Available at: doi: https://doi.org/10.1136/bmj.l15 [Accessed 29.01.2020].

Crown Prosecution Service (CPS). 2020. *HBV and Forced Marriage*. Available at: www.cps. gov.uk/publication/honour-based-violence-and-forced-marriage [Accessed 10.01.2020].

Department of Health. n.d. Female Genital Mutilation (FGM) Mandatory Reporting Duty. Available at: https://assets.publishing.service.gov.uk/government/uploads/system/uploads/attachment_data/file/525405/FGM_mandatory_reporting_map_A. pdf [Accessed 25.03.2022].

Department of Health. 2015. *FGM Prevention Programme: Understanding the Enhanced Dataset – Updated Clarification and Guidance to Support Implementation*. Available at: https://assets.publishing.service.gov.uk/government/uploads/system/uploads/attachment_data/file/461524/FGM_Statement_September_2015.pdf [Accessed 30.01.2020].

Dias, D., Gerry, F., Burrage, H. 2014. 10 reasons why our FGM has failed – and 10 ways to improve it. *The Guardian*. 7 February 2014.

Dixon, S., Duddy, C., Harrison, G., Papoutsi, C., Ziebland, S., Griffiths, F. 2021. Conversations about FGM in primary care: a realist review on how, why and in what circumstance FGM is discussed in primary care consultations. *BMJ Open*. Available at: https://pubmed.ncbi.nlm.nih.gov/33753429/ [Accessed 12.03.2022].

Dixon, S., Shacklock, J., Leach, J. 2019. Rapid response: re: tackling Female Genital Mutilation in the UK. *BMJ*; February. Available at: www.bmj.com/content/364/bmj. l15/rapid-responses [Accessed 20.08.2021].

Eshareturi, C., Lyle, C., Morgan, A. 2014. Policy issues and responses to violence: a cultural or national problem? *Journal of Aggression, Maltreatment & Trauma*; 23, 369–382.

Evans, C., Tweheyo, R., McGarry, J., Eldridge, J., Albert, J., Nkoyo, V., Higgenbottom, G. 2019. Seeking culturally safe care: a qualitative systematic review of the healthcare experiences of women and girls who have undergone female genital mutilation/cutting. *BMJ Open Access*, 2019-9: e027452. doi: 10.11.36/bmjopen-2018-027452

Forced Marriage (Civil Protection) Act. 2017. Available at: www.legislation.gov.uk/ukpga/2007/20/section/1 [Accessed 16.10.2020].

FORWARD. 2020. *Community Engagement*. Available at: www.forwarduk.org.uk/how-we-work-for-women-and-girls/community-engagement [Accessed 30.01.2020].

Gill, A.K., Begikani, N., Hague, G. 2012. HBV in Kurdish communities. *Women's Studies International Forum*; 35, 75–85.

Hemming, J. 2011. *The FGM Initiative Interim Report*. Available at: www.rosauk.org/wp-content/uploads/2015/10/FGM-Interim-Report-Nov-2011.pdf [Accessed 30.01.2020].

Helba, C., Bernstein, M., Leonard, M., Bauer, E. 2014. *Report on Exploratory study into Honor Violence Measurement Methods*. Available at: https://www.ojp.gov/ncjrs/virtual-library/abstracts/report-exploratory-study-honor-violence-measurement-methods-0 [Accessed 18.04.2022].

HM Government. 2014. *Female Genital Mutilation Declaration*. Available at: www.gov.uk/government/publications/female-genital-mutilation-declaration [Accessed 30.01.2020].

Home Affairs Committee. 2014. *Female Genital Mutilation: The Case for a National Action Plan*. Available at: https://publications.parliament.uk/pa/cm201415/cmselect/cmhaff/201/20102.htm [Accessed 17.04.22].

Home Office. 2020. *Statistics on So-called 'Honour-based' Abuse Offences Recorded by the Police*. Available at: www.gov.uk/government/statistics/statistics-on-so-called-honour-based-abuse-offences-england-and-wales-2019-to-2020/statistics-on-so-called-honour-based-abuse-offences-recorded-by-the-police [Accessed 3.01.2022].

Home Office. 2022. *Statistics on So-called 'Honour-based' Abuse Offences Recorded by the Police*. Available at: www.gov.uk/government/statistics/statistics-on-so-called-honour-based-abuse-offences-england-and-wales-2020-to-2021/statistics-on-so-called-honour-based-abuse-offences-england-and-wales-2020-to-2021 [Accessed 03.01.2022].

Iranian and Kurdish Women's Rights Organisation (IKWRO). 2017. *Honour Killing is Preventable*. Available at: http://ikwro.org.uk/2017/07/honour-killing-preventable/ [Accessed 15.10.2020].

Johnsdotter, S. 2009. *Discrimination of Certain Ethnic Groups? Ethical Aspects of Implementing FGM Legislation in Sweden*. Faculty of Health and Society, Malmo University: Malmo.

Karlson, S., Carver, N., Mogilnika, M., Pantazis, C. 2019. *When Safeguarding Becomes Stigmatising*. University of Bristol: Bristol. Available at: https://research-information.bris.ac.uk/files/187177083/Karlsen_et_al_2019_When_Safeguarding_become_Stigmatising_Final_Report.pdf [Accessed 30.01.2020].

Karma Nirvana. 2021. *Shining the Spotlight: Bringing Honour-based Abuse into the Mainstream. 3 Year Strategy 2021–2024.* Available at:. https://s40641.pcdn.co/wp-content/uploads/KN-Spotlight-2021-V4.pdf [Accessed 18.04.2022].

Kelly, B. 2019. Rapid response: re: tackling Female Genital Mutilation in the UK. *BMJ*; January. Available at: www.bmj.com/content/364/bmj.l15/rapid-responses [Accessed 31.01.2020].

Khalifa, S., Brown, E. 2016. *Communities Tackling FGM in the UK: Best Practice Guide.* The Tackling Female Genital Mutilation Initiative and Options Consultancy Services: London. Available at: https://esmeefairbairn.org.uk/userfiles/Documents/Publications/Communities_Tackling_FGM_in_the_UK_-_Best_Practice_Guide.pdf. [Accessed 30.01.2020].

MacFarlane, A., Dorkenoo, E. 2015. *Prevalence of Female Genital Mutilation in England and Wales: National and Local Estimates.* City of London University: London. Available at: www.city.ac.uk/__data/assets/pdf_file/0004/282388/FGM-statistics-final-report-21-07-15-released-text.pdf [Accessed 30.01.2020].

Mather, N., Rymer, J. 2015. Editorial: mandatory reporting of female genital mutilation by healthcare professionals. *British Journal of General Practice*; June. Available at: https://bjgp.org/content/65/635/282 [Accessed 30.01.2020].

NHS Digital. 2018. *Patients – Your FGM Information and How We Use It.* Available at: https://digital.nhs.uk/data-and-information/clinical-audits-and-registries/female-genital-mutilation-datasets/patients-your-fgm-information-and-how-we-use-it [Accessed 30.01.2020].

Pirie, A. 2015. *Together We Can Stop It. Community Engagement in FGM: Learning from Midaye's FGM Forums.* The Midaye Somali Development Network: London. Available at: http://midaye.org.uk/wp-content/uploads/2015/07/MIDAYE_FGM_Report-Together_We_Can_Stop_It.pdf [Accessed 30.01.2020].

Plugge, E., Adam, S., El Hindi, L., Gitau, J., Shokunde, N., Mohamed-Ahmed, O. 2018. The prevention of female genital mutilation in England: what can be done? *Journal of Public Health*; 30, 41(3), e261–e266. doi: 10.1093/pubmed/fdy128

RCM, RCN, RCOG, Equality Now, UNITE. 2013. *Tackling FGM in the UK: Intercollegiate Recommendations for Identifying, Recording, and Reporting.* Royal College of Midwives: London. Available at: www.rcog.org.uk/globalassets/documents/news/tackingfgmuk.pdf [Accessed 30.01.2020].

Royal College of Obstetrics and Gynaecology. 2015. *Female Genital Mutilation and its Management: Green Top Guideline no. 53.* Available at: www.rcog.org.uk/globalassets/documents/guidelines/gtg-53-fgm.pdf [Accessed 30.01.2020].

Safeguarding Hub. 2020. *Forced Marriage, Signs and Tactics.* Available at: https://safeguardinghub.co.uk/forced-marriage-signs-and-tactics/ [Accessed 15.10.2020].

SafeLives. 2017. *Your Choice: Honour-based Violence, Forced Marriage and Domestic Abuse.* Available at: https://safelives.org.uk/sites/default/files/resources/Spotlight%20on%20HBV%20and%20forced%20marriage-web.pdf [Accessed 15.10.2020].

Serious Crime Act 2015. Available at: www.legislation.gov.uk/ukpga/2015/9/part/5/crossheading/female-genital-mutilation/enacted [Accessed 29.01.2020].

UNICEF. 2013. *Female Genital Mutilation/Cutting: A Statistical Overview and Exploration of the Dynamics of Change.* Available at: https://data.unicef.org/resources/fgm-statistical-overview-and-dynamics-of-change/ [Accessed 12.03.2022].

United Nations. 1948. *The Universal Declaration of Human Rights*; Article 16(2). Available at: www.un.org/en/universal-declaration-human-rights/ [Accessed 15.10.2020].

Van Baelen, L., Ortensi, L., Leye, E. 2016. Estimates of first-generation women and girls with female genital mutilation in the European Union, Norway and Switzerland. *Eur. J. Contracept. Reprod. Health Care*; 21, 474–82. doi:10.1080/13625187.2016.1234597

World Health Organization. 2018. *Care of Girls and Women Living with Female Genital Mutilation: A Clinical Handbook.* World Health Organization: Geneva.

World Health Organization. 2021. *Types of Female Genital Mutilation.* Available at: https://www.who.int/news-room/fact-sheets/detail/female-genital-mutilation [Accessed 17.04.2022].

Section 5:

CULTURE, EQUALITY AND DIVERSITY

19

HOMELESSNESS

LORRAINE JOOMUN

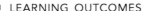 LEARNING OUTCOMES

By the end of this chapter you will be able to:

- Be aware of the causes of homelessness that can be varied and complex, the differing classifications of homelessness and why the statistical data is not an accurate account of the prevalence of homelessness.
- Have an understanding of the health needs of the homeless across the lifespan. The implications for their health and wellbeing including physical, psychological, social and mental health.
- Recognise the importance of attitudes, values and judgements when working with homeless individuals or any marginalised group of people. How poor communication can lead to disengagement, exclusion and lead to worsening health outcomes.
- Discuss the barriers and implications to accessing health and social care services for homeless individuals and how these could be overcome.

Introduction

Homelessness is a major public health issue that has received more Government and media attention over the last decade than it has in previous decades. Homelessness has been a problem for many years and it is estimated that around 227,000 people were experiencing homelessness across the UK in 2021. Homeless people are one of the most marginalised groups in society. Their health and wellbeing is significantly affected because of their homeless status. Not only physical and mental health, but emotional wellbeing, identity and loss. Their wellbeing is aggravated by the stigmatising views of society including attitudes of healthcare professionals. These attitudes contribute to non-engagement by homeless people and forms a barrier to the uptake of health and social care services.

Causes of homelessness

The word 'homeless' is interpreted as being without a home, so if taken literally according to what constitutes a home, a person may have some form of shelter but not necessarily a home. The notion of walls and a roof will not be a 'home' as previously defined. Therefore, a person living in temporary accommodation with none of the comfort of being a 'home' is constitutionally classed as homeless (Kellett and Moore 2003). So contextually according to this definition, they are homeless. There are many interpretations of the meaning of homeless, and some people's understanding is being without a home, therefore living on the streets, which in some cases is true but not in all situations.

Shelter (2017), the housing and homelessness charity, establishes the legal definition of being homeless as not having a home in the UK or anywhere else in the world. Shelter also identify other situations of homelessness, which does not necessarily mean living on the streets. Such as victims of domestic abuse where it is unsafe for the person to stay in the home or where the condition of the home is damaging to their health. Local councils also class persons as homeless if they have no home where the family can live together, or the accommodation is on a temporary basis (Shelter-Cymru 2018). These definitions change the perception of homelessness and can attribute this to the high percentage of people deemed as homeless.

The European Typology on Homelessness and Housing Exclusion (ETHOS) classifies homeless people according to their living situation; for example, rooflessness, without a shelter of any kind, sleeping rough on the streets (FEANTSA 2015). 'Houselessness' is where there is a place to sleep which is temporary or living in a homeless shelter or institution. Other categories are: living in insecure housing; threatened with eviction; a victim of domestic abuse; or living in inadequate housing. These types of inadequate housing are caravans, housing that is in a poor state of repair or where there is severe overcrowding. The media often use the term 'homeless' to describe individuals sleeping rough on the streets. However, the term has a much broader meaning than that. Shelter (2017) differentiates between the 'street homeless' and those living in 'temporary accommodation'. The single homeless are those frequently living on the streets, whereas women with dependent children who become homeless are placed in temporary accommodation. The types of accommodation vary according to the association who is housing the women and consists of voluntary agencies, local authority, housing associations or bed and breakfast accommodation. These do not include those who live in squats or as travellers (Vostanis 2002). Riggs and Coyle (2002) refer to 'hearthlessness' as the absence of any home-like ethos within an accommodation. The hearth represents the focal point of a room that emits warmth and cosiness, which is akin to the feeling of home that this depicts. People living in temporary accommodation, although they have a roof over their head, depict this feeling of hearthlessness as they refer to the accommodation as a house or four walls, but not a home as it lacks this quality. Many individuals and families 'sofa surf'; they reside with family and friends, staying for short periods before moving on to another friend or family member (Clarke 2016). These are the hidden homeless; they are not counted in the homeless data therefore it is difficult to ascertain how many people are actually without a permanent home (Clarke 2016).

Being homeless refers to many different concepts: some would argue that having a roof over your head does not equate to homelessness, while others would challenge this notion. For people living in temporary accommodation the insecurity of moving to different accommodation has the same consequences of being homeless.

Person(s) can be defined homeless for various reasons, for example, those who live in a caravan or boat and are unable to site it, or who have accommodation that is uninhabitable due to poor conditions (Shelter 2017). This can also apply to households unable to live together or with a family member at risk of abuse or violence if they remain in the accommodation. Homelessness is not a choice, it can be the result of rent arrears or flight because of legal or social issues (Daiski 2007). The reasons why people become homeless are often complex and multifaceted; the probable factors include housing arrears, or poor housing drugs and alcohol, mental health issues, relationship breakdown and domestic and neighbour violence. Many studies argue that the majority of women with dependent children are homeless because of relationship breakdown, domestic violence or neighbour violence (Anderson et al. 2006, Axelson and Dail 1988, Tischler and Vostanis 2007, Tischler et al. 2004, 2007, Vostanis 2002).

In today's economic climate, structural factors are principally a cause of homelessness, especially with changes within the labour market such as redundancies and austerity policies. More and more families are losing their homes because of the job situation, being unable to continue mortgage repayments and having their homes repossessed (Queens Nursing Institute 2010). In recent years the cost of housing has increased which makes it even more difficult to find affordable housing as there is an insufficient supply of low-cost housing. Rae and Rees (2015) raises other factors that can predispose to homeless situations, these being poverty, ethnicity, substance misuse and mental health issues. A third factor is housing, which is dependent on supply and financial circumstances of the individual. Eviction from their homes due to mortgage or rental arrears, which can be a subsequent factor of loss of job or income, is a frequent cause of homelessness.

Health needs of women

The impact of homelessness can affect people's sense of autonomy and control over their lives and may lead to poor health outcomes for themselves and their children. Sociological factors include several health outcomes such as mental and physical ill health, drug and alcohol dependence and domestic abuse.

Poor mental health is a well-known risk factor for homeless people (Lauber 2006) and has also been associated with homeless women with dependent children (Tischler 2000, Tischler et al. 2007, Tischler and Vostanis 2007). A study undertaken in the UK using the general health questionnaire reported that the rate of mental illness in homeless mothers was three times higher in the homeless sample compared to those who were housed (Vostanis et al. 1998). A further study undertaken by Vostanis (2002) stated that mental illness in mothers was the strongest predictor of child mental illness. Homeless mothers had similar rates of mental illness to that of single homeless women. Similar results have been reported internationally, many of these studies focused on single homeless adults (Cougnard et al. 2006). There appears to be a higher increase in mental illness among the homeless than among the population in general. It is unclear whether mental illness was a precursor to becoming homeless or whether being homeless led to mental illness. However, several studies identify that homelessness exacerbates mental illness with it being a cycle where one perpetuates (Taylor et al. 2007, Tischler 2000, Tischler and Vostanis 2007, Tischler et al. 2007, Vostanis 2002).

Homeless families are more likely to report substance misuse than low-income families, but less likely than the single homeless. Heavy alcohol intake was also found to be a risk factor. The Fragile Families Dataset proposes that substance abuse is a risk factor for homelessness, with families who have recently become homeless having higher rates than families who are in stable housing (Rog et al. 2008). It is reported that homeless women with dependent children have history of abuse, been in foster care, and substance misuse. Although not all homeless families practise substance misuse, those that do have an added health need which impacts on their mental health.

Pregnant homeless women are also at risk of mental illness and the rate of depression in these women is high (D'Souza and Garcia 2004). Pregnant women who are homeless have an increased risk of poor maternal and child health as there is no guarantee that a permanent home will be found before the baby is born. These women will move frequently and there is no continuity of care during pregnancy (D'Souza and Garcia 2004). Babies may be born preterm of low birth weight and often suffering from the effects of substance misuse or alcohol when born. Once again, the rate of depression in these women is high.

Parents may have already experienced relationship problems between themselves and their children which are then further exacerbated by becoming homeless. The stress of living in temporary accommodation affects the physical, social and psychological ability to cope in this situation, and can lead to unintentional neglect as a result of underestimating the needs of their children. This can lead to a range of parenting issues which, if not identified and appropriate interventions put in place, can compound the situation by causing more distress and dysfunctionalism. A study undertaken by the Scottish

Executive Central Research Unit in 2002 identified that physical and mental health of families deteriorated while in temporary accommodation. Poverty has also been associated with poor mental health in women (Weinreb et al. 2006). Slesnick et al. (2012) suggest that homeless women with dependent children have double the incidence of ill health and hunger than non-homeless families. The relationship between mother and child is often impaired while these families are in temporary accommodation. A study by Tischler et al. (2007) discovered that parenting was being observed by other residents and staff at the hostel, therefore the actions and decisions they took were often judged which consequently influenced their parenting. In such circumstances women felt they lost parental authority which gave way to feelings of hopelessness and failure. 'Public parenting' where shelter staff or others interfere with the discipline of a child can provoke distress, fear and anxiety. Another factor that is influenced by homelessness is the daily routine, which is often controlled by the shelter staff, and mothers report that they have no control over what time the children eat or go to bed. Many of these relationships between mother and child are 'fractured' while they are living in homeless accommodation. So not only are these women traumatised by being homeless, they are also unable to function as parents. The physical and mental health of women who are homeless is of concern especially with the rise in the homeless population. Their health needs are not being addressed adequately, which is likely to have an adverse effect on their children.

These can lead to poor health outcomes in children, including behavioural and emotional disorders and mental ill health. Further evidence shows that children who are exposed to adverse childhood experiences are likely to have poor educational attainment and can become involved in anti-social behaviour and crime, which can lead to these children becoming homeless adults (Public Health Wales 2015).

Children's health

Impairment in parental functioning often occurs when parents have mental health issues, sleep deprivation or other stressors that affect their ability to care for their children adequately. This results in an inability to respond to children's needs or offer protection and can lead to children being unsupervised. Children who are deprived of attention or support can be psychologically affected, and they may have already witnessed domestic abuse or even been physically abused (Hardcastle and Bellis 2019). Women with dependent children who are victims of domestic abuse find themselves in refuges or other homeless accommodation as a means of escaping from a life of abuse or even death. Anooshian (2005) argues that children's behaviour was more aggressive when exposed to domestic violence alongside homelessness. Children then become even more isolated and the incidence of anti-social behaviour increases especially in older children. This study also suggests that parent–child interaction shows aggressive tendencies and therefore demonstrates less warmth in the relationship between parent and child. It is understandable that these children become isolated from peers and use aggression as a form of expression. Another study showed it can also be attributed to modelling where children who have witnessed or experienced violence will copy this behaviour (Bandura 1995).

An earlier study by Vostanis et al. (2001) undertaken with homeless mothers and children found that mental health problems were greater in children who experienced neighbourhood violence or domestic abuse compared to children who were homeless for other reasons. The study found that social, professional or family support had a protective element in relation to mental illness.

Harpaz-Rotem et al. (2006) indicated that housing status such as homelessness in particular was not significantly associated with poor mental health in children. There was a higher incidence of emotional problems such as depression and anxiety in the child if the mother identified as having emotional problems or suffered from mental illness. Children who suffered from physical abuse and had low self-esteem also showed symptoms of depression and anxiety. Children who were homeless presented with behavioural and emotional disorders (Vostanis 2004) and children's behavioural problems were seen to improve once the children were re-housed in a more stable environment, although children showed no improvement in mental health issues after being re-housed. Up to 39% of children had higher levels of mental health problems one year after being re-housed compared to children who were in stable housing but were socio-economically disadvantaged (Vostanis et al. 1998).

Single homeless health needs

Single homeless people often sleep rough, or 'street sleeping' as it is often portrayed by the media. Many sofa surf for a period of time with families or friends until they are encouraged to leave and then find themselves on the street. Living rough leaves them open to the elements, often wet and cold and fearing for their safety. Their health deteriorates over time, often leading to poor mental health including depression, substance misuse and suicide (Riggs and Coyle 2002), higher rates of smoking and increased levels of tuberculosis (TB) (Wright 2014). The incidence of physical illness and non-communicable diseases are higher for individuals who are living rough than for the non-homeless, such as vitamin deficiency, gastrointestinal and cardiac, cancers and hepatitis (Wright and Tompkins 2006). Their early mortality rates are higher as well as accelerated ageing and an increase in long-term health issues (Bradley 2018). They develop respiratory conditions due to sleeping in the cold and wet and have a higher incidence of infections because of the lack of hygiene facilities and the re-using of dirty needles and syringes (John and Law 2011). They also suffer complications of injecting substances, blood-borne viruses, DVT, abscesses and septicaemia (Wright and Tompkins 2006). The list of possible health needs is endless, not discounting infestations such as lice and scabies. Injury and foot problems due to ill fitting shoes, walking, uncut toenails, frostbite, lack of hygiene all contribute to the misery of being homeless.

Older person health needs

The age attributed to homeless people classed as elderly is 50+ years; although this is younger than the more nominal age of 65 it is the marker of old age in the homeless population (Grenier et al. 2016). Homelessness in older people seems to be a growing global problem as a result of population ageing, or natural disasters such as floods, wars, tsunamis and fires. Many other reasons for homelessness in this population are intensified by poverty, rising housing costs, loss of home, death of a spouse, domestic abuse, family breakdown, gambling and alcohol misuse (Crane and Warnes 2010). The health of the older person is akin to other homeless people already discussed in this chapter with the addition of more chronic diseases. Their lifestyle, living conditions and age are compounded by arthritis, diabetes, hypertension, chronic respiratory disease and dental problems. Those living on the streets in damp and wet conditions are prone to leg ulcers, cellulitis exacerbated by poor nutrition (Grenier et al. 2016). Like all homeless people, depression, anxiety and alcohol consumption is also a common theme for the older homeless population. Older people tend to be more unsteady on their feet and prone to fall, and of course this is no different for those who are homeless, often neglecting hygiene and self-care and incontinent when drunk. Although drug misuse is less in this age range, there has been a steady increase in drug taking over the last 10–15 years (Crane and Warnes 2010). Homeless hostels, shelters and B&Bs are often unable to meet the needs of the older person, and they are more at risk of assault, violence and an unsafe environment.

Social exclusion

Homeless people are often discriminated against as they become marginalised and are often excluded by society. Burton and Kagan (2003, p. 5) define marginalisation as 'the state of being excluded from society and classed as an outsider', homeless individuals experience social exclusion like so many other disadvantaged groups such as gypsy travellers and asylum seekers. All these groups are actively mobile and normally have no permanent address. People who are homeless often feel they are being judged by society and professionals alike (Wen et al. 2007). Therefore the attitudes of health professionals are important factors as to whether people access healthcare services or engage with professionals.

Chaturvedi (2014) proposes that negative values and stereotyping portrayed by society on homelessness can impact on the homeless person's self-worth and identity. Homeless people felt they were treated as second-class citizens because of their homeless situation, their care was often compromised and they were disrespected by staff. Negative attitudes from nurses, of not being listened to, was a cause of disempowerment for these people and they became disenchanted with health and social care services and often disengaged. These negative attitudes can act as a barrier to accessing healthcare services.

Barriers to accessing healthcare services

Tischler et al. (2007) found that homeless women with dependent children have difficulty in accessing health, social and educational services. Homeless women and their children usually present at accident and emergency departments for their health care needs rather than accessing primary care services. They are unlikely to take up screening or immunisations and usually access healthcare when symptomatic (Vostanis 2002). Disengagement, especially for women who are suffering from mental health problems, may be the ultimate coping mechanism when they feel out of control (Tischler and Vostanis 2007).

Adverse experiences such as homelessness, family breakdown, abuse, poor education or being in care as a child increases the likelihood of mental health issues, which in turn hinder the individual's ability to cope and to a greater or lesser degree cause difficulties of engagement with social, health and housing agencies (Taylor et al. 2007). The barriers to accessing services are many, such as mobility of homeless people and the lack of flexibility of services across different boroughs and NHS services. The lack of communication and collaboration between professionals hinder access to services for these vulnerable people and therefore resources are not effectively targeted.

Reid and Klee (1999) focused on young homeless people aged between 16–25 years. This age group tended to seek out GP services, however, accident and emergency departments were also used intensively. Reasons why access to GP services were problematic included cost of travel or GP located near family members that caused the homelessness. Deception was sometimes used, such as giving a false address or not stating they were homeless. Many homeless people felt they were discriminated against because of their homeless situation and preventative health services were rarely taken up such as health checks, cervical smears or vaccinations.

Parents who were homeless were fearful of accessing GP services; their perception was that their children would be taken into care. Other barriers were related to time and cost that involved travelling to and from health and social care services and the limited access to telephones making it difficult to make appointments. The high mobility of these people moving from one temporary accommodation to another often resulted in missed appointments. The appointment notification would not always be received as it was usually sent to their previous address. As a result appointments were missed and they were removed from the waiting list. Homeless people had the same issues with social services so were reluctant to contact social services again as they felt they were too 'heavy handed' (Neale et al. 2008, p. 152) and would remove the children.

Other barriers that were a cause for concern for the homeless were lack of money for transport and medication, discrimination by health care professionals, reasons for disengaging with services. When they became sick they were fearful of visiting the hospital or family physician because of the way they were spoken to and judged. Homeless people were reluctant to use the services therefore this affected their health and wellbeing. When health professionals were helpful and compassionate, homeless people returned to use these services as they felt they were not being judged (Reid et al. 2005). Homeless women with dependent children were identified as being the most in need of healthcare. The barriers that were found pertaining to accessing health care services were the mistrust of professionals, financial problems and access to a primary care provider (Hwang et al. 2010).

Barriers to accessing mental health services by homeless people suggests that their needs are not being addressed adequately. The access to medication is one such example, where the need to continue with medication already prescribed is essential. Delays in repeat prescribing occur where GPs need to confirm that the drug had previously been prescribed. This sometimes takes a period of time where GPs need to contact previous primary care services. Women often have a battle where GPs misbelieve the women and are challenged when requesting a repeat prescription. Even providing a previous copy of a prescription is not always proof enough of their honesty, so there seems to be a definite mistrust between the health professional and homeless people. Raising awareness and better communication seems to be the key to working with homeless people in helping them engage with health and social care services.

Conclusion

The health outcomes of the homeless are poor compared to the remainder of the population who are in stable housing. The rates of mental ill health are three times higher than those who are permanently housed. Women are often victims of domestic abuse and users of drugs and alcohol. The dependent children of homeless women also suffer from mental ill health, especially when they have witnessed domestic abuse or neighbourhood violence. Where the mother has emotional problems there is a higher incidence of emotional problems in the child. People who are homeless become socially excluded and they have a sense of not belonging. Homeless people are often victims of negative attitudes and responses from service providers and healthcare professionals are often perceived as not being caring or compassionate, which impacts on the homeless person's self-esteem and self-worth. There appear to be many barriers in accessing healthcare services, which encompass the lack of flexibility of services, communication and collaboration between professionals and mobility of homeless people. These lead to health needs often not being adequately addressed for the homeless population.

Consider the following questions

1. What are the causes of homelessness and why is the rate increasing year on year?
2. Adverse childhood experiences (ACEs) can be compounded by homelessness. Why is this?
3. How can communication be improved to prevent missed appointments by homeless people?
4. As a health professional you have a duty of care for all patients/clients regardless of their social situation. How will you ensure that homeless individuals will get the respect and care they need by you and your colleagues?
5. Mental health issues are a growing concern for adults and children who are homeless. What are the important factors for consideration?

Key terms

Homeless: Being without a home, in temporary accommodation or a victim of domestic abuse where it is unsafe for the person to stay in the home or where the condition of the home is damaging their health where family relationships have become strained and difficult, resulting in a person becoming evicted for non-payment of rent, mortgage or other reasons.

Homelessness: Rough sleeping, no permanent housing and lack of a right to secure housing.

Domestic abuse: An incident or pattern of incidents of controlling, coercive, threatening, degrading and violent behaviour, including sexual violence, in the majority of cases by a partner or ex-partner, but also by a family member or carer.

Houselessness: Where there is a place to sleep which is temporary or living in a homeless shelter or institution. Living in insecure housing, threatened with eviction, domestic abuse or living in inadequate housing such as caravans, unfit housing or severe overcrowding.

Rooflessness: Without a shelter of any kind, sleeping rough on the streets, classifies homeless people according to their living situation.

Hearthlessness: Absence of any home-like ethos within a place of abode.

Sofa surf: Staying with friends or relatives, moving around staying for short periods with either friends or family.

Substance misuse: The use of psychoactive substances in a way that is harmful or hazardous to health. This includes alcohol and illicit drugs.

Adverse childhood experiences (ACEs): Potentially traumatic events that occur in childhood (0–17 years), for example experiencing violence, abuse or neglect. Witnessing violence in the home or community. Having a family member attempt or die by suicide.

Anti-social behaviour: Acting in a way that causes or is likely to cause alarm or distress to one or more people in another household. To be antisocial, the behaviour must be persistent.

Socio-economically disadvantaged: Living in less favourable social and economic circumstances than others in the same society; can include low income and living in a deprived area.

Disempowerment: To take away someone's confidence and feeling of being in control of their life.

Further reading

Crisis. 2018. *Everybody In: How to End Homelessness in Great Britain.* Available at: www.crisis.org.uk/ending-homelessness/homelessness-knowledge-hub/international-plans-to-end-homelessness/everybody-in-how-to-end-homelessness-in-great-britain-2018/ [Accessed 24.06.2018].

Johnson, G., Ribar, D. C., Zhu, A. 2017. *Women's Homelessness: International Evidence on Causes, Consequences, Coping and Policies.* Available at: http://ftp.iza.org/dp10614.pdf [Accessed 24.06.2018].

Tischler, V., Rademeyer, A., Vostanis, P. 2007. Mothers experiencing homelessness: mental health, support and social care needs. *Health and Social Care in the Community*; 15(3), 246–253.

References

Anderson, L., Stuttaford, M., Vostanis, P. 2006. A family support service for homeless children and parents: user and staff perspectives. *Child and Family Social Work*; 11(2), 119–127.

Anooshian, L. 2005. Violence and aggression in the lives of homeless children. *Journal of Family Violence*; 20(6), 373–387.

Axelson, L., Dail, P. 1988. The changing character of homelessness in the United States. *Family Relations*; 37(4), 463–469.

Bandura, A. 1995. Exercise of personal and collective efficacy in changing societies. In A. Bandura (Ed.), *Self-efficacy in Changing Societies*. Cambridge University Press: New York.

Bradley, J. 2018. There is no excuse for homelessness in Britain in 2018. *The BMJ*. Available at: bmj.com/content/360/bmj.k902/rr [Accessed 12.03.2022].

Burton, M., Kagan, C. 2003. Marginalization. In I. Prilleltensky, G. Nelson (Eds), *Community Psychology: In Pursuit of Wellness and Liberation*. MacMillan/Palgrave: London.

Chaturvedi, S. 2014. Homelessness, identity and the therapeutic space. *BACP Children and Young People and Families Journal*; Sept., 26–29.

Clarke, A. 2016. The prevalence of rough sleeping and sofa surfing amongst young people in the UK. *Social Inclusion*; 4(4), 60–72.

Cougnard, A., Grolleau, S., Lamarque, F., Beitz, C., Brugère, S., Verdoux, H. 2006. Psychotic disorders among homeless subjects attending a psychiatric emergency service. *Social Psychiatry and Psychiatric Epidemiology*; 41(11), 904–910.

Crane, M., Warnes, A. 2010. Homelessness among older people and service responses. *Reviews in Clinical Gerontology*; 20(4), 354–363.

D'Souza, L., Garcia, J. 2004. Improving services for disadvantaged childbearing women. *Child Care, Health and Development*; 30(6), 599–611.

Daiski, I. 2007. Perspectives of homeless people on their health and health needs priorities. *Journal of Advanced Nursing*; 58(3), 273–281.

FEANTSA. 2015. *ETHOS – European Typology of Homelessness and Housing Exclusion*. Available at: www.feantsa.org/spip.php?article120 [Accessed 06.01.2016].

Grenier, A., Sussman, T., Barken, R., Bourgeois-Guérin, V., Rothwell, D. 2016. Growing old in shelters and on the street; experiences of older homeless people. *Journal of Gerontological Social Work*; 59(6), 458–477.

Hardcastle, K., Bellis, M. 2019. *Asking About Adverse Childhood Experiences (ACEs) in Health Visiting: Findings from a Pilot Study*. Public Health Wales NHS Trust: Wrexham.

Harpaz-Rotem, I., Rosenheck, R. A., Desai, R. 2006. The mental health of children exposed to maternal mental illness and homelessness. *Community Mental Health Journal*; 42(5), 437–448.

Hwang, S., Ueng, J. J. M., Chiu, S., et al. 2010. Universal health insurance and health care access for homeless persons. *American Journal of Public Health*; 100(8), 1454–1461.

John, W., Law, K. 2011. Addressing the health needs of the homeless. *British Journal of Community Nursing*; 16(3), 134–139.

Kellett, P., Moore, J. 2003. Routes to homelessness and home-making in contrasting societies. *Habitat International*; 27(1), 123–141.

Lauber, C. 2006. Homeless people at disadvantage in mental health services. *European Archives of Psychiatry and Clinical Neuroscience*; 256(3), 138–145.

Neale, J., Tompkins, C., Sheard, L. 2008. Barriers to accessing generic health and social care services: a qualitative study of injecting drug users. *Health and Social Care in the Community*; 16(2), 147–154.

Public Health Wales. 2015. *Adverse Childhood Experiences and their Impact on Health-harming Behaviours in the Welsh Adult Population*. Stationery Office: Cardiff.

Queens Nursing Institute. 2010. *Briefing: Assessing Homeless Families' Health Needs*. Queens Nursing Institute: London.

Rae, B., Rees, S. 2015. The perceptions of homeless people regarding their healthcare needs and experiences of receiving healthcare. *Journal of Advanced Nursing*; 71(9), 2096–2107.

Reid, K., Flowers, P., Larkin, M. 2005. Exploring lived experience. *The Psychologist*; 18(1), 20–23.

Reid, P., Klee, H. 1999. Young homeless people and service provision. *Health and Social Care in the Community*; 7(1), 17–24.

Riggs, E., Coyle, A. 2002. Young people's accounts of homelessness: a case study analysis of psychological well-being and identity. *Counselling Psychology Review*; 17(3), 5–15.

Rog, D. J., Houlpka, C. S., Patton, L. C. 2008. *Characteristics and Dynamics of Homeless Families with Children*. Available at: http://aspe.hhs.gov/hsp/homelessness/improving-data08/report [Accessed 03.07.18].

Scottish Executive Central Research Unit. 2002. *Homeless Families*. Edinburgh: Scottish Government.

Shelter. 2017. *Far from Alone: Homelessness in Britain in 2017*. Available at: https://england.shelter.org.uk/__data/assets/pdf_file/0017/1440053/8112017_Far_From_Alone.pdf [Accessed 20.06.2020].

Shelter-Cymru. 2018. *What is the Legal Definition of Homelessness?* Available at: https://sheltercymru.org.uk/get-advice/homelessness/help-from-the-council/what-will-the-council-check/what-is-the-legal-definition-of-homelessness/ [Accessed 07.02.20].

Slesnick, N., Glassman, M., Katafiasz, H., Collins, J. C. 2012. Experiences associated with intervening with homeless, substance-abusing mothers: the importance of success. *Social Work*; 57(4), 343–352.

Taylor, H., Stuttaford, M. C., Broad, B., Vostanis, P. 2007. Listening to service users: young homeless people's experiences of a new mental health service. *Journal of Child Health Care*; 11(3), 221–230.

Tischler, V. 2000. Service innovations: a mental health service for homeless children and families. *Psychiatric Bulletin*; 24(9), 339–341.

Tischler, V., Karim, K., Rustall, S., Gregory, P., Vostanis, P. 2004. A family support service for homeless children and parents: users' perspectives and characteristics. *Health and Social Care in the Community*; 12(4), 327–335.

Tischler, V., Rademeyer, A., Vostanis, P. 2007. Mothers experiencing homelessness: mental health, support and social care needs. *Health and Social Care in the Community*; 15(3), 246–253.

Tischler, V., Vostanis, P. 2007. Homeless mothers: is there a relationship between coping strategies, mental health and goal achievement. *Journal of Community and Applied Social Psychology*; 17(2), 85–102.

Vostanis, P. 2002. Mental health of homeless children and their families. *Advances in Psychiatric Treatment*; 8(6), 436–469.

Vostanis, P. 2004. The impact, psychological sequelae and management of trauma affecting children. *Child and Adolescent Psychiatry*; 17(4), 269–273.

Vostanis, P., Grattan, E., Cumella, S. 1998. Mental health problems of homeless children and families: longitudinal study. *British Medical Journal*; 316(7135), 899–902.

Vostanis, P., Tischler, V., Cumella, S., Bellerby, T. 2001. Mental health problems and social supports among homeless mothers and children victims of domestic and community violence. *International Journal of Social Psychiatry*; 47(4), 30–40.

Weinreb, L., Buckner, J. C., Williams, V., Nicholson, J. 2006. A comparison of the health and mental health status of homeless mothers in Worcester, Mass: 1993 and 2003. *American Journal of Public Health*; 96(8), 1444–1448.

Wen, C., Hucak, P. L., Hwang, S. W. 2007. Homeless people's perceptions of welcomeness and unwelcomeness in healthcare encounters. *Journal of General Internal Medicine*; 22(7), 1011–1017.

Wright, J. 2014. Health needs of the homeless. *InnovAiT: Education and Inspiration for General Practice*; 7(2), 91–98.

Wright, N., Tompkins, C. 2006. How can health services effectively meet the health needs of homeless people? *The British Journal of General Practice*; 56(525), 286–293.

20

GYPSIES AND TRAVELLERS

DEB MCNEE

━━━━━━━━━━━━━━━ LEARNING OUTCOMES ━━━━━━━━━━━━━━━

- Recognise the specific health needs of Gypsy and Traveller children.
- Appreciate that poverty, discrimination, culture and health beliefs are important determinants of health for this community.
- Identify some of the barriers and facilitators to accessing services.
- Recognise that each family and child is an individual within that community and their unique culture should be supported as such, avoiding stereotyping.

Introduction

It has long been recognised that certain populations have poorer health than others. Governments have sought to tackle this difficult issue; from the Black Report (1980) to the Acheson Report (1998) concluding that health inequalities, including poverty, may be due to culture, socioeconomic status and differing health behaviours. Poverty alone has such a detrimental effect on children, disadvantaging their development, their education, their future relationships and the trajectory of their life course (Marmot et al. 2008). Gypsies and Travellers not only experience poverty but also discrimination, social exclusion, poor health and difficulties accessing services (Smith and Ruston 2013). In fact, health across the life course is generally much poorer when compared to other similar lower socioeconomic population groups (Parry et al. 2007) with increased experiences of long-term illness, disability, anxiety and depression (Cemlyn at el. 2009). The explanations behind these stark health inequalities can be attributed to several multifaceted socioeconomic determinants of health like poverty, poor housing, fewer employment options and lack of education (Marmot et al. 2008), but they may also be a consequence of deeper and more complex cultural issues (Dion 2008).

Gypsies and Travellers are often referred to as a 'hard to reach population' (Goward et al. 2006), making limited use of much-needed health care provision (Van Cleemput et al. 2007). Tudor Hart's (1971) inverse care law exemplifies their predicament in relation to accessing health; he describes how the most needy and vulnerable in society often have the least availability or access to health services. Barriers are complex, but include difficulties with location, provision and health literacy (McFadden et al. 2018), as well as limited cultural understanding and inappropriateness from health professionals (Francis 2013). Smith and Ruston (2013) agree that there is a combined correlation between cultural identity, socioeconomic position and racial discrimination when accessing services. The perceived threat from the outside world described as being the cause for further withdrawal into their own community, thus reducing the access to health information and services.

Defining 'Gypsy and Traveller'

Before defining this population, it is important to remember that every child and every family are different, they have their own identities, beliefs and experiences. The identification of certain characteristics between cultures is useful in understanding opinions, barriers and perceptions; these are essential in providing a culturally competent healthcare support for the community and *with* the community (Francis 2013). In contrast, categorisation of a community or group can potentially risk stereotyping and neglecting intersectionality. Therefore, professionals must be cognisant of this and avoid making presumptions based on a particular site, community or minority group (Cattanach 2020).

The definition describes the largest and most marginalised ethnic minority group in Europe, which includes Romany English Gypsies, Irish Travellers, Welsh Gypsies, Scottish

Gypsies, New Travellers (post-1960s) and Roma migrants from Eastern Europe, in addition to other smaller travelling groups such as Showpeople (Richardson and Ryder 2012). They share similar practices, beliefs, traditions and often their own unique language (Ryder 2011). These significant commonalities in terms of culture and lifestyle are the centrality of family, extended family and community networks; the nomadic way of life; and a strong self-governing work ethic (The Traveller Movement 2021).

The umbrella term often used now is 'Gypsy, Roma and Traveller', recognising the ever-increasing numbers of the Roma community migrating to the UK from Eastern European countries. However, it is imperative that terminology is used with caution and best practice is to ask for preferences when supporting these individual groups. Some are offended by the term 'Gypsy', seeing it as abusive or derogatory, and others are proud to acknowledge their heritage (Bhopal and Myers 2016). Many British communities prefer not to be identified as the generic 'Roma' (House of Commons 2019), presumably due to the desire for recognition of both their individual heritage and birthplace.

There is often a reluctance to self-identify as Gypsy or Traveller to unfamiliar people or on official data collections; this is essentially due to the fear of discrimination and mistrust (Van Cleemput 2018). This adds to the already problematic process of population estimates, with difficulties surrounding poor literacy, language barriers and the logistics of collecting data from both settled and nomadic families. Hence the reason the numbers are thought to be underestimated across the globe. In Europe there are thought to be around 10–12 million Roma (European Commission 2020). In England and Wales the 2011 Census revealed statistics for the first time: 58,000 people identified as Gypsy or Irish Traveller accounting for just 0.1% of the resident population (Office for National Statistics (ONS) 2014). However, this gross underestimation is thought to be well over 400,000 in the UK (McFadden et al. 2018).

Gypsies and Travellers are a recognised ethnic minority group protected under the Race Relations (Amendment) Act 2000 and the Equality Act 2010. As such, an essential requirement when writing about this community is the capitalisation of Gypsy and Traveller, acknowledging their distinct identity and ethnicity (Cromarty 2019).

History, discrimination and nomadism

The history of the Gypsy and Traveller community dates back to the medieval period when records identify the first migration of Gypsies from India into Europe (Marushiakova and Popov 2001). It is impossible to know why they first fled their homelands and historians have many theories including war, famine and epidemics. These dark-skinned and colorfully dressed people brought interest and an air of secrecy wherever they went. In fact their darker complexions led to misperceptions of origin being Egypt, which then prompted the derivation of the term 'Gypsy' (Taylor 2014). In truth, it is more likely that they originated from India as linguistic analysis of the Romani language indicates this. Prejudice appears to have been incipiently evident with few reasons for this but their lifestyle. 'The secret people' may have acquired their reputation of mystery and distrust due to their affinity for fortune-telling and their swift arrival and departure within villages (Keet-Black 2013).

Irish Travellers are thought to have originated in Ireland and have travelled within the UK since the 19th century (Niner 2002). They are a distinctly different group from Gypsies but have some very similar beliefs and traditions.

In contrast, Roma have mostly migrated to the UK since the 1990s. Initially they were seeking asylum from poverty, persecution and racism in Eastern Europe. Later, due to changes in the EU law, many Roma families exercised their legal right to travel and settle in the UK (Brown et al. 2013). Although their desire was for a better quality of life, the stark reality is that many live in poverty and face similar disadvantages to the Gypsy and Traveller populations who were born in the UK (Cook et al. 2010).

Longstanding discrimination has been evident since the 16th century when legislation was passed to remove Gypsies from England; refusal lead to imprisonment, deportation or death. During World War II an unfathomable half a million were murdered, having been escorted to the concentration camps, sometimes in their own caravans (Kenrick 2010).

Contextually, and from a constructivist perspective, it is important to have an awareness of these historical discriminatory events as it exposes some causality regarding trust and privacy. Regrettably this prejudice continues today with reports of bullying in schools, non-inclusive practices and negative attitudes from teaching staff (Bhopal 2011), along with online hate speech via social media where the attacks are often incited by mainstream media (Thompson and Woodger 2020). The launch of the television documentary *My Big Fat Gypsy Wedding* in 2010 promised the viewer an insight into this very secret community; instead, it delivered a far from realistic portrayal and resulted in long-term quantifiable harm including reports of physical and sexual assault, racist abuse and intimidation (Foster 2012). Whilst this is deplorable, it is inconceivable that within the health service where inclusivity is fundamental to the core values, there too are reports of abuse, hostility and judgemental approaches from healthcare staff (McFadden et al. 2018).

Much public and bureaucratic disapproval of the community stems from their travelling lifestyle and inability to find legitimate transitory places to stop (Shubin 2011) with political and legal legislations in place requiring them to move on. This impacts on their traditional nomadic desire which for some is seen more as a psychological and cultural state of mind rather than an act of physically travelling (Liegeois 1986). Some families continue to travel, some live permanently on council or private sites and others are housed (Cromarty 2019).

Housing and family

As the 2011 census evidenced, just over three-quarters of Gypsies and Irish Travellers were living in *conventional* housing and only one-quarter in caravans or temporary structures (ONS 2014). Many feel that the lack of culturally appropriate accommodation provision and restrictions on traditional stopping places has forced them into houses, breaching their cultural identity (Sweeney and Dolling 2021) and directly impacting their physical and mental health, isolating them away from their community networks (Smith and Greenfields 2013). Environmentally, the positive factors of a permanent address include improved living and sanitary conditions, as well as better access to health and education; but the downside is the social segregation and negative impact on health. Compounding this, higher incidence of stress and depression are reported due to permanent relocation, and very often due to the fact that families are moved into deprived estates where discrimination is widespread (Cemlyn et al. 2009). Furthermore, living on an overcrowded 'slab' on a site with inadequate facilities can ecologically impede health. An increased prevalence of infectious diseases and respiratory conditions may be linked to the locations of both unauthorised and authorised sites, which are typically situated alongside busy roads or heavy industrial sites (Greenfields and Brindley 2016).

Gypsy and Traveller culture epitomise all that encompasses the family, children, home and community. Family is fundamental to their identity with expectations that they will be cared for intergenerationally (McCaffery 2014). Births, weddings and funerals are highly celebrated events with many extended family members travelling to attend and fulfilling their role as a member of their distinct ethnic group (Allen and Adams 2012). The population is ever increasing, with higher averages of children born at around four per family (Greenfields 2008). Gender roles tend to be task-specific: the men are responsible for financially supporting the family and will actively search for self-employed work, whilst the women tend to care for the home and family (Cemlyn et al. 2009). These dichotomous constructions may elicit higher expectations on the women who are then responsible for taking care of the children and looking after the home (Levinson and Sparkes 2003). Nonetheless, socialisation of children is restricted to the community, but mainly to the women who view it as an honour as well as an obligation in maintaining cultural heritage (Casey 2014). Children are the centre of the family and for many mothers a 'raison d'être' or reason for existence (Parry et al. 2004). They are prioritised, seldom chastised physically, and independence is encouraged from an early age (Smith 1997). Many mothers find it difficult to even say 'no' to their children, often giving in and complying to their requests in the form of sweets or snacks (Dion 2008). Ominously, this reluctance to set boundaries at an early age, accompanied by the large amount of freedom the children enjoy, could potentially lead to unruly and disruptive behaviour (Reid and Taylor 2007). It could also be indicative of the higher rates of accidents and obesity.

Education and literacy

Within education, Gypsy, Roma and Traveller children are the most at-risk group with the lowest attainment figures and highest number of exclusions (Equality and Human Rights Commission 2019). Explanations for this include withdrawal from school at an early age and high levels of absenteeism (Myers and Bhopal 2009). Primary education is generally more accepted, but things change as the child reaches the age of 'cultural adulthood' by 14 years (Bhopal 2011); there is then an expectation that self-governance is developed and gender becomes more defined. Whereas boys may be required to leave school to follow in their father's trade, it is anticipated that girls should marry young and assume domestic and childcare responsibilities (Hamilton 2016). This pubertal stage of development intensifies cultural concerns from the community around exposure to drugs, alcohol and sexual activity in school, not to mention their assimilatory fear that their child's cultural identity and morals are being eroded (Cudworth 2015). For many families it may be considered that school is no longer a necessity if the child has met a basic level of literacy and numeracy, especially if they perceive education to be dissonant to their culture. Encouragingly though, evidence is emerging that parental attitudes towards continued schooling are changing, particularly for girls (Hamilton 2016).

It appears that while consecutive UK governments have made commitments to improve education provision, they have failed to deliver and the focus now needs to be on the inclusivity, cultural appropriateness and involvement of the family (Hamilton 2016).

Mortality and health

Gypsies and Travellers are believed to have the lowest life expectancy of any group in the UK, at 10–12 years lower than the national average for men and women respectively (Department for Communities and Local Government 2012). Mortality rates in Irish Travellers were nearly three and a half times higher compared to that of the general population. Positively, it was acknowledged that this was a decline of 13% over the previous 20 years, except that the general population dropped by 35% (Abdalla et al. 2010).

Similarly, migrant Roma have a life expectancy 10 years lower than other European citizens, and their child mortality rates are between two and six times higher than the general population of Europe (Migration Yorkshire 2014). The European Commission found health inequalities akin to Gypsies and Travellers with a high prevalence of diabetes, cardiovascular disease, premature myocardial infarction, obesity, asthma and mental health issues (European Commission 2014).

In relation to self-evaluation of general health Gypsies and Irish Travellers rated the lowest (ONS 2014). This is supported by the largest epidemiological study of health by Parry et al. in 2004, confirming that Gypsies and Travellers are known to have the worst health outcomes of all other ethnic groups in the UK (Parry et al. 2004, 2007). Lifestyle behaviours were observed to be unhealthier with higher levels of smoking and therefore, unsurprisingly, higher levels of respiratory and cardiovascular issues.

There is no surprise that mental health is a serious concern within the community as discrimination and racism are known to be causative factors related to depression, anxiety and a higher incidence of substance misuse (Todorova et al. 2010). Suicide is sadly a more common phenomenon among men and some women, with Irish Travellers being three times more likely to take their own lives (Department for Communities and Local Government 2012). These health inequalities are significant, and yet Gypsies and Travellers are omitted from NHS ethnic monitoring codes, resulting in loss of meso-level health data (Millan and Smith 2019) which then impacts on any policy development at macro level.

Children's health

Poorer outcomes exist for birth and maternal health for Gypsies and Travellers, with an excess prevalence of miscarriages, stillbirths, neonatal deaths and infant mortality (Aspinall 2014). The cultural norm of consanguinity continues to be practised and may be the reason for some of these neonatal deaths; it is certainly known to be the cause of some congenital abnormalities (Kalaydjieva et al. 2001).

Obesity is a serious health concern (McGorrian et al. 2012) and 'big' children are often seen as healthy children (Parry et al. 2004). Breastfeeding has many known health benefits as well as reducing the risk of obesity later in life (Zheng et al. 2020) but within this community the rates appeared anecdotally to be extremely low (Dion 2008). Explanations are certainly assumed to be cultural with mothers describing the concept as 'filthy' or 'shameful' referring to the taboo around modesty for women (Dion 2008). In a study by Pinkney (2012) a disappointing 3% of Gypsy and Traveller mothers had breastfed as opposed to 69% of their comparators. Optimistically though were the attitudes of Gypsy and Traveller mothers in their feeding choices with 50% of mothers favouring formula feeding, 45% impartial and 5% favouring breastfeeding. This indicated that a high proportion of mothers appear undecided and therefore could have been potentially influenced to breastfeed their infants. Surprisingly, this study did not consider any cultural barriers that may inhibit breastfeeding uptake, but it did recommend further research in light of this surprising result (Pinkney 2012).

Historically, there has been evidence of vaccination refusal by the community, chiefly in relation to the Pertussis vaccine (Van Cleemput 2000). A lower uptake of immunisations is believed to be due to issues around preference, education, accessibility, literacy and data capture (Dar et al. 2013). More recent studies, however, demonstrated that families do want their children to be immunised to ensure optimum health (Ellis et al. 2020) but with a caveat that they delay the MMR – alluding to the historical unsubstantiated autism scandal.

Child abuse is not specific to certain cultures or ethnicity, but acknowledging the risk in this community is vital due to their minimal exposure to the general population (Van Cleemput 2000) and the inequalities they encounter. Statistics around child protection and care proceedings are again limited, however, there does seem to be a disproportionate growth of children entering state care. Consequently it is imperative that children's services work in partnership with families and are cognisant of the causal factors together with the protective cultural ones (Allen and Riding 2018).

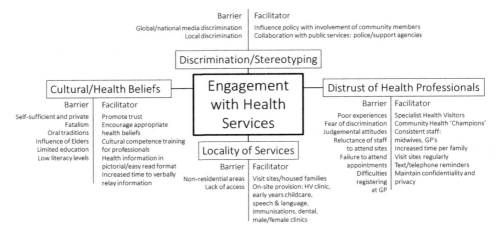

Figure 20.1   Barriers and facilitators to engagement with health services

The role of the health care professional in engaging the community

Deep-seated cultural beliefs and attitudes underpin Gypsy and Traveller health-related behaviours, with the perception that ill health and early death is inevitable (Van Cleemput et al. 2007). This fatalistic approach appears to be perpetuated through oral traditions about health and a lack of empowerment (Dion 2008). Whilst there is a degree of fatalism, Forster (2017) found that this may be accompanied by personal health accountability and self-determination. An inability to access or engage with health services is impacted by social exclusion and discrimination (Van Cleemput 2018). In acknowledging and understanding these barriers, health care professionals have a duty of care in facilitating appropriate and individualised healthcare provision (see Figure 20.1).

Barriers are considerable and complex; they include difficulties registering with GP practices; negative attitudes from staff; reluctance of healthcare professionals to visit sites; lack of continuity of staff; location of services; previous poor experiences of healthcare; and low levels of health literacy (McFadden et al. 2018). Health professionals' failure to understand the cultural needs of the community is also exacerbating these barriers; addressing this through cultural competence training will potentially improve uptake of services (Francis 2013).

Privacy is one of the main concerns for families, requiring sensitive conversations around mental health, sexuality, childbirth and substance misuse (McFadden et al. 2018) and normally with same-gender professionals. This dialogue will sometimes take a degree of trust to be established before any information is given, a prerequisite to successful engagement (Greenfields 2017).

Over the years, key public health strategies aimed at reducing these health inequalities have been implemented to empower communities. Wales took the lead in 2011 with the first national strategy 'Travelling to a Better Future' (Welsh Government 2011).

This comprised of guidance for public services in relation to improved health, education and accommodation. 'Enabling Gypsies, Roma and Travellers' followed in 2018 (Welsh Government 2018) with a greater emphasis on site provision and financial inclusion. This approach has been reflected across the nations with Public Health England publishing their 'NHS Long Term Plan' in 2019, which promises to embed the needs of the Gypsy and Traveller community into policymaking whilst guaranteeing resources being available (NHS England 2019).

Best-practice initiatives that improve uptake of services involve close collaboration with communities, with consistent teams building trust with service users (Greenfields 2017). Provision delivered on site alleviates the issues with access as well as promoting this trust between the family and the health care professional. Provision includes services such as well baby clinics, immunisations and dental care (McFadden et al. 2018). Specialist health visitors are in the privileged position of facilitating this trust as well as being culturally aware of the barriers and facilitators for engagement. Health champions from the community are proven to be trusted mentors and are also able to support families in accessing health, education and housing services (Lally 2014).

Conclusion

Having an awareness of the health and social inequalities experienced by the Gypsy and Traveller community can help to influence inclusive services and future policy, but it is imperative that the community are involved with the planning and that any public health strategies or interventions are culturally appropriate and accessible. By then increasing the uptake of maternity and early years services will certainly improve the health and future outcomes for children, reducing their inequities across the life course. Engagement between families and professionals is only successful if trust is established.

To reflect on Marmot's vision of a fairer world, it should not matter where a child is born, to whom, the colour of their skin or their lack of opportunities; all children should be awarded the right to a healthy life free from discrimination and poverty.

Consider the following questions

When supporting a family in the future:

1. Would you feel confident in recognising and understanding the complex factors preventing them from accessing services?
2. Would you feel empowered to recognise their health needs and implement initiatives to promote health and aid engagement?
3. Would you feel better prepared in reducing the discrimination and stereotyping that exists?

Key terms

Poverty: An inability to afford the basic needs of life, for example food, clothing or shelter.

Discrimination: Treating a person unfairly because of who they are or because they possess certain characteristics.

Health inequalities: The preventable and unfair differences in people's health across the population and between specific communities.

Culture: The ideas, customs and social behaviours of a particular group of people or community.

Ethnic minority: A group of people with a shared culture, tradition, language or history.

Health beliefs: An individual's perception of both their health and illness which ultimately influences their behaviour or lifestyle.

Nomadism: A traditional way of life for some communities where they choose to move from place to place with no permanent settlement.

Privacy: A right to be left alone, a wish to be allowed to enjoy a specific space either on their own or with others.

Social exclusion: The process of isolating and excluding certain groups of people from participating in social, economic, political or cultural life.

Further reading

Allen, D., Adams, P. 2012. *Social Work with Gypsy, Roma and Traveller Children.* CoramBAAF: London.

Friends, Families and Travellers. 2022. *Getting a Fair Deal for Gypsies, Roma and Travellers: Working Towards Equality*. Available at: www.gypsy-traveller.org/ [Accessed 12.03.2022].

Parry, G., Van Cleemput, P., Peters, J., Walters, S., Thomas, K., Cooper, C. 2007. Health Status of Gypsies and Travellers in England. *Journal of Epidemiology and Community Health*; 61(3), 198–204.

References

Abdalla, S., Quirke, B., Daly, L., Fitrzpatrick, P., Kelleher, C. 2010. All Ireland Traveller Health Study: increasing gap in mortality between Traveller and general populations in the Republic of Ireland over two decades. *Journal of Epidemiology & Community Health*; (Sup1), A23.

Acheson, D. 1998. *Independent Inquiry into Inequalities in Health*. Stationery Office: London.

Allen, D., Adams, P. 2012. *Social Work with Gypsy, Roma and Traveller Children.* CoramBAAF: London.

Allen, D., Riding, S. A. 2018. *The Fragility of Professional Competence. A Preliminary Account of Child Protection Practice with Romani and Traveller Children in England*. European Roma Rights Centre: Brussels.

Aspinall, P. J. 2014. *Hidden Needs Identifying Key Vulnerable Groups in Data Collections: Vulnerable Migrants, Gypsies and Travellers, Homeless People, and Sex Workers.* University of Kent: Canterbury.

Bhopal, K. 2011. 'This is a school, it's not a site': teachers' attitudes towards Gypsy and Traveller pupils in schools in England, UK. *British Educational Research Journal*; 37(3), 465–483.

Bhopal, K., Myers, M. 2016. Marginal groups in marginal times: Gypsy and Traveller parents and home education in England, UK. *British Educational Research Journal*; 42(1), 5–20.

Black, D., Morris, J.N., Smith, C. and Townsend, P. 1980. *Inequalities in Health: Report of a Research Working Group.* Department of Health and Social Security: London.

Brown, P., Scullion, L., Martin, P. 2013. *Migrant Roma in the United Kingdom: Population Size and Experiences of Local Authorities and Partners.* Available at: https://pure.hud.ac.uk/en/publications/migrant-roma-in-the-united-kingdom-population-size-and-experience [Accessed 10.04.2021].

Casey, R. 2014. 'Caravan wives' and 'decent girls': Gypsy-Traveller women's perceptions of gender, culture and morality in the North of England. *Culture, Health & Sexuality*; 16(7), 806–819.

Cattanach, J. 2020. Reducing child health inequality among Gypsy Travellers. *Community Practitioner*; 93(1), 45–47.

Cemlyn, S., Greenfields, M., Burnett, S., Matthews, Z., Whitwell, C. 2009. *Inequalities Experienced by Gypsy and Traveller Communities: A Review.* Equality and Human Rights Commission: Manchester.

Cook, J., Dwyer, P., Waite, L. J. 2010. The experiences of Accession 8 migrants in England: motivations, work and agency. *International Migration*; 49(2), 54–79.

Cromarty, H. 2019. *Gypsies and Travellers.* House of Commons Library: London.

Cudworth, D. 2015. Schooling, space and social justice. *Power and Education*; 7(1), 73–89.

Dar, O., Gobin, M., Hogarth, S., Lane, C., Ramsay, M. 2013. Mapping the Gypsy Traveller community in England: what we know about their health service provision and childhood immunization uptake. *Journal of Public Health*; 35(3), 404–412.

Department of Communities and Local Government. 2012. *Progress Report by the Ministerial Working Group on Tackling Inequalities Experienced by Gypsies and Travellers.* Crown: London.

Dion, X. 2008. Gypsies and Travellers: cultural influences on health. *Community Practitioner*; 81(6), 31–34.

Ellis, N., Walker-Todd, E., Heffernan, C. 2020. Influences on childhood immunisation decision-making in London's Gypsy and Traveller communities. *British Journal of Nursing*; 29(14), 822–826.

Equality and Human Rights Commission. 2019. *Is Britain Fairer? The State of Equality and Human Rights 2018.* HMSO: London.

European Commission. 2014. *Roma Health Report Health Status of the Roma Population.* European Union: Brussels.

European Commission. 2020. *EU Roma Strategic Framework for Equality, Inclusion and Participation for 2020–2030.* Available at: https://ec.europa.eu/info/sites/info/files/eu_roma_strategic_framework_for_equality_inclusion_and_participation_for_2020_-_2030_0.pdf [Accessed 9.04.2021].

Forster, N. 2017. Knocking on wood and bucking up your ideas: control and fatalism in Gypsy and Traveller health. *European Journal of Public Health;* 27(3).

Foster, B. 2012. *Bigger Fatter Gypsier.* Report to the Advertising Standards Authority: London.

Francis, G. 2013. Developing the cultural competence of health professionals working with Gypsy Travellers. *Journal of Psychological Issues in Organizational Culture;* 3(S1), 64–77.

Goward, P., Repper, J., Appleton, L., Hagan, T. 2006. Crossing boundaries. Identifying and meeting the mental health needs of Gypsies and Travellers. *Journal of Mental Health;* 15(3), 315–327.

Greenfields, M. 2008. Accommodation needs of Gypsies/Travellers: new approaches to policy in England. *Social Policy and Society;* 7(1), 73–89.

Greenfields, M. 2017. Good practice in working with Gypsy, Traveller and Roma communities. *Primary Health Care;* 27(10), 24–29.

Greenfields, M., Brindley, M. 2016. *Impact of Insecure Accommodation and the Living Environment on Gypsies' and Travellers' Health.* Traveller Movement: London.

Hamilton, P. 2016. School books or wedding dresses? Examining the cultural dissonance experienced by young Gypsy/Traveller women. *Gender and Education;* 30(7), 829–845.

Hart, J. T. 1971. The Inverse Care Law. *The Lancet;* 297(7696), 405–412.

House of Commons. 2019. *Tackling Inequalities Faced by Gypsy, Roma and Traveller Communities.* House of Commons: London.

Kalaydjieva, L., Gresham, D., Calafell, F. 2001. Genetic studies of the Roma (Gypsies): a review. *BMC Medical Genetics;* 2(5).

Keet-Black, J. 2013. *Gypsies of Britain.* Shire: Colchester.

Kenrick, D. 2010. *The A to Z of the Gypsies (Romanies).* Rowman & Littlefield: Plymouth.

Lally, S. 2014. The role of the specialist health visitor when working with Gypsy and Traveller families. *Journal of Health Visiting;* 2(4), 208–213.

Levinson, M., Sparkes, A. 2003. Gypsy masculinity and the home–school interface. *British Journal of Sociology of Education;* 24(5), 587–603.

Liegeois, J. 1986. *Gypsies: An Illustrated History.* Al Saqui Books: London.

Marmot, M., Freil, S., Bell, R., Houweling, T. A. J., Taylor, S. 2008. Closing the gap in a generation: health equity through action on the social determinants of health. *The Lancet;* 372(9650), 1661–1669.

Marushiakova, E., Popov, V. 2001. *Gypsies in the Ottoman Empire.* University of Hertfordshire Press: Hatfield.

McCaffery, J. 2014. Identities, roles and iterative processes: methodological reflections from research on literacy among Gypsies and Travellers. *Research in Comparative and International Education;* 9(4), 375–386.

McFadden, A., Siebelt, L., Jackson, C., Jones, H. et al. 2018. *Enhancing Gypsy, Roma and Traveller Peoples' Trust: Using Maternity and Early Years' Health Services and Dental Health Services as Exemplars of Mainstream Service Provision*. University of Dundee: Dundee. Available at: https://doi.org/10.20933/100001117 [Accessed 12/03/2022].

McGorrian, C., Frazer, K., Daly, L., Moore, R. G., et al. 2012. The health care experiences of Travellers compared to the general population: the All-Ireland Traveller Health Study. *Journal of Health Services Research & Policy*; 17(3), 173–180.

Migration Yorkshire. 2014. *Providing an Effective Health Service for Roma Women in Yorkshire*. Romamatrix: Leeds.

Millan, M., Smith, D. 2019. A comparative sociology of Gypsy Traveller health in the UK. *International Journal of Environmental Research and Public Health*; 16(3), 379.

Myers, M., Bhopal, K. 2009. Gypsy, Roma and Traveller children in schools: understandings of community and safety. *British Journal of Educational Studies*; 57(4), 417–434.

NHS England. 2019. *The NHS Long Term Plan*. Available at: www.longtermplan.nhs.uk/publication/nhs-long-term-plan/ [Accessed 23.04. 2021].

Niner, P. 2002. *The Provision and Condition of Local Authority Gypsy and Traveller Sites in England*. University of Birmingham: Birmingham.

Office for National Statistics. 2014. *2011 Census Analysis: What Does the 2011 Census Tell Us About the Characteristics of Gypsy or Irish Travellers in England and Wales?* Available at: www.ons.gov.uk/peoplepopulationandcommunity/culturalidentity/ethnicity/articles/whatdoesthe2011censustellusaboutthecharacteristicsofgypsyoririshtravellersinenglandandwales/2014-01-21 [Accessed 03.04.2021].

Parry, G., Van Cleemput, P., Peters, J., Moore, J., Walters, S., Thomas, K., Cooper, C. 2004. *The Health Status of Gypsies and Travellers in England*. University of Sheffield: Sheffield.

Parry, G., Van Cleemput, P., Peters, J., Walters, S., Thomas, K., Cooper, C. 2007. Health status of Gypsies and Travellers in England. *Journal of Epidemiology and Community Health*; 61(3), 198–204.

Pinkney, K. 2012. The practice and attitudes of Gypsy and Traveller women towards early infant feeding. *Community Practitioner*; 85(7), 26–29.

Reid, B., Taylor, J. 2007. A feminist exploration of Traveller women's experiences of maternity care in the Republic of Ireland. *Midwifery*; 23(3), 248–259.

Richardson, J., Ryder, A. 2012. *Gypsies and Travellers: Empowerment and Inclusion in British Society*. Policy Press: Bristol.

Ryder, A. 2011. *UK Gypsies and Travellers and the Third Sector*. University of Birmingham: Birmingham.

Shubin, S. 2011. 'Where can a Gypsy stop?' Rethinking mobility in Scotland. *Antipode*; 43(2), 494–524.

Smith, D., Greenfields, M. 2013. *Gypsies and Travellers in Housing: The Decline of Nomadism*. Bristol: Policy Press.

Smith, D., Ruston, A. 2013. 'If you feel that nobody wants you you'll withdraw into your own': Gypsies/Travellers, networks and healthcare utilisation. *Sociology of Health & Illness*, 35(8), 1196–1210.

Smith, T. 1997. Recognising difference: the Romani 'Gypsy' child socialisation and education process. *British Journal of Sociology of Education*; 18(2), 243–256.

Sweeney, S., Dolling, B. 2021. *Last on the List: An Overview of Unmet Need for Pitches on Traveller Sites in England*. Friends, Families and Travellers: Brighton.

Taylor, B. 2014. *Another Darkness, Another Dawn: A History of Gypsies, Roma and Travellers*. Reaktion Books: London.

The Traveller Movement. 2021. *Gypsy Roma Traveller History and Culture*. The Traveller Movement: London. Available at: https://travellermovement.org.uk/about/gypsy-roma-traveller-history-and-culture [Accessed 03.04.2021].

Thompson, N., Woodger, D. 2020. 'I hope the river floods': online hate speech towards Gypsy, Roma and Traveller communities. *British Journal of Community Justice*; 16(1), 41–63.

Todorova, I., Falcón, L. M., Lincoln, A., K., Price, L. L. 2010. Perceived discrimination, psychological distress and health. *Sociology of Health & Illness*; 32(6), 843–861.

Van Cleemput, P. 2000. Health care needs of Travellers. *Archives of Disease in Childhood*; 82(1), 32–37.

Van Cleemput, P. 2018. Health needs of Gypsy Travellers. *InnovAiT*; 11(12), 681–688.

Van Cleemput, P., Parry, G., Thomas, K., Peters, J., Cooper, C. 2007. Health-related beliefs and experiences of Gypsies and Travellers: a qualitative study. *Journal of Epidemiology and Community Health*; 61(3), 205–210.

Welsh Government. 2011. *'Travelling to a Better Future': Gypsy and Traveller Framework for Action and Delivery Plan*. Welsh Government: Cardiff.

Welsh Government. 2018. *Enabling Gypsies, Roma and Travellers*. Welsh Government: Cardiff.

Zheng, M., Cameron, A. J., Birken, C. S., et al. 2020. Early infant feeding and BMI trajectories in the first 5 years of life. *Obesity*; 28(2), 339–346.

21

CULTURE COMPETENCE IN CARE: WORKING WITH BLACK, ASIAN, MINORITY ETHNIC AND FAITH FAMILIES

FATIMA HUSAIN

LEARNING OUTCOMES

By the end of this chapter you will be able to:

* Understand how cultural competence is conceptualised and why it is important.
* Reflect on your own practice and on how to become more culturally competent.
* Understand why cultural competence requires systemic changes.

Introduction

This chapter provides the reader with an understanding of cultural competence and reflects on what it means to be a culturally competent practitioner. Its aim is to help practitioners think through what they and their organisations may need to do to 'respect the inherent dignity and worth of the person' and 'recognize the central importance of human relationships' (National Association of Social Workers (NASW) 2008).

It is important to remember that although this chapter refers to cultural competence in the context of the UK's Black and minority ethnic (BME) communities, the concept and associated frameworks have the potential for much wider application and across a range of sectors, not just health or social care.

Black, Asian and minority ethnic is used instead of the acronym BAME. It is important to note that both acronyms – BME and BAME – are highly problematic and reduce diverse communities into a monolith which is precisely what the cultural competence model seeks to challenge.

Background

The writing of this chapter is foregrounded by an unprecedented pandemic caused by the COVID-19 virus, which has cost many lives worldwide and led to exceptional policy responses: quarantine, self-isolation, lockdown, social distancing and effectively shut down the world's economy and placed intense pressure on healthcare systems. One issue the pandemic has highlighted is persistent inequalities of outcome and the disproportionate impact of the virus.

In any discussion on cultural competence or any similar framework in health and social care there are three issues to think about: the paradigm or model of healthcare; the relationship between health and inequality; and the response of the system in tackling these inequalities.

The current pandemic highlights two of the above, first, that the medical model to intervene and prevent serious illness or death pre-empts everything so any framework to support diverse communities within healthcare settings will be disregarded at some point. This means that a cultural competence framework may be considered by healthcare professionals as an 'add-on' or a 'nice to have' rather than an integral way of operating within a medical model of care.

The second is reflected in a government review which found that the rates of death due to COVID-19 were higher for those from Black, Asian and minority ethnic groups in comparison to white ethnic groups. The review further states that

> the relationship between health and ethnicity is complex and flags that the increased risk of acquiring the infection is linked to people of BAME backgrounds being more likely to live in urban areas, overcrowded households, in deprived areas or work in job roles that could expose them to higher risk. (NHS Confederation 2020)

As a response to this, the NHS Confederation has set up an NHS Race and Health Observatory stating that the impact the pandemic has had on Black, Asian and minority ethnic communities and healthcare staff has highlighted racial inequalities and its root causes (NHS Confederation 2020). However, it is of critical importance to remember that what has been highlighted is not unique to the COVID-19 pandemic but is another reminder of the persistent health disparities experienced by Black people specifically.

The associations between race/ethnicity and health inequalities are complex and a suitable way to understand this complexity is to consider the interaction of socio-economic and individual factors (including help-seeking behaviours, socio-cultural factors and biology/genetics). Socio-economic factors require reflection on individual, family or community journeys of forced movement or planned migration (and possible dislocation) and settlement which may result in socio-economic deprivation such as poor housing, overcrowded living conditions, precarious work and financial disadvantage, all stressors on the mind and body. We know that Black, Asian and minority ethnic groups experience higher rates of poverty than the general population (Parliamentary Office of Science & Technology (POST) 2007), with British Bangladeshi groups experiencing the highest level of socio-economic disadvantage. The evidence indicates that South Asians have been found to have lower access to care for coronary heart disease but are 50% more likely to have a heart attack or angina. Grey et al.'s (2013) review on mental health inequalities found that in comparison to white people, more BME people are diagnosed with mental health issues every year.

Ethnic and racial inequalities in health outcomes in the UK broadly reflect racial biases in the USA healthcare system. It suffices to say that the evidence presents a stark picture of deficient health care through the life course: maternity care (Anekwe 2020), peri-natal depression (Edge 2011) mental health support (Bignall et al. 2019) and old age (Evandrou et al. 2016). The key issue of concern is to how the system responds to (and redresses) these. By 'the system' we mean all the institutions, their policies and procedures that are used to implement a service that is publicly available. This concerns primarily organisations and entities supported by the state through public funds but may include private sub-contractors within the system. Although this chapter focuses on health and social care, it can be applied to education, policing, welfare and employment support, and the range of preventative support services that are available to children, young people and their families. Grey et al. (2013) state that barriers to accessing services include a lack of cultural understanding, poor communication about where and how to seek help, and inadequate referrals. For example, we know that Black and Asian groups access primary care at rates as high as the general population (in relation to need) but access to hospital care is lower (King's Fund 2006). Thornton (2000) reports that disparities between Black and minority ethnic patients and their white counterparts are evident in the mental health care they receive – from assessment, diagnosis through to treatment.

It is important to note the systemic nature of these disparities. The King's Fund (2006) states that there is evidence which indicates that the NHS has not catered well to Britain's 'diverse' population. The Department of Health's patient surveys (2009, 2021) reveal a consistent pattern of higher levels of dissatisfaction amongst minority ethnic groups when compared with the white majority. Blake et al. (2016) noted unresponsive services, staff who feel ill-equipped to address diversity, and the application of cultural assumptions in the provision of care, resulting in Black, Asian and minority ethnic service users feeling unheard or seemingly invisible within systems of care.

An overview of anti-discriminatory practice

Any discussion of cultural competence (first developed as a concept within social work practice in the USA) needs to be considered in the context of the UK's approach to addressing diversity and difference. The first point to consider is legal protection under the Equality Act 2010, which consolidated and supersedes all previous anti-discrimination legislation (Sex Discrimination Act 1975, Race Relations Act 1976, and the Disability Discrimination Act 1995) and protects a set of characteristics. Because this chapter focuses on cultural competence as it relates to Black, Asian and minority ethnic communities, the protected characteristics of interest are race including colour, nationality, ethnic or national origin and religion or belief. This does not preclude the reader from incorporating other protected characteristics in their reflections and practice.

The second point is the history of anti-discriminatory practice based on different theoretical approaches, primarily in the context of social work education and social care provision. These approaches ranged from an assimilationist approach which resulted in a cultural deficit model being used, to a Black professional model which combined an understanding of lived experiences, power relationships and discriminatory practice. Ely and Denney (1987) provide an excellent overview.

However, Williams and Bernard (2018) observe that from the late 1990s anti-racist practice came under criticism for its focus on race and Black perspectives, with calls for a more encompassing conceptualisation of anti-discriminatory practice. Some argued that cultural beliefs and practices needed more emphasis whilst others such as Mullaly (2002) contended that theoretical frameworks need to consider multiple forms of oppressions including sex, class, age and disability.

Barriers to care

Practice, however, has tended to remain in a 'multi-cultural limbo' (Becher and Husain 2003), acknowledging the importance of 'culture' but unable to build skills in analysing cultural information and relating it directly to a family's lived experiences. Additionally, practice labelled 'culturally sensitive' often fails to account for the diverging biographies and distinct value systems of individuals and families as distinct units within their community. Critically, such services have often relied on an essentialist notion of cultural values and practices. Veering towards a cultural deficit model (i.e. the problem lies in people's cultural values and practices), this approach assumes that individuals passively receive and incorporate a fixed set of normative practices and 'culture' into their every-day life. This has frequently resulted in 'culturally' inappropriate service interventions with little reflection on systemic disparities.

Evidence suggests that some of these barriers in service provision persist despite developments in theory and policy, due to:

- A lack of agreement and a unified understanding of what needs to happen at every level of service delivery.
- Uncertainty about who should act and when.
- Existing tools and processes within a service not being appropriate.
- An unwillingness or inability to promote organisational cultural change.

More recent evidence, based on research conducted at a regional or local authority level, suggests that some of the longstanding barriers have yet to be adequately addressed. These include limited access to interpretation services and information, problems with intercultural understanding (Chantkowski 2014) and issues such as cultural naivety, insensitivity and discrimination towards 'BME' service users (Memon et al. 2016). With reference to mental health services (although this can be applied more widely) Edge and MacKian (2010) suggest that to reduce inequalities, more responsive and culturally appropriate approaches are needed. A conclusion of an EHRC review is stark: 'without a major re-think by new health bodies on how they tackle discrimination and advance equality some groups will continue to experience poorer health' (Widger et al. 2011).

It is within the context of existing frameworks not being wholly suitable, the narrative shift from 'anti-discriminatory' practice to 'culture', and the persistence of barriers to care experienced by BME communities that the concept of cultural competence (Cross et al. 1989; Campinha-Bacote 1999) initially started gaining favour in the UK. And it may yet, if properly operationalised with institutional or systemic cultural competence at its core, present a way to adjust systems of care and professional practice so that Black, Asian and minority ethnic groups are seen and heard.

Unpacking the cultural competence model

Arising out of cultural pluralism (multi-cultural theories in the UK), the underlying premise of the cultural competence model (Cross et al. 1989) is that how people live their lives is shaped by their specific beliefs, values and cultural practices. The additional premise is that this applies equally to practitioners (as individuals) and to the systems within which they practise. Kohli et al. (2010) traced the historical development of cultural competence and assert that the key to this framework is a reflexive-dialectic stance which involves carefully examining multiple perspectives and experiences and acknowledging that no one is born culture-less or identity-less.

Within this model, culture is broadly defined by Cross et al. (1989) as

> the integrated pattern of human behaviour that includes thoughts, communications, actions, beliefs, customs, values, and institutions of a racial, ethnic, religious or social group.

It is important to note that 'culture' is a highly problematic concept which can lead to interpretations of behaviours among groups and individuals as fixed over time. As a catch-all concept, it can hide differences of faith and the practice of religious and cultural rituals. Importantly, it deflects from systemic anti-blackness and embedded racial discrimination by de-emphasising structural biases which are persistently experienced by Black and Asian people. A contemporary related issue is that of discussions and narratives about a problematic 'Muslim community'. This leads to people making assumptions about Muslims in relation to how they behave and what they practise – about 'Islamic culture' – which leads a highly diverse community to be treated as one group with the same practices. This then means that structural biases in relation to race and ethnicity are ignored, and a fixed concept of a problematic culture becomes embedded in people's thinking and practice. This positions Black and Asian groups in particular as the 'other' with institutional normative practice viewed as a culture and ethnicity-free frame of reference. A persistent example of this relates to women's bodies and the stigmatisation of clothing (rooted also in cultural practices) worn by some Muslim women. UK Prime Minister Boris Johnson referred to women who wear the *niqab* (a flowing robe including a head and face covering with only the eyes visible) as 'letter boxes' (Daily Mail, August 6, 2018) and brushed aside accusations of racism and Islamophobia, or the curious situation in France where politicians spent a substantial amount of public resources to legislate against the clothing of a few hundred women so that Muslim women who wear a *niqab* in public are fined while other people (due to coronavirus measures) are fined for not wearing a face covering (masks) (Euronews 28 September, 2020). These types of actions essentialise socio-religious practices by a minority and create an environment where prejudiced speech and actions against Muslims are considered acceptable and the systemic nature of discrimination (and misogyny) is ignored.

Critical to the conceptualisation of 'cultural competence' is that culturally prescribed behaviour is situational rather than static and can be modified by individual characteristics as well as contextual social factors (Lynch and Hanson 2003). Within the model, it then becomes the responsibility of practitioners to dissect what culture may mean and then assess the salience of different aspects of 'culture' in people's lives. The Merriam Webster Dictionary defines competence as 'the quality or state of being competent: such as the quality or state of having sufficient knowledge, judgment, skill, or strength' (https://www.merriam-webster.com/dictionary/competence). Lum (2000) cited in Kohli et al. (2010) suggests that competence in the context of this model relates to capability, sufficiency and adequacy in how practitioners relate to and support those from cultural backgrounds that are different from their own. In relation to professional practice, competence can be described as the capacity to function appropriately as an individual, and as an organisation by taking into account clients' lived experiences to meet the demands of a particular situation (Smith 1998).

When defining cultural competence, it is fair to acknowledge that there is no standard or widely accepted definition of cultural competence. One of the earliest definitions set out by Cross et al. (1989) states:

> Cultural competence is a set of congruent behaviors, attitudes, and policies that come together in a system, agency or among professionals and enable that system, agency or those professions to work effectively in cross-cultural situations.

Subsequently, cultural competence was defined in the broadest terms as the ability to respond to the unique needs of individuals and families and thus support and sustain clients within their appropriate cultural context (McPhatter 1997). A more encompassing definition set out by the Council on Social Work Education and quoted by Kohli et al. (2010) defines it as

> the ability of professionals to function successfully with people from different cultural backgrounds including, but not limited to, race, ethnicity, culture, class, gender, sexual orientation, religion, physical or mental ability, age, and national origin.

What these definitions do is place the responsibility squarely on the shoulders of professionals to engage in reflexive-dialectic practice, requiring practitioners to think about how one's own positioning shapes practitioner–service user interactions. Kholi et al. (2010) explain that this type of approach would enable practitioners to more easily work with diverse individuals and families.

Although the literature on cultural competence in social work is more extensive, it has also been promoted within healthcare settings (Campinha-Bacote 1999, Betancourt et al. 2002). For healthcare, Betancourt et al. (2002) describe cultural competence as the ability of providers and organisations to effectively deliver health care services that meet the social, cultural and linguistic needs of patients. Irrespective of the definitions used, cultural competence is described as a process or a journey of 'becoming', not as a state of 'being' (Cross et al. 1989, Campinha-Bacote 1999).

The basic cultural competence model as conceptualised by Cross et al. (1989) comprises three components – knowledge, awareness and sensitivity – each of which is briefly explained below.

Cultural knowledge

This component of the model requires organisations and practitioners to familiarise themselves with the background, practices and values of the individuals and families they serve and the communities within which they work. As a starting point, the acquisition of cultural knowledge requires the collation of local cultural, linguistic and demographic profiles. It entails seeking information about culturally patterned behaviours, values, belief systems and the migration and settlement histories of communities. It includes knowledge and understanding of the dynamic nature of cultural interaction. Acquiring cultural knowledge in itself can be highly problematic as it can lead to essentialist stereotyping of individual, families and communities. An example of the problematic nature is the labelling of communities and families as 'hard to reach' or 'they take care of their own' which may lead to little or no effort on the part of professionals to adapt practices to include these groups.

Cultural awareness

This second component needs to be developed alongside the acquisition of cultural knowledge. Cultural awareness is about challenging the notion of static cultures and using one's own cultural practices as a fixed frame of reference from which to view and potentially judge others. This requires awareness of one's own cultural beliefs and practices, biases or prejudices, and is rooted in respect, validation and openness toward differences among people. Acquiring cultural awareness means recognising that there is more than one way of doing things and that others may believe in different truths/realities (Kholi et al. 2010). The notion of reflexivity is critical to the development of cultural awareness.

Reflexivity can be described as the ability to think critically about one's own assumptions and values and monitor our own actions. By thinking about and questioning these assumptions, values and actions it is possible to become open to other, alternative possibilities. A reflexive approach can be applied at:

- An individual professional level, by acknowledging that what we know about ourselves and about other people may not be objective fact but comprises constructed social realities that can change.
- An organisational level, by questioning policies and practices and devise constructive ways to develop and modify organisational structures.
- The level of practitioner–client interaction, by practitioners thinking about their assumptions of a particular situation, and how these might affect the intervention process and influence health and/or social care outcomes.

It is important to note that reflexivity differs from reflection in that reflection is about assessing and understanding a situation 'from a distance'. Reflexivity, on the other hand, is about being an 'active subject' and critically examining how one's own social realities affected that situation. Cultural awareness, underpinned by the notion of reflexivity, is therefore considered essential for developing a sensibility to diversity and difference that questions ethno-centrism (see Key Terms at the end of the chapter).

Cultural sensitivity

The third component, cultural sensitivity, is the ability to change working practices and develop skills and strategies to work positively with cultural differences. At the organisational level this relates primarily to customising services to reflect diversity within and between cultures. Sensitivity refers also to a practitioner's attitude to each client's cultural uniqueness and the ability to 'relate to clients in culturally relevant and appropriate ways' (Cummins 2003). In relation to working with Black, Asian and minority ethnic families, it involves understanding the complexity and contradictions inherent in people's lives and requires a determination not to assign judgemental values (good/bad; right/wrong).

Cultural competence model as a system of care

As depicted in Figure 21.1 it is at the intersection of these three components – knowledge, awareness and sensitivity – that cultural competence practice is achieved.

As a system of care, the literature suggests that cultural competence requires the integration and transformation of knowledge about individuals and groups of people into specific standards, policies and practices that are used in appropriate cross-cultural settings to increase the quality of services so that better outcomes may be achieved for those in need. At the organisational level applying a cultural competence model would require not just an interrogation of existing strategies, policies, operational plans and professional training but also the adaption of these into a system of practice. The measures put in place, such as interpretation services or community mentors, is likely to vary by the types of services available and the groups and families served. Each measure put in place has to be interrogated to assess the risks – and operationalising a culturally competent model means that 'practice is driven in service delivery systems by client preferred choices, not by culturally blind or culturally free interventions' (NCCC 2017).

It is important to note that cultural competence is not an individual task that a practitioner undertakes on their own, it is both a collective (organisational) and individual effort. It requires training and organisational support, and a commitment to reflect the diversity of the communities being served. However, ethnic matching of client to practitioner can be problematic and is no substitute for training and embedding cultural competence practice within a system of care.

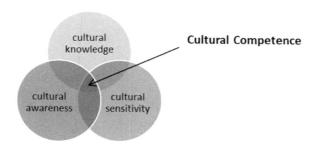

Figure 21.1 The cultural competence model

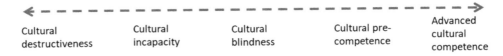

| Cultural destructiveness | Cultural incapacity | Cultural blindness | Cultural pre-competence | Advanced cultural competence |

Figure 21.2 Achieving cultural proficiency by applying the cultural competence model (adapted from Cross 2012)

As indicated earlier in the chapter, cultural competence needs to be considered a process in which 'the practitioner continuously strives to achieve the ability to effectively work within the cultural context of an individual family or community with a diverse cultural or ethnic background' (Campinha-Bacote et al. 1996). Cross (2012) articulates this process as a five-stage continuum (see Figure 21.2) which applies equally to organisations and individual practitioners. Referring back to the concept of reflexivity, it is important to note that Cross (2012) describes this as an on-going, continuous process of striving for competence: 'No matter how proficient an agency may become, there will always be room for growth'.

Adding to the model: additional concepts

Having described the three core components of the cultural competence model above, there are additional aspects which have more recently been referred to in relation to the model: cultural respect, cultural humility and linguistic competence. Any model would need to incorporate anti-racist practice and, more specifically, address anti-Black racism. A full discussion of these is beyond the scope of this chapter, however Figure 21.3 shows how these can be incorporated into the core model.

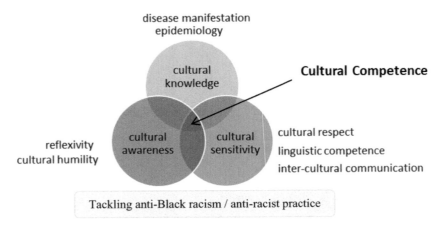

Figure 21.3 Expanding the cultural competence model

Discussion

In the previous sections we summarised how the theoretical approach to social work practice has developed in the UK, from a cultural deficit model through to Black perspectives and more recently cultural competence. The different approaches and the evolution of practice is influenced by political theory and policy formulations of the type of diverse and inclusive society we want to live in. Cultural competence in healthcare mirrors the developments in social care, with the added complexity of the medical model of care which focuses on the absence of illness and disease as overriding all other ways of supporting and caring for diverse groups.

In considering the three components of the cultural competence framework, four key assumptions stand out for the individual practitioner. First, systemic change, which examines the cultural premises upon which practices and organisations are built and maintained, is needed. Second, diverse worldviews need to be incorporated into practice too because reality is socially constructed based on individual experiences and established cultural practices. Third, practitioner–service user interactions are underpinned by a relationship of power which needs to be challenged. For practitioners, the concept of cultural awareness can guide a critical exploration of their social and professional positioning. Kohli et al. (2010) assert that the socio-cultural realities of both practitioners and service users are integral to culturally acceptable service delivery. Fourth, the cultural competence model requires collective actions to change culture and learning at an organisational level. Seeleman et al. (2009) suggest that the cultural competence model can be incorporated into healthcare settings and should include knowledge of epidemiology and disease manifestation in diverse groups. To counter criticism of the shift to culture, Abrams and Moio (2009) suggest incorporating concepts from Critical Race Theory, the core premise of which is that even though there is equality legislation, outcomes for racialised groups are different and require concerted effort to recognise this and not subsume 'difference' within a colour-blind 'culture' category. For example, we know that the experiences and outcomes for a Black British woman (of Kenyan background) are different from those of an Asian woman of Indian background (originally from Kenya also). The reason for this is that approaches to practice are formed within systems and structures built on anti-Black racism and racialised oppression.

Brach and Fraser (2000) note that while there is substantial research evidence to suggest that the cultural competence framework should in fact work, there is little evidence about which cultural competency techniques are effective and when and how to implement them properly.

A range of tools to measure aspects of cultural competence both at practitioner and organisational level are available in the USA where the cultural competence framework has been implemented in many social and health care settings. However, the lack of evidence on 'what works' may hinder a wider adoption of the approach. In the UK cultural competence remains largely conceptual and few attempts have been made to develop specific tools, such as the family support toolkit by Husain (2007). Moreover, there is little evidence to show whether it improves social and health care outcomes for Black,

Asian and minority ethnic groups. It is therefore fair to say that until the cultural competence model is applied systematically, and different variations tested, it will likely remain as a concept people refer to but are unwilling or unable to fully put into practice.

Conclusion

This chapter has taken the reader on a conceptual journey to explain the foundations of cultural competence. It provides a basis for students and practitioners to reflect on their own cultural positioning and how they interact with those considered 'different' and supports critical reflection of how their teachers, mentors and supervisors approach practice with diverse racialised and ethnic groups. Its core intent has been to build understanding of the ethos, values and attitudes needed to place a service user or patient fully at the centre of the care offered.

Consider the following questions

To consolidate and extend your learning from this chapter consider these questions:

1. Why are the terms Black and minority ethnic (BME) and Black, Asian and minority ethnic (BAME) problematic?
2. Why is the notion of 'culture' problematic?
3. What are the issues in moving from anti-racist approaches to the concept of culture?
4. What is needed for services to tackle systemic anti-Black racism and become more culturally competent?
5. Reflecting on the stages to achieving cultural competence, where would you place yourself?

Key terms

BME: Black and minority ethnic

BAME: Black, Asian and minority ethnic

Ethno-centrism: Viewing and judging other cultures based on preconceptions originating in the standards and customs of one's own culture. These preconceptions can be supported by wider public discourses, whereas cultural pluralism recognises the strengths of other cultures or cultural practices in their own right and values the differences.

Critical Race Theory: A framework to examine racialised systems based on a reflection that although Black people are equal under the law, they experience worse outcomes across a range of systems than their white 'equal' counterparts.

Further reading

Aymer, C., Okitikpi, T. 2009. *Key Concepts in Anti-discriminatory Social Work*. Sage: London.

Bronheim, S. n.d. *Cultural Competence: It All Starts at the Front Desk*. National Center for Cultural Competence: Washington, DC. Available at: https://nccc.georgetown.edu/documents/FrontDeskArticle.pdf [Accessed 12.03.2022].

Garran, A., Werkmeister Rozas, L. 2013. Cultural competence revisited. *Journal of Ethnic and Cultural Diversity in Social Work*; 22(2), 97–111. doi: 10.1080/15313204.2013.785337

Sharifia, N., Adib-Hajbaghery, M., Najafic, M. 2019. Cultural competence in nursing: a concept analysis. *International Journal of Nursing Studies*; 99. doi.org/10.1016/j.ijnurstu.2019.103386www.gov.uk/discrimination-your-rights

References

Abrams, L., Moio, J. 2009. Critical race theory and the cultural competence dilemma in social work education. *Journal of Social Work Education*; 45(2), 245–261. doi: 10.5175/JSWE.2009.200700109

Anekwe, L. 2020. Ethnic disparities in maternal care. *BMJ*; 368. doi: m442

Becher, H., Husain, F. 2003. *South Asian Hindus and Muslims in Britain: Developments in Family Support*. NFPI: London.

Betancourt, J., Green, A., Carrillo, J. 2002. *Cultural Competence in Health Care: Emerging Frameworks and Practical Approaches*. The Commonwealth Fund: New York.

Bignall, T., Jerai, S., Helsby, E., Butt, J. 2019. *Racial Disparities in Mental Health: Literature and Evidence Review*. The Race Equality Foundation: London. Available at: https://raceequalityfoundation.org.uk/wp-content/uploads/2020/03/mental-health-report-v5-2.pdf [Accessed 12.03.2022].

Blake, M., Bowes, A., Gill, V., Husain, F., Mir, G. 2016. A collaborative exploration of the reasons for lower satisfaction with services among Bangladeshi and Pakistani social care users. *Health and Social Care in the Community*; 25, 1090–1099. doi.org/10.1111/hsc.12411

Brach, C., Fraser, I. 2000. Can cultural competency reduce racial and ethnic health disparities? A review and conceptual model. *Medical Care Research and Review*; 57 (Supp. 1), 181–217. doi: 10.1177/107755870005700109

Campinha-Bacote, J. 1999. A model and instrument for addressing cultural competence in health care. *Journal of Nursing Education*; 38(5), 203–207. doi.org/10.3928/0148-4834-19990501-06

Campinha-Bacote J., Yahle T., Langenkamp M. 1996. The challenge for cultural diversity for nurse educators. *The Journal of Continuing Education in Nursing*; 27, 59–64.

Chantkowski, M. 2014. *BME People and Access to Health and Wellbeing Services in Sunderland: A Report from BME Engagement Events*. North East Community Solutions CIC, on behalf of Healthwatch Sunderland.

Cross, T. 2012. Cultural competence continuum. *Journal of Child and Youth Care Work*; 24, 83–86.

Cross, T., Bazron, B., Dennis, K., Isaacs, M. 1989. *Towards a Culturally Competent System of Care, Volume 1*. Georgetown University Child Development Center: Washington, DC.

Cummins, L. 2003. *Multicultural Competence in Social Work Practice*. Allyn and Bacon: Toronto.

Daily Mail (6 August, 2018) https://www.dailymail.co.uk/news/article-6030927/Boris-Johnson-says-burka-makes-women-look-like-bank-robbers-letter-boxes.html

Department of Health. 2009. *Report on the Self-reported Experience of Patients from Black and Minority Ethnic Groups*. Department of Health: London. Available at: https://assets.publishing.service.gov.uk/government/uploads/system/uploads/attachment_data/file/213375/BME-report-June-09-FINAL3.pdf

Department of Health. 2021. https://www.ethnicity-facts-figures.service.gov.uk/health/patient-experience/inpatient-satisfaction-with-hospital-care/latest

Edge, D. 2011. It's leaflet, leaflet, leaflet then, 'see you later': Black Caribbean women's perceptions of perinatal mental health care. *British Journal of General Practice*; 61(585), 256–262.

Edge, D., MacKian, S. 2010. Ethnicity and mental health encounters in primary care: help-seeking and help-giving for perinatal depression among Black Caribbean women in the UK. *Ethnicity and Health*; 15(2), 93–111.

Ely, P., Denney, D. 1987. *Social Work in a Multiracial Society*. Gower: Aldershot.

Euronews (28 September, 2020) https://www.euronews.com/my-europe/2020/09/23/has-covid-19-destroyed-the-case-for-banning-the-burqa-in-europe

Evandrou, M., Falkingham, J., Feng, Z., Vlachantoni, A. 2016. Ethnic inequalities in limiting health and self-reported health in later life revisited. *Journal of Epidemiology and Community Health*; 70(7), 653–662. doi:10.1136/jech-2015-206074

Grey, T., Sewell, H., Shapiro, G., Ashraf, F. 2013. Harnessing diversity: mental health inequalities facing UK minority ethnic populations causal factors and solutions. *Journal of Psychological Issues in Organizational Culture*; 3(S1), 146–157. doi: 10.1002/jpoc.21080

Husain, F. 2007. *Cultural Competence in Family Support: A Toolkit for Working with Black, Minority Ethnic and Faith Families*. NFPI: London.

King's Fund. 2006. *Briefing: Access to Health Care and Minority Ethnic Groups*. Available at: www.kingsfund.org.uk/sites/default/files/field/field_publication_file/access-to-health-care-minority-ethnic-groups-briefing-kings-fund-february-2006.pdf [Accessed 01.07.2020].

Kohli, H., Huner, R., Faul, A. 2010. Historical and theoretical development of culturally competent social work practice. *Journal of Teaching in Social Work*; 30, 252–271. doi.org/10.1080/08841233.2010.499091

Lum, D. 2000. *Social Work Practice and People of Color: A Process Stage Approach*. Wadsworth: Belmont, CA.

Lynch, E., Hanson, M. 2003. *Developing Cross-cultural Competence: A Guide for Working with Children and Their Families.* Paul Brookes Publishing: Baltimore, MD.

McPhatter, A. R. 1997. Cultural competence in child welfare: What is it? How do we achieve it? What happens without it? *Child Welfare*; 76(1), 255–278.

Memon, A., Taylor, K., Mohebati, L., Sundin, J., Cooper, M., Scanlon, T., de Visser, R. 2016. Perceived barriers to accessing mental health services among black and minority ethnic (BME) communities: a qualitative study in southeast England. *BMJ Open*; 6(11), e012337.

Mullaly, B. 2002. *Challenging Oppression: A Critical Social Work Approach.* Oxford University Press Canada: Don Mills.

National Association of Social Workers (NASW). 2008. *Code of Ethics.* NASW: Washington, DC.

NCCC. 2017. *Developing Organizational Policies that Reflect the Values of Cultural and Linguistic Competence.* Available at: https://nccc.georgetown.edu/leadership/documents/2017April13ForumPPT.pdf [Accessed 01.07.2020].

NHS Confederation. 2020. PHE 2020 Disparities in risks and outcomes of Covid-19. Available at: www.nhsconfed.org/resources/2020/06/phe-review-disparities-in-risk-and-outcomes-of-COVID19 [Accessed 01.12.2020].

Parliamentary Office of Science and Technology (POST). 2007. *Ethnicity and Health, Post Note No. 276.* Available at: https://post.parliament.uk/research-briefings/post-pn-276/ [Accessed 01.01.2021].

Seeleman, C., Suurmond, J., Stronks, K. 2009. Cultural competence: a conceptual framework for teaching and learning. *Medical Education*; 43, 229–237. doi:10.1111/j.1365-2923.2008.03269.x

Smith, L. 1998. Concept analysis: cultural competence. *Journal of Cultural Diversity*; 5(1), 4–10.

The Equality Act. 2010. https://www.legislation.gov.uk/ukpga/2010/15/contents

Thornton, J. 2020. Ethnic minority patients receive worse mental healthcare than white patients, review finds. *BMJ*; 368. doi: m1058

Widger, T., Prosser, S., Rogers, S., Hutton, C., 2011. *The Performance of the Health Sector in Meeting the Public Sector Equality Duties: Moving Towards Effective Equality Outcomes.* A Focus Consultancy Report. Equality and Human Rights Commission: London.

Williams, C., Bernard, C. 2018. Black history month: a provocation and a timeline. *Critical and Radical Social Work*; 6(3), 391–406.

22

PUBLIC HEALTH AND THE LGBTQ+ COMMUNITY

DAVE CLARKE

━━━━━━━━━━ LEARNING OUTCOMES ━━━━━━━━━━

By the end of this chapter you will be able to:

- Be aware of LGBTQ+ history and rights campaigning.
- Understand the legal and political position of LGBT people in society.
- Develop awareness of LGBT health inequalities.
- Consider how health and social care practice for LGBT people can be inclusive.

Introduction

The lives of lesbian, gay, bisexual, transgender, queer + (LGBTQ+) people have changed extraordinarily over the last 50 years as society's awareness of and attitudes towards those who identify as LGBTQ+ have changed and become more accepting. The European Social Survey (2020) found that between 2002 and 2014 the proportion of respondents who agreed or strongly agreed that those who identify as lesbian or gay should be free to live as they wish increased from 73% to 81.1%. Analysis of the data revealed that the change was more significant in the attitudes of older adults, with those aged 75 and above increasing by 10% and those aged 65–74 increasing by 17% in the 2002 to 2014 timeframe. Notably, changing societal attitudes have resulted in societal change, an example being same-sex marriage becoming commonplace in many Western countries. In the UK same-sex marriage became legal in England, Wales and Scotland in 2014, and Northern Ireland in 2020. However, worldwide there continues to be 72 countries that criminalise LGBTQ+ people (Human Dignity Trust 2020) and health inequalities continue to exist for LGBTQ+ people. Additionally, in recent years there has been increasing anti-trans activity in the UK in response to the Gender Recognition Act 2004 reform consultation, which had predominantly been led by feminist opposition to trans rights (Armitage 2020).

This chapter will explore the historical, political, legislative context of LGBTQ+ lives and illuminate the health inequalities seen within the LGBTQ+ community, bringing to life an inclusive understanding and approach to public health.

What is the LGBT community?

The LGBTQ+ community is a loosely defined grouping which includes individuals who identify as LGBTQ+ (see boxed text below), LGBTQ+ organisations and businesses, campaigning groups and geographical areas such as LGBTQ+ villages. The trans community has not always been included or wished to be included as they are concerned with gender identity and not sexuality. It was not until 2015 that Stonewall, the largest LGBTQ+ campaigning organisation in Europe, included campaigning for transgender equality. The letter Q can also be added; LGBTQ includes queer or questioning and other sexuality and gender identities (see Key terms at the end of the chapter).

This is an easy read guide to LGBT; see also Key terms at the end of the chapter.

LGBTQ+ stands for Lesbian, Gay, Bi, Transgender, Queer or Questioning.
Lesbians are women who are attracted to women.
Gay men are attracted to men. Gay can also be used to describe lesbians.
Bi people are attracted to more than one gender.
Trans means that the gender you were given as a baby doesn't match the gender you feel yourself to be.

(Stonewall.org.uk)

The Pride flag has become a symbol of the LGBTQ+ community and was designed by Gilbert Baker in 1978. Gilbert was an openly gay man and drag queen in the USA and the first versions of the flag were flown at the San Francisco Freedom Day Parade (Gonzalez, n.d.). The flag has been redesigned over time and now has six coloured stripes rather than the original eight. The red strip is at the top of the flag, followed by orange, yellow, green, blue and violet. Each stripe has its own meaning: red for life, orange for healing, yellow for sunlight, green for nature, blue for harmony and violet for spirit. The Pride flag now has many variations, more recently adding colours for trans and LGBTQ+ people who are from Black Asian or minority ethnic groups. The trans flag represents the transgender community, and consists of five horizontal stripes: two light blue, two pink, and one white in the centre. A guide to LGBTQ+ flags and their meaning can be found at https://flagmakers.co.uk/blog/resources/a-guide-to-lgbtq-pride-flags-and-their-meanings/.

Although LGBTQ+ people may identify as belonging to the LGBTQ+ community, some will not. There are also many intersections for LGBTQ+ people which need to be considered as LGBTQ+ people may also have a religious belief, Black, Asian or minority ethnic heritage, be disabled and so on. Intersectionality is an important aspect of an individual's life that will impact on how they live in society and may lead to belonging to friendship/community groups that will not overlap/interact: for example, someone who identifies as gay may also be a practising Catholic and have friends in each group who may not interact.

One example of how the LGBT community has an impact in society is the campaigning for equal rights that has influenced societal attitudes towards LGBT people and led to changes in the UK law. The box below gives a brief overview of the timeline and key milestones from 1951 to 2020.

LGBT rights timeline of major events

1951: The first known case of sex reassignment surgery was Roberta Cowell.

1966: Formation of the Beaumont Society, a trans support group.

1967: The Sexual Offences Act decriminalises sex between two men over 21 'in private'.

1969: The Stonewall Riots take place in New York City.

1972: The Gay Liberation Front (GLF) first London Pride event.

1988: Introduction of Section 28 of the Local Government Act which stopped the promotion of 'homosexuality' in schools.

1992: The World Health Organization (WHO) declassifies homosexuality as a mental illness.

1994: The age of consent for same-sex relations between men is lowered to 18.

2001: Ban lifted on LGBT people serving in the armed forces.

2002: Gender Recognition Act passed.

2014: Same-sex marriage legalised in England, Wales and Scotland.

2019: WHO declassifies transgender health issues as a mental illness.

2020: Same-sex marriage legalised in Northern Ireland.

While it may seem that LGBT people have equal rights, especially now that same-sex marriage is legal in the UK, LGBT people continue to fear discrimination, harassment and hate crimes in their everyday lives. The 2018/2019 police hate crimes data for England and Wales recorded 14,491 offences committed against people due to their sexual orientation and 2,333 offences against people due to their gender identity (Home Office 2019). Hate crime includes verbal abuse, intimidation, threats, harassment, assault and bullying, as well as damage to property (Crown Prosecution Service 2020). For many LGBT people society is not as accepting as we might assume; LGBT people continue to live in fear of rejection by family, friends and colleagues, violence and harassment and loneliness. These negative experiences have a direct effect on health inequalities, as explored later in this chapter.

The Equality Act 2010

The Equality Act 2010 brings together a number of laws related to equality into one act and became UK law on 1st October 2010. The Act identifies nine 'protected characteristics' which are covered by the law: age, disability, gender reassignment, marriage and civil partnership, pregnancy and maternity, race, religion or belief, sex, and sexual orientation. As part of the Act individuals who have a protected characteristic are assumed to or are perceived to have a protected characteristic or are connected with someone who has a protected characteristic cannot be discriminated against, victimised or harassed. The Equality Act 2010 offers protection to LGBT people so that they are not discriminated against, especially in the provision of services. This includes health and social care services, and as such practitioners need to have an awareness of the Act and protected characteristics, and consider how their practice is non-discriminatory. However, the Stonewall *LGBT in Britain – Health Report* (2018a) identified that nearly one-quarter of the 5,000 people surveyed had heard healthcare staff making negative remarks about LGBT people. The survey also reported that 13% of respondents had received unequal treatment from healthcare staff because they identified as LGBT, while 25% have experienced inappropriate curiosity. Considering these findings, it is essential that all health and social care staff receive training on the Equality Act 2010 and working with LGBT+ identifying people.

Health inequalities and LGBTQ+ people

The health and wellbeing of people from LGBT communities in the UK has become a topical issue, for example: Department of Health advisory groups; the launch of a Public Health England initiative for Black minority ethnic men who have sex with men; and the LGBT Action Plan (Government Equalities Office 2018a). Belonging to a minority sexual group in itself was historically characterised as an illness and although this is no longer the case, research suggests that LGB individuals are more likely to report fair or poor health in comparison to heterosexual people (Elliott et al. 2014) and experiences of healthcare are negative for some LGB people (13%) and trans people (40%), as identified in the *LGBT Survey Research Report* (Government Equalities Office 2018b). There are significant differences between the health needs of those from sexual and gender minority communities and those of heterosexual people. LGBTQ+ people report that they have experienced or fear discrimination because of identifying as LGBTQ+ and this creates a barrier to receiving appropriate care and treatment (e.g. Connolly and Lynch 2016, Elliott et al. 2014, Lick et al. 2016, Stonewall 2008, 2015). An illuminative report, *Unhealthy Attitudes* (Stonewall 2015), suggests that one in ten health and social care workers directly involved in patient care have witnessed colleagues expressing the belief that someone can be 'cured' of being lesbian, gay or bisexual, and that workplace bullying is frequent in health and social care workers, with one-quarter of LGB staff stating that they experienced homophobic and bi-phobic abuse from colleagues.

Health inequalities are the result of a complicated set of social, cultural and political influences, and for those who identify as LGBTQ+ it is thought the causes are linked to:

- Cultural and social norms that favour and rank heterosexuality over other forms of sexuality.
- Minority stress related to sexual orientation/gender identity.
- Victimisation.
- Discrimination.
- Stigma.

(Zeeman et al. 2019)

Inequalities are not isolated to health alone and the box below lists a number of broader areas, including health, where LGBT people are disproportionately affected in comparison to heterosexual people.

Areas of LGBT inequality

Family rejection

Homelessness

Health, including alcohol, smoking, mental health and suicide, long-term conditions and cancers

Risk-taking behaviour

Domestic violence

Isolation

Hate crime

Being an older LGBT person

The next section will explore the impact of identifying as LGBT for young people, adults and older people and conclude by examining the impact of the COVID-19 epidemic for LGBT people.

LGBTQ+ young people

Health inequalities for LGBT people can begin at an early age and can have detrimental and lasting effects on a young person's health and wellbeing. Adolescence can be a challenging time for young people as they develop their individual identities and make decisions around education and careers. Identifying as an LGBT young person can have negative consequences on home and school life at a time when support is required. LGBT young people face a 'hostile' environment and can be exposed to homophobia, biphobia, transphobia, greater mental ill health and unwanted and risky sex (Hudson-Sharp and Metcalf 2016, p. iv). One study in Scotland revealed that almost half of LGB school students felt that they did not belong/fit in at school and 21% felt unsafe at school (Guasp 2012). In 2017 the Stonewall *School Report* described how anti-LGBT bullying and language has decreased in Britain's schools since 2012; however, school continued to be a difficult place for some LGBTQ+ young people with almost half of all LGBTQ+ pupils surveyed still facing bullying at school, with more than two in five trans young people having tried to take their own life. There is little evidence at this time of how these issues affect educational attainment for LGBTQ+ young people, however Guasp's (2012) study found a higher percentage of LGBT students struggling to study in comparison to non-LGBT students. Conversely, an examination of a representative survey of the UK population revealed that more gay men and lesbians had university degrees as compared to heterosexual people (Powdthavee and Wooden 2014). However, evidence suggests that negative experiences in education for LGBT people continue into higher education. Stonewall *University Report* (2018b) identified two in five LGBT students (42%) responding to the survey having hidden their identity at university for fear of discrimination and 7% of trans students being physically attacked by another student or member of university staff.

LGBTQ+ adulthood and growing older

LGBT inequalities continue into adulthood and continue to be multifaceted and include: family rejection, homophobia/biphobia/transphobia, hate crime, victimisation, harassment, domestic violence. Health inequalities include: substance misuse, smoking, increased mental health issues and suicide, long-term conditions and specific cancers. Further exploration of health inequalities reveals that substance misuse is a particular issue for LGB people. Public Health England (2014) found double the rate of alcohol dependency for gay and bisexual men compared with heterosexual men, with those aged 18–19 twice as likely to drink twice a week or more. The same review revealed higher rates of smoking compared to heterosexual people and Stonewall (2018a) found that one in eight LGBT people aged 18–24 (13%) take drugs at least once a month, which is higher than the general population (9%). The *Trans Research Review* (Mitchell and Howarth 2009) reported the risk of substance misuse for trans people was high.

In relation to physical health, a review of the evidence relating to inequality in LGBT groups (Hudson-Sharp and Metcalf 2016) stated that evidence existed in relation to physical health demonstrating that gay men were more likely than heterosexual men to develop anal and prostate cancer; HIV medication could cause blood disorders; renal problems and sexual dysfunction; and that there was contradictory evidence in relation to the prevalence of diabetes among lesbians and gay men. There is little evidence available that reports the physical health of trans people in comparison to the general population.

Adverse mental health is reported as being worryingly high amongst LGBT people. Stonewall (2018a) found that half of LGBT people (52%) said they had experienced depression in the last year; another 10% saying they think they might have experienced depression; two–thirds of trans people (67%) reported having experienced depression in the last year and more than half of LGBT women (55%) reported the same experience.

Growing older as a LGBT person raises specific issues relating to needing care, independence and mobility. Stonewall's (2011) survey of LGB people aged over 55 revealed that they were more likely to be single; live alone; three in five were not confident in social care; and four in ten of gay and bisexual men over 55 are single compared with just 15% of heterosexual men who reported growing old alone as much more difficult.

As LGBTQ+ people grow older accessing health and social care services may become essential for daily living, as it is for many older people in the UK. However, for LGBTQ+ people having health or social care professionals in your own home or living in a residential or nursing home can be difficult unless these services strive for an inclusive environment and practice for LGBTQ+ people. Age UK have produced *Safe to Be Me: A Resource Pack for Professionals* (2017) that is not only informative but also tells the stories of individuals.

LGBTQ+ people and the impact of COVID-19

The COVID-19 pandemic has impacted everyone in our society and it is widely accepted that those from a BAME background are disproportionately affected by the virus and have adverse health outcomes (Bhatia 2020a), also that the burden of care for women has dramatically increased during lockdown (Power 2020a). However, the effect of the pandemic on LGBT people has been largely unreported. A survey of 550 LGBT people, undertaken by the LGBT Foundation (2020a), revealed that the pandemic was having a negative impact on LGBT people and exacerbating existing LGBT inequalities. The report suggested that LGBT people are being disproportionately affected by the pandemic in the following areas: mental health, isolation, substance misuse, eating disorders, safety, finances, homelessness, access to support and access to healthcare. With the lack of routine epidemiological monitoring of sexual orientation or gender minorities it is unlikely that the number of LGBT people who die of COVID-19 will be known.

Specific findings from the survey include: 42% of respondents would like to access support for their mental health at this time; 30% are living alone at this time (this rises to 40% of LGBT people aged 50+); 25% would like support to reduce their isolation, such as a befriending service; 18% are concerned that this situation is going to lead to substance or alcohol misuse or trigger a relapse; 8% do not feel safe where they are currently staying; 16% had been unable to access healthcare for non-COVID related issues. This rises to 22% of BAME LGBT people, 26% of disabled LGBT people, 27% of trans people, 27% of non-binary people and 18% of LGBT people aged 50+ (LGBT Foundation 2020). Although this survey is not representative due to a relatively low response rate it does identity some startling findings and implies that LGBT people could have long-term effects from the COVID-19 pandemic and specifically lockdowns.

Promoting LGBTQ+ health through non-discriminatory practice

Working with LGBTQ+ patients and clients in a manner which is not only non-discriminatory but also inclusive often only needs subtle differences in our approach and some knowledge of LGBTQ+ health inequalities, such as those discussed earlier in this chapter. It is essential that as health and social wellbeing professionals we reflect on and re-tune our approach to working with LGBTQ+ patients and clients so that the barriers to accessing health and social care are reduced for individuals.

An area of practice that is important when working with LGBTQ+ patients and clients is communication. Being aware of and using neutral gender pronouns, using language our patients and clients use (e.g. 'gay', not 'homosexual') and reducing wherever possible non-inclusive language (e.g. asking if someone is 'in a relationship' rather than 'married') are all good ways to be inclusive. Asking a client their preferred name or pronoun can be helpful if you are unsure.

A non-judgemental attitude is essential and being able to recognise your own non-verbal cues and ensuring these are not sending unintended messages of surprise or negativity is important to build trust. If you make a mistake, apologise. This useful guide from the US National LGBTQIA+ Health Education Centre contains excellent advice and a case study: www.lgbtqiahealtheducation.org/wp-content/uploads/Providing-Inclusive-Services-and-Care-for-LGBT-People.pdf

Tuller (2020) developed a set of actions which can ensure a welcoming environment for LGBTQ+ people, which is adapted below for use in the UK:

- Advertise health and social care services as accepting of members of the LGBTQ+ community by displaying positive images online and in the physical environment.
- Be part of national and local LGBTQ+ initiatives such as the NHS Rainbow Badge Scheme.
- Educate staff and providers to be comfortable in discussing the lives and health inequalities of LGBTQ+ people.

- Include in staff training to refer to all patients by their name and chosen descriptive pronoun.
- Maintain an open mind and avoid judgement regarding sexual orientation and practices.
- On forms include the term 'partner' in addition to the spouse; include 'transgender' as an option.
- Provide waiting room magazines from the LGBTQ+ community and leaflets to services and charities linked to LGBTQ+ health inequalities.
- Support of LGBTQ Pride Day, World AIDS Day and International Transgender Day of Remembrance.
- Train staff and provide continuing education on working with LGBTQ+ patients and clients and the Equality Act 2010.

As individuals and health and social care teams we can make relatively easy changes to our approach and services to help make them accessible to the LGBTQ+ community.

Conclusion

The rights of LGBTQ+ people in the UK and other Western countries has, over the past 50 years, progressed from a place where homosexuality was illegal to all four countries of the UK legalising same-sex marriage. However, the everyday experience of many LGBTQ+ people is not one of acceptance, but enduring discrimination, harassment and victimisation. It is through understanding the inequalities that LGBTQ+ people endure that we can understand the effect of discrimination. The inequalities LGBTQ+ people face are multifaceted and while in this chapter there has been a specific focus on health inequalities, it is important that health and social care practitioners develop an awareness of the broader issues when working with LGBTQ+ clients. Finally, when working with LGBTQ+ clients it is important that we have open and honest conversations to understand their needs but not to be overly inquisitive. What is important is recognising the issue/problem an LGBTQ+ client wishes to discuss and where appropriate referring to a relevant service.

Consider the following questions

Having read the chapter take time to think about the following:

1. What inequalities might a same-sex couple who adopt a child encounter?
2. What could be the barriers for LGBTQ+ people accessing health and social care?
3. How can you ensure that your own practice is inclusive of LGBTQ+ people?
4. Does heteronormativity exist in your area of practice? What examples are there of this?

Key terms

Taken from LGBT Foundation/Stonewall; a full glossary of LGBT-related terms can be found at www.stonewall.org.uk/help-advice/faqs-and-glossary/glossary-terms.

Biphobia: Prejudice and discrimination towards, fear and/or dislike of someone who is bisexual or who is perceived to be bisexual, based on their sexual orientation.

Bisexual/Bi: Someone who is attracted to people of the same gender and other genders.

Cis/Cisgender: Someone who identifies with the gender they were assigned at birth; someone who is not transgender.

Coming out: The disclosure of one's LGBTQ+ identity to someone else. Coming out is rarely a once-in-a-lifetime event as many LGBTQ+ people may want or need to come out to each new person they meet or may realise different facets of their LGBTQ+ identity over time which they might then choose to disclose.

Gay: Someone who is almost exclusively romantically, emotionally or sexually attracted to people of the same gender. The term can be used to describe anyone regardless of gender identity but is more commonly used to describe men.

Gender: The socially constructed and reinforced divisions between certain groups (genders) in a culture including social norms that people in these different groups are expected to adhere to, and a person's sense of self relating to these divisions.

Gender assigned at birth: The gender that a person is assumed to be at birth, usually based on the sex assigned at birth.

Gender fluid: Someone whose gender is not fixed; their gender may change slowly or quickly over time and can switch between any number of gender identities and expressions, as each gender fluid person's experience of their fluidity is unique to them.

Gender identity: A person's internal feelings and convictions about their gender. This can be the same or different to the gender they were assigned at birth.

Gender neutral: Something that has no limitations to use that are based on the gender of the user.

Genderqueer: Someone whose gender is outside or in opposition to the gender binary. Often viewed as a more intentionally political gender identity than some other non-binary genders, through the inclusion of the politicised 'queer'.

Gender reassignment: The protected characteristic which trans people are described as having, or protected characteristic group they are described as being part of, with reference to the Equality Act 2010. A person has the protected characteristic of gender reassignment if the person is proposing to undergo, is undergoing or has undergone a process (or part of a process) for the purpose of reassigning the person's sex by changing physiological or other attributes of sex.

Heterosexual: Someone who is romantically or sexually attracted to someone of a different gender, typically a man who is attracted to women or a woman who is attracted to men.

Homosexual: A term used to describe someone who is almost exclusively attracted to people of the same gender. Some consider this word too medical and prefer the terms 'gay', 'lesbian' or 'queer'.

Homophobia/Homophobic: Prejudice and discrimination towards, fear and/or dislike of someone who is, or who is perceived to be attracted to people of the same gender as themselves, based on their sexual orientation.

Intersex: A person whose biological sex characteristics don't fit into the binary medical model of male and female. This can be due to differences in primary and secondary sex characteristics including external and internal genitalia, hormones and/or chromosomes.

Lesbian: A woman who is largely or exclusively emotionally, sexually and/or physically attracted to other women.

LGBTphobic: Prejudice and discrimination towards, fear and/ or dislike of someone who is LGBT or who is perceived to be LGBT, that is based on their LGBT identity.

Misgender: The act of referring to someone as the wrong gender or using the wrong pronouns (he, she, boy, sister etc.). This usually refers to intentionally or maliciously referring to a trans person incorrectly, but of course can also be done accidentally.

Non-binary: Used to describe those whose gender does not fit into the gender binary. The term can be used by some as an identity in itself and is also used as an overarching term for genders that don't fit into the gender binary, such as genderqueer, bigender and gender-fluid.

Outing/Out: Disclosing someone else's sexual orientation or gender identity without their consent.

Pansexual/Pan: Someone who is emotionally, sexually and/or physically attracted to others regardless of gender identity.

Protected characteristic: Under the Equality Act 2010 it is against the law to discriminate against someone because they have a protected characteristic. These are outlined under the Act and comprise: age, disability, gender reassignment, marriage and civil partnership, pregnancy and maternity, race, religion or belief, sex, sexual orientation.

Queer: An overarching or umbrella term used by some to describe members of the LGBTQ+ community. The term has been reclaimed by members of the community from previous derogatory use, and some members of the community may not wish to use it due to this history. When Q is seen at the end of LGBTQ+, it typically refers to 'queer' and, less often, 'questioning'.

Key websites

This list of websites is not exhaustive and is intended to be a place to start exploring LGBT-related resources for yourself and your clients. A comprehensive list of resources is provided by The Be You Project: https://thebeyouproject.co.uk/resources/

FFLAG: Supports friends and family members of LGBTQ people. www.fflag.org.uk

Galop: If you've experienced hate crime, sexual violence or domestic abuse, Galop is there for you. They also support lesbian, gay, bi, trans and queer people who have had problems with the police or have questions about the criminal justice system. www.galop.org.uk/

Mermaids UK: Family and individual support for gender diverse and transgender children and young people. Mermaids is passionate about supporting children, young people and their families to achieve a happier life in the face of great adversity. www.mermaidsuk.org.uk/

Stonewall: The largest LGBT charity in the UK providing information, training and campaigning for LGBT rights. www.stonewall.org.uk

Switchboard: Switchboard is an LGBT+ helpline – a place for calm words when you need them most. They're here to help you with whatever you want to talk about. Nothing is off limits and conversations are 100% confidential. Call 0300 330 0630 (10.00am–10.00pm daily). https://switchboard.lgbt

References

Age UK. 2017. *Safe to Be Me: A Resource Pack for Professionals*. Age UK: London. Available at: www.ageuk.org.uk/globalassets/age-uk/documents/booklets/safe_to_be_me.pdf [Accessed 26.03.2022].

Armitage, L. 2020. Explaining backlash to trans and non-binary genders in the context of the UK Gender Recognition Act reform. *Journal of the International Network for Sexual Ethics*; 8, 11–35.

Bhatia, M. 2020. COVID-19 and BAME Group in the United Kingdom. *The International Journal of Community and Social Development*; 2(2), 269–272.

Connolly, M., Lynch, K. 2016. Is being gay bad for your health and wellbeing? Cultural issues affecting gay men accessing and using health services in the Republic of Ireland. *Journal of Nursing Research*; 21(3), 177–196.

Crown Prosecution Service. 2020. *Hate Crime*. Available at: www.cps.gov.uk/crime-info/hate-crime [Accessed 09.12.2020].

Elliott, M., Kanouse, D., Burkhart, Q., Abel, G., Lyrat-Zopoulos, G., Beckett, M., Schuster, M., Roland, M. 2014. Sexual minorities in England have poorer health and worse health care experiences: a national survey. *Journal of General Internal Medicine*; 5(301), 9–16.

European Social Survey. 2020. Exploring Public Attitudes, Informing Public Policy. *Selected Findings From the First Seven Rounds*. City University: London.

Gonzalez, N. n.d. How did the rainbow flag become a symbol of LGBTQ Pride? *Britannica*. Available at: www.britannica.com/story/how-did-the-rainbow-flag-become-a-symbol-of-lgbt-pride [Accessed 20.12.2000].

Government Equalities Office. 2018a. LGBT Action Plan. *Improving the Lives of Lesbian, Gay, Bisexual and Transgender People*. Government Equalities Office: London.

Government Equalities Office. 2018b. *LGBT Survey Research Report*. Government Equalities Office: London.

Guasp, A. 2012. *The School Report: The Experiences of Gay Young People in Scotland's Schools*. Available at: www.stonewallscotland.org.uk/scotland/at_school/secondary_schools/7966.asp [Accessed 08.12.2020].

Home Office. 2019. Home Office Statistical Bulletin 24/19. *Hate Crime England and Wales, 2018 to 2019*. Home Office: London.

Hudson-Sharpe, N., Metcalf, H. 2016. *Inequality Among Lesbian, Gay, Bisexual and Transgender Groups in the UK: A Review of Evidence*. National Institute of Economic and Social Research: London.

Human Dignity Trust. 2020. *Map of Countries that Criminalise LGBT People*. Available at: www.humandignitytrust.org/lgbt-the-law/map-of-criminalisation/ [Accessed 08.12.2020].

LGBT Foundation. 2020. *Hidden Figure: The Impact of the COVID-19 Pandemic on LGBT Communities in the UK. LGBT Foundations*. (3rd edn). Available at: https://s3-eu-west-1.amazonaws.com/lgbt-website-media/Files/7a01b983-b54b-4dd3-84b2-0f2ecd72be52/Hidden%2520Figures-%2520The%2520Impact%2520of%2520the%2520COVID-19%2520Pandemic%2520on%2520LGBT%2520Communities.pdf [Accessed 03.01.2021].

Lick, D., Durso, L., Johnson, K. 2016. Minority stress and physical health among sexual minorities. *Perspectives on Psychological Science*; 8(5), 521–548.

Mitchell, M., Howarth, C. 2009. *Trans Research Review. Equality and Human Rights Commission Research Report 27*. Available at: https://itgl.lu/wp-content/uploads/2015/04/SB-2009-3-pdf.pdf [Accessed 03.01.2021].

Powdthavee, N., Wooden, M. 2014. *What Can Life Satisfaction Data Tell us About Discrimination Against Sexual Minorities? A Structural Equation Model for Australia and the United Kingdom*. IZA Discussion Paper No. 8127. Institute for the Study of Labor: Bonn.

Power, K. 2020. The COVID-19 pandemic has increased the care burden of women and families. *Sustainability: Science, Practice and Policy*; 16(Special Edn.), 1.

Public Health England. 2014. *Promoting the Health and Wellbeing of Gay, Bisexual and Other Men Who Have Sex With Men*. Public Health England: London.

Stonewall. 2008. *Prescription for Change: Lesbian and Bisexual Women's Health Check*. Available at: www.stonewall.org.uk/sites/default/files/prescription_for_change_scotland_final.pdf [Accessed 08.12.2020].

Stonewall. 2011. *Lesbian, Gay and Bisexual People in Later Life*. Available at: www.stonewall.org.uk/system/files/LGB_people_in_Later_Life__2011_.pdf [Accessed 08.12.2020].

Stonewall. 2015. *Unhealthy Attitudes: The Treatment of Lesbian, Gay, Bisexual and Transgender People Within Health and Social Services*. Available at: www.stonewall.org.uk/sites/default/files/unhealthy_attitudes.pdf [Accessed 08.12.2020].

Stonewall. 2017. *School Report: The Experiences of Lesbian, Gay, Bi and Trans Young People in Britain's Schools in 2017*. Available at: www.stonewall.org.uk/system/files/the_school_report_2017.pdf [Accessed 08.12.2020].

Stonewall. 2018a. *LGBT in Britain – Health Report*. Available at: www.stonewall.org.uk/system/files/lgbt_in_britain_health.pdf [Accessed 08.12.2020].

Stonewall. 2018b. *LGBT in Britain – University Report*. Available at: www.stonewall.org.uk/system/files/lgbt_in_britain_universities_report.pdf [Accessed 08.12.2020].

Tuller, D. 2020. For LGBTQ patients, high-quality care in a welcoming environment. *Health Affiliations (Millwood)*; 39(5), 736–739.

UK Parliament. 2010. *Equality Act 2010*. www.legislation.gov.uk/ukpga/2010/15/pdfs/ukpga_20100015_en.pdf [Accessed 09.12.2020].

Zeeman, L., Sherriff, N., Browne, K., McGlynn, N., Mirandola, M., Gios, L., Davis, R., Sanchez-Lambert, J., Aujean, S., Pinto, N., Farinella, F., Donisi, V., Niedźwiedzka-Stadnik, M., Rosińska, M., Pierson, M., Amaddeo, F. 2019. Health4LGBTI Network 2019: a review of lesbian, gay, bisexual, trans and intersex (LGBTI) health and healthcare inequalities. *European Journal of Public Health*; 29(5), 974–980.

INDEX

Page numbers in *italic* indicate figures and in **bold** indicate tables.